T0348603

The Endoscopic Hepatologist

Editor

CHRISTOPHER J. DIMAIO

GASTROINTESTINAL ENDOSCOPY CLINICS OF NORTH AMERICA

www.giendo.theclinics.com

Consulting Editor
CHARLES J. LIGHTDALE

April 2019 • Volume 29 • Number 2

ELSEVIER

1600 John F. Kennedy Boulevard • Suite 1800 • Philadelphia, Pennsylvania, 19103-2899

http://www.theclinics.com

GASTROINTESTINAL ENDOSCOPY CLINICS OF NORTH AMERICA Volume 29, Number 2 April 2019 ISSN 1052-5157, ISBN-13: 978-0-323-67793-6

Editor: Kerry Holland

Developmental Editor: Donald Mumford

© **2019 Elsevier Inc. All rights reserved.**

This periodical and the individual contributions contained in it are protected under copyright by Elsevier, and the following terms and conditions apply to their use:

Photocopying

Single photocopies of single articles may be made for personal use as allowed by national copyright laws. Permission of the Publisher and payment of a fee is required for all other photocopying, including multiple or systematic copying, copying for advertising or promotional purposes, resale, and all forms of document delivery. Special rates are available for educational institutions that wish to make photocopies for non-profit educational classroom use. For information on how to seek permission visit www.elsevier.com/permissions or call: (+44) 1865 843830 (UK)/(+1) 215 239 3804 (USA).

Derivative Works

Subscribers may reproduce tables of contents or prepare lists of articles including abstracts for internal circulation within their institutions. Permission of the Publisher is required for resale or distribution outside the institution. Permission of the Publisher is required for all other derivative works, including compilations and translations (please consult www.elsevier.com/permissions).

Electronic Storage or Usage

Permission of the Publisher is required to store or use electronically any material contained in this periodical, including any article or part of an article (please consult www.elsevier.com/permissions). Except as outlined above, no part of this publication may be reproduced, stored in a retrieval system or transmitted in any form or by any means, electronic, mechanical, photocopying, recording or otherwise, without prior written permission of the Publisher.

Notice

No responsibility is assumed by the Publisher for any injury and/or damage to persons or property as a matter of products liability, negligence or otherwise, or from any use or operation of any methods, products, instructions or ideas contained in the material herein. Because of rapid advances in the medical sciences, in particular, independent verification of diagnoses and drug dosages should be made.

Although all advertising material is expected to conform to ethical (medical) standards, inclusion in this publication does not constitute a guarantee or endorsement of the quality or value of such product or of the claims made of it by its manufacturer.

Gastrointestinal Endoscopy Clinics of North America (ISSN 1052-5157) is published quarterly by Elsevier Inc., 360 Park Avenue South, New York, NY 10010-1710. Months of issue are January, April, July, and October. Business and Editorial Offices: 1600 John F. Kennedy Blvd., Suite 1800, Philadelphia, PA, 19103-2899. Periodicals postage paid at New York, NY and additional mailing offices. Subscription prices are $359.00 per year for US individuals, $624.00 per year for US institutions, $100.00 per year for US students and residents, $399.00 per year for Canadian individuals, $737.00 per year for Canadian institutions, $476.00 per year for international individuals, $737.00 per year for international institutions, and $245.00 per year for Canadian and international students/residents. To receive student/resident rate, orders must be accompanied by name of affiliated institution, date of term, and the *signature* of program/residency coordinator on institution letterhead. Orders will be billed at individual rate until proof of status is received. Foreign air speed delivery is included in all *Clinics* subscription prices. All prices are subject to change without notice. **POSTMASTER:** Send address change to *Gastrointestinal Endoscopy Clinics of North America*, Elsevier Health Sciences Division, Subscription Customer Service, 3251 Riverport Lane, Maryland Heights, MO 63043. **Customer Service: 1-800-654-2452 (US). From outside the United States, call 1-314-447-8871. Fax: 1-314-447-8029. E-mail: JournalsCustomerService-usa@elsevier.com (for print support) or JournalsOnlineSupport-usa@elsevier.com (for online support)**.

Reprints. For copies of 100 or more, of articles in this publication, please contact the Commercial Reprints Department, Elsevier Inc., 360 Park Avenue South, New York, NY 10010-1710. Tel. 212-633-3874; Fax: 212-633-3820; E-mail: reprints@elsevier.com.

Gastrointestinal Endoscopy Clinics of North America is covered in *Excerpta Medica, MEDLINE/PubMed (Index Medicus), and MEDLINE/MEDLARS.*

Contributors

CONSULTING EDITOR

CHARLES J. LIGHTDALE, MD
Professor of Medicine, Division of Digestive and Liver Diseases, Columbia University Medical Center, New York, New York

EDITOR

CHRISTOPHER J. DIMAIO, MD, AGAF, FASGE
Associate Professor of Medicine, Dr. Henry D. Janowitz Division of Gastroenterology, Icahn School of Medicine at Mount Sinai, Director, Mount Sinai Pancreas Center, Director of Therapeutic Endoscopy, Mount Sinai Hospital, New York, New York

AUTHORS

JAWAD AHMAD, MD, FRCP, FAASLD
Professor of Medicine, Recanati/Miller Transplantation Institute, Icahn School of Medicine at Mount Sinai, New York, New York

HARRY R. ASLANIAN, MD
Professor of Medicine, Section of Digestive Diseases, Yale School of Medicine, New Haven, Connecticut

JASON G. BILL, MD
Advanced Endoscopy Fellow, Instructor of Medicine, Washington University School of Medicine, St Louis, Missouri

KENNETH F. BINMOELLER, MD
Director, Interventional Endoscopy Services, California Pacific Medical Center, San Francisco, California

ROSS C.D. BUERLEIN, MD
Fellow, Division of Gastroenterology and Hepatology, University of Virginia, Charlottesville, Virginia

JONATHAN M. BUSCAGLIA, MD, FASGE, AGAF
Chief, Division of Gastroenterology and Hepatology, Associate Professor of Medicine, Renaissance School of Medicine at Stony Brook University, Stony Brook University Hospital, Stony Brook, New York

DAVID CARR-LOCKE, MD, FRCP, FACG, FASGE, AGAF, NYSGEF
Department of Gastroenterology and Hepatology, Weill Cornell Medicine, The Center for Advanced Digestive Care, NewYork-Presbyterian Hospital, New York, New York

KENNETH J. CHANG, MD, FASGE, FACG
Chief, Gastroenterology and Hepatology, Director, H. H. Chao Comprehensive Digestive Disease Center, University of California, Irvine Medical Center, Orange, California

TIFFANY CHUA, MD
Division of Gastroenterology and Hepatology, Mayo Clinic, Phoenix, Arizona

JAMES F. CRISMALE, MD
Assistant Professor of Medicine, Recanati/Miller Transplantation Institute, Icahn School of Medicine at Mount Sinai, New York, New York

DAVID L. DIEHL, MD, FACP, FASGE
Clinical Professor of Medicine and Pathology, Department of Gastroenterology and Nutrition, Geisinger Medical Center, Danville, Pennsylvania

CHRISTOPHER J. DIMAIO, MD, AGAF, FASGE
Associate Professor of Medicine, Dr. Henry D. Janowitz Division of Gastroenterology, Icahn School of Medicine at Mount Sinai, Director, Mount Sinai Pancreas Center, Director of Therapeutic Endoscopy, Mount Sinai Hospital, New York, New York

LIONEL S. D'SOUZA, MD
Director, Endoscopic Surgery, Division of Gastroenterology and Hepatology, Assistant Professor of Medicine, Renaissance School of Medicine at Stony Brook University, Stony Brook University Hospital, Stony Brook, New York

DOUGLAS O. FAIGEL, MD
Professor of Medicine, Division of Gastroenterology and Hepatology, Mayo Clinic, Phoenix, Arizona

PRASHANT KEDIA, MD
Division of Gastroenterology, Department of Medicine, Methodist Dallas Medical Center, Dallas, Texas

THOMAS E. KOWALSKI, MD
Associate Professor, Director, Pancreaticobiliary and Advanced Endoscopy Section, Division of Gastroenterology and Hepatology, Sidney Kimmel College of Medicine, Thomas Jefferson University, Philadelphia, Pennsylvania

NIKHIL A. KUMTA, MD, MS
Director of Surgical and Bariatric Endoscopy, Dr. Henry D. Janowitz Division of Gastroenterology, Icahn School of Medicine at Mount Sinai, Mount Sinai Hospital, New York, New York

ANDREW LANGE, MD
Resident, Department of Internal Medicine, Yale School of Medicine, Yale Primary Care Center, New Haven, Connecticut

DAVID E. LOREN, MD, FASGE
Associate Professor, Associate Director, Pancreaticobiliary and Advanced Endoscopy Section, Division of Gastroenterology and Hepatology, Sidney Kimmel College of Medicine, Thomas Jefferson University, Philadelphia, Pennsylvania

SAURABH MUKEWAR, MD
Department of Gastroenterology and Hepatology, Weill Cornell Medicine, Center for Advanced Digestive Care, NewYork-Presbyterian Hospital, New York, New York

DANIEL K. MULLADY, MD
Professor of Medicine, Director, Interventional Endoscopy, Washington University School of Medicine, St Louis, Missouri

THIRUVENGADAM MUNIRAJ, MD
Assistant Professor of Medicine, Section of Digestive Diseases, Laboratory for Medicine and Pediatrics, Yale School of Medicine, New Haven, Connecticut

ANDREW NETT, MD
Interventional Endoscopy Services, California Pacific Medical Center, San Francisco, California

ALEKSEY NOVIKOV, MD
Advanced Endoscopy Fellow, Division of Gastroenterology and Hepatology, Department of Medicine, Thomas Jefferson University Hospital, Philadelphia, Pennsylvania

JEREMY S. NUSSBAUM, BS
Dr. Henry D. Janowitz Division of Gastroenterology, Icahn School of Medicine at Mount Sinai, Mount Sinai Hospital, New York, New York

HABEEB SALAMEH, MD, MS
Advanced Endoscopy Fellow, Icahn School of Medicine at Mount Sinai, New York, New York

JASON B. SAMARASENA, MD, FACG
Associate Professor, H. H. Chao Comprehensive Digestive Disease Center, University of California, Irvine Medical Center, Orange, California

PAUL R. TARNASKY, MD
Division of Gastroenterology, Department of Medicine, Methodist Dallas Medical Center, Dallas, Texas

ANDREW Y. WANG, MD, AGAF, FACG, FASGE
Associate Professor of Medicine, Director of Interventional Endoscopy, Division of Gastroenterology and Hepatology, University of Virginia, Charlottesville, Virginia

Contents

Foreword: The Endoscopic Hepatologist: Not an Oxymoron xiii

Charles J. Lightdale

Preface: The Endoscopic Hepatologist xv

Christopher J. DiMaio

The Use of Endoscopic Ultrasound in the Evaluation of Unexplained Biliary Dilation 161

Lionel S. D'Souza and Jonathan M. Buscaglia

Isolated biliary dilation, as an incidental diagnosis, is increasing owing to an increase in the use of noninvasive abdominal imaging and poses a diagnostic challenge to physicians especially when further noninvasive diagnostic testing fails to reveal an etiology. This article reviews available data describing the natural history of this clinical scenario and the impact of endoscopic ultrasound examination in the evaluation of unexplained dilation of the common bile duct.

Endoscopic Ultrasound–guided Liver Biopsy 173

David L. Diehl

There remains an important role for liver biopsy in the management of liver disorders. Image-guided liver biopsy can be obtained with percutaneous or transjugular approaches. Real-time image-guided liver biopsy can be accomplished with endoscopic ultrasound (EUS). EUS-guided liver biopsy (EUS-LB) has emerged as a safe means of obtaining liver biopsy. EUS-LB confers several advantages over other methods, including the ability to target both lobes of the liver, increased patient comfort and decreased apprehension during the procedure, and shorter recovery time after the biopsy. Future development of technology that allows for EUS-guided portal pressure measurement could further drive EUS-LB use.

Advances in Endoscopic Imaging of the Biliary Tree 187

Saurabh Mukewar and David Carr-Locke

Direct endoscopic imaging of the biliary tree is increasingly performed by endoscopists since the introduction of digital single-operator cholangioscopy. In parallel, there have been several advances to overcome the challenges associated with direct peroral cholangioscopy with development of multibending cholangioscopes and new devices to enable direct placement of an endoscope into the biliary tree without a supporting duodenoscope. The indications for cholangioscopy are also evolving with newer indications, such as intraductal lithotripsy, foreign body (mostly stent) removal, guide wire cannulation of specific ducts, photodynamic therapy for cholangiocarcinoma, and performance of fluoroscopy-free cholangiography. There has also been progress in image enhancement during cholangioscopy and additional imaging techniques, such as intraductal ultrasound, confocal laser endomicroscopy, and optical coherence tomography.

Practical Management of Indeterminate Biliary Strictures **205**

Aleksey Novikov, Thomas E. Kowalski, and David E. Loren

Indeterminate biliary strictures pose a diagnostic and therapeutic challenge. Although underlying malignancy is a primary concern, biliary strictures may result from benign processes. An accurate diagnosis is paramount to define the treatment strategy and minimize morbidity. The limitations of traditional endoscopic retrograde cholangiopancreatography-based tissue acquisition with cytology brushings are well-documented. Endoscopic retrograde cholangiopancreatography is generally unable to determine a stricture's etiology. Complementary advanced endoscopic imaging and multimodal tissue acquisition have evolved. Careful consideration of the clinical presentation, location of the stricture, and interpretation of imaging constitute the most optimal approach for diagnosis and management.

Stenting for Benign and Malignant Biliary Strictures **215**

Jason G. Bill and Daniel K. Mullady

Benign and malignant biliary strictures are common indications for endoscopic retrograde cholangiopancreatography. Diagnosis involves high-quality cross-sectional imaging and cholangiography with various endoscopic sampling techniques. Treatment options include placement of plastic biliary stents and self-expanding metal stents, which differ in patency duration and cost effectiveness. Whether the etiology is benign or malignant, a multidisciplinary strategy should be implemented. This article will discuss general principles of biliary stenting in both benign and malignant conditions.

Endoscopic Management of Biliary Issues in the Liver Transplant Patient **237**

James F. Crismale and Jawad Ahmad

Biliary complications remain a common problem after liver transplantation (LT). The therapeutic endoscopist encounters a variety of situations in LT including strictures at the duct-to-duct biliary anastomosis, strictures elsewhere in the biliary tree caused by an ischemic injury, and bile leaks at the anastomosis or from the cut surface and stone disease. Biliary complications lead to significant morbidity and occasionally reduced graft and patient survival. Several factors increase the risk of strictures and leaks. Endoscopic intervention in experienced hands is successful in the management of biliary complications following LT and percutaneous or surgical correction should seldom be required.

Endoscopic Management of Complex Biliary Stone Disease **257**

Prashant Kedia and Paul R. Tarnasky

Video content accompanies this article at http://www.giendo.theclinics.com/.

Choledocholithiasis is a common disorder that is managed universally by endoscopic retrograde cholangiopancreatography (ERCP). For difficult or complex stones, ERCP with conventional techniques may fail to achieve biliary clearance in 10% to 15% of cases. This review summarizes the literature regarding the current available endoscopic techniques for complex stone disease, including mechanical lithotripsy, endoscopic papillary large balloon dilation, cholangioscopy-guided lithotripsy, and endoscopic ultrasound-guided biliary access.

Endoscopic Ultrasound-Guided Biliary Drainage **277**

Jeremy S. Nussbaum and Nikhil A. Kumta

Endoscopic retrograde cholangiopancreatography is the preferred procedure for biliary drainage in benign and malignant obstructions. Endoscopic ultrasound-guided biliary drainage is an emerging technique for when endoscopic retrograde cholangiopancreatography fails. It is a highly versatile procedure with several options of access point, stent direction, and drainage route. Based on the current literature, the cumulative success rate is 88% to 93%, with an overall complication rate of 13% to 20%. Endoscopic ultrasound-guided biliary drainage seems to be an effective and valuable alternative technique after failed endoscopic retrograde cholangiopancreatography when performed by highly skilled endoscopists.

Endoscopic Retrograde Cholangiopancreatography and Endoscopic Ultrasound-Guided Gallbladder Drainage **293**

Habeeb Salameh and Christopher J. DiMaio

Gallbladder disease is one of the most common gastrointestinal diseases encountered in clinical practice. Surgical removal and percutaneous drainage are both widely available and effective in the management of acute cholecystitis. Several endoscopic approaches exist as an alternative to these interventions. These include transpapillary approaches via endoscopic retrograde cholangiopancreatography (ERCP), transmural drainage and access approaches via endoscopic ultrasound (EUS), and endoscopic surgical approaches using natural orifice transluminal endoscopic surgery (NOTES) techniques. This article reviews the epidemiology and pathophysiology of gallbladder diseases and discusses the various percutaneous, surgical, and endoscopic approaches to managing gallbladder disease.

Endoscopic Ultrasound-Guided Interventions for the Measurement and Treatment of Portal Hypertension **311**

Jason B. Samarasena and Kenneth J. Chang

The number of endoscopic ultrasound (EUS)-guided interventions is rapidly growing within advanced endoscopy. EUS offers high-resolution imaging of mediastinal and intra-abdominal vasculature, which can be targeted for various interventions, hence a growing number of studies have explored EUS-guided vascular catheterization. Potential clinical applications of EUS-guided portal venous access include angiography, measurement of the portosystemic pressure gradient, and EUS-guided transhepatic intrahepatic portosystemic shunt creation. This article reviews different devices and techniques used in these applications.

liver are under development. The literature has shown that many percutaneous ablative techniques are readily adaptable for EUS. In this review, the authors discuss the current developments on EUS-guided ablation of liver tumors, including injection of sclerosants, thermal therapy, and EUS-guided portal injection of chemotherapy.

GASTROINTESTINAL ENDOSCOPY CLINICS OF NORTH AMERICA

FORTHCOMING ISSUES

July 2019
Inflammatory Bowel Disease
Simon Lichtiger, *Editor*

October 2019
Colonoscopic Polypectomy
Douglas K. Rex, *Editor*

January 2020
Endoscopic Closures
Roy Soetikno and Tonya Kaltenbach, *Editors*

RECENT ISSUES

January 2019
Gastroparesis: Current Opinions and New Endoscopic Therapies
Qiang Cai, *Editor*

October 2018
Management of Benign Pancreatic Disease
John M. Poneros, *Editor*

July 2018
Endoscopic Management of Gastrointestinal Bleeding
Ian M. Granlek, *Editor*

RELATED CLINICS SERIES

Gastroenterology Clinics
Clinics in Liver Disease

THE CLINICS ARE AVAILABLE ONLINE!
Access your subscription at:
www.theclinics.com

Foreword

The Endoscopic Hepatologist: Not an Oxymoron

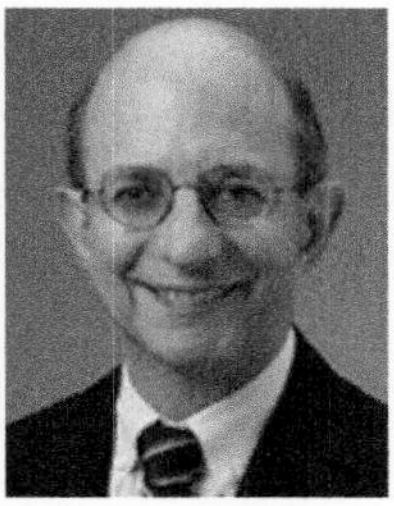

Charles J. Lightdale, MD
Consulting Editor

Endoscopists have long had an impact in the management of pancreatobiliary disease and esophageal and gastric varices secondary to cirrhosis, but the use of endoscopic methods in diagnosis and management of primary liver disease has been modest to nil. This is changing. With the use of new instruments and techniques, mostly based on progress in endoscopic retrograde cholangiopancreatography and more importantly in endoscopic ultrasonography (EUS), advanced endoscopists have recently shown the capability to carry out procedures that have the potential to compete successfully with interventional radiologists.

Liver biopsies for assessment of benign liver disease are easily and safely accomplished and are comparable in quality to those obtained by percutaneous and transjugular methods. Elastography is available to measure liver stiffness and fibrosis. Focal hepatic lesions can be targeted for biopsy using EUS, and contrast-enhanced harmonic EUS can be used to better define subtle abnormalities. EUS-guided ablation of primary and metastatic liver cancer has become a reality. EUS-guided puncture of portal and hepatic veins can be safely accomplished to measure portal-hepatic gradients often critical in management of cirrhosis. This evaluation of portal-systemic gradients can be carried out with liver biopsy during the same EUS session. Even EUS-directed intrahepatic portal-systemic shunts have been successfully performed.

The integration of endoscopy with hepatology is a major advance and certain to grow. The endoscopic hepatologist is no longer an oxymoron (defined as a figure of speech in which apparently contradictory terms are linked). I am truly pleased that Dr Christopher DiMaio, a skilled and thoughtful leader in interventional endoscopy, agreed to be the Editor for this issue of *Gastrointestinal Endoscopy Clinics of North America.* He has gathered a remarkable group of authors, who together have

Gastrointest Endoscopy Clin N Am 29 (2019) xiii–xiv
https://doi.org/10.1016/j.giec.2019.02.002
1052-5157/19/© 2019 Elsevier Inc. All rights reserved.

presented a comprehensive state-of-the-art issue on this subject that should be of great interest to interventional endoscopists and hepatologists alike.

Charles J. Lightdale, MD
Department of Medicine
Columbia University Medical Center
161 Fort Washington Avenue
New York, NY 10032, USA

E-mail address:
CJL18@columbia.edu

Preface
The Endoscopic Hepatologist

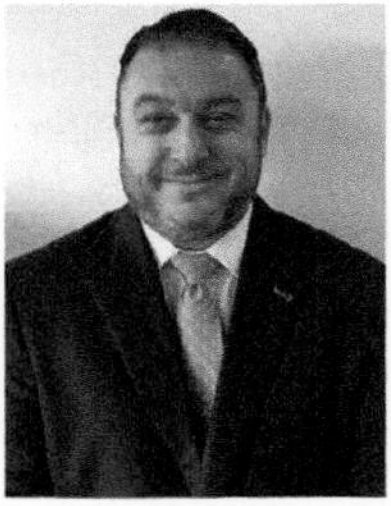

Christopher J. DiMaio, MD, AGAF, FASGE
Editor

The role of advanced endoscopic techniques, such as endoscopic ultrasound (EUS) and endoscopic retrograde cholangiopancreatography (ERCP), continues to evolve in the diagnosis and management of a variety of gastrointestinal (GI) conditions. ERCP has traditionally been a "plumbers" tool, a minimally invasive intervention to manage obstruction and leaks of the pancreaticobiliary tree, all with the assistance of 2-dimensional black-and-white fluoroscopic images. EUS, in its infancy, was used as a tool to identify and stage GI malignancies and eventually perform fine-needle aspirates of tumors. Further advances in tools and techniques led to newer applications for the "Endoscopic Oncologist," such as EUS-guided celiac plexus neurolysis and EUS-guided fiducial placement. The next wave of innovation centered on diseases of the pancreas. The "Endoscopic Pancreatologist" could now offer minimally invasive procedures for drainage of inaccessible pancreatic or biliary ducts or drainage and debridement of periluminal collections. Further advances have led to the development of EUS-guided ablation techniques for solid and cystic pancreatic neoplasms.

In 2019, we are at the dawn of the next phase of evolution of ERCP and EUS. Introduction of improved and novel imaging devices, new techniques in tissue acquisition and endovascular access, and the introduction of dedicated devices for transluminal drainage and tumor ablation has created an opportunity for the advanced endoscopist to diagnose and manage the heretofore largely ignored areas of primary liver disease and its complications. This new wave marks the beginning stages of the "Endoscopic Hepatologist."

In this issue of *Gastrointestinal Endoscopy Clinics of North America*, we have assembled a collection of review articles written by a fantastic group of leaders in the field of advanced endoscopy, many of whom are pioneers in the development and study of these novel techniques. Their insight and expertise will provide clarity for current applications of EUS and ERCP in liver disease, while simultaneously revealing what

Gastrointest Endoscopy Clin N Am 29 (2019) xv–xvi
https://doi.org/10.1016/j.giec.2019.02.001
1052-5157/19/© 2019 Elsevier Inc. All rights reserved.

the not-too-distant future holds in terms of what may soon be the new standard of care for the diagnosis and management of a variety of liver diseases.

I am extremely indebted to the authors for crafting these outstanding reviews, and I thank them for their time and efforts. I am also fortunate to have spent my formative years as a GI fellow over a decade ago working with and learning from Dr Lightdale and would like to thank him for the opportunity to serve as editor for this issue.

Christopher J. DiMaio, MD, AGAF, FASGE
The Dr. Henry D. Janowitz Division of Gastroenterology
Icahn School of Medicine at Mount Sinai
One Gustave L. Levy Place, Box 1069
New York, NY 10029, USA

E-mail address:
Christopher.DiMaio@MountSinai.org

The Use of Endoscopic Ultrasound in the Evaluation of Unexplained Biliary Dilation

Lionel S. D'Souza, MD*, Jonathan M. Buscaglia, MD

KEYWORDS

- Biliary dilation • Endoscopic ultrasound • Abnormal liver tests
- Magnetic resonance cholangiopancreatography

KEY POINTS

- With the increase in the use of noninvasive imaging tests, incidental findings such as isolated bile duct dilation have become increasingly common.
- Transabdominal ultrasound examination, computed tomography scans, and MRI have limitations in the identification of pathology in the periampullary region.
- Asymptomatic biliary dilation with normal liver tests is less likely to yield significant pathology on endoscopic ultrasound evaluation.
- The presence of symptoms and/or abnormalities in liver tests increases the pretest probability of finding significant pathology on endoscopic ultrasound examination.
- An individualized diagnostic approach to patients with isolated biliary dilation is necessary to avoid missed diagnoses and minimize unnecessary health care use.

INTRODUCTION

The use of endoscopic ultrasound (EUS) examination in the diagnosis of pancreaticobiliary disease has grown to become common place over the past few decades with a wealth of data describing its efficacy in the evaluation of this region of the gastrointestinal tract. The biliary tree is an intricate and adaptive system whose function is to maintain the flow of bile from the liver to the intestinal tract, where bile acids assist in the absorption of fat and fat-soluble nutrients. This flow is also crucial in the excretion of toxins and metabolites that are cleared by the liver. Bile flow occurs through the sphincter of Oddi and the ampulla of Vater, which functions as a valve to prevent reflux

The authors have no relevant disclosures to declare.
Division of Gastroenterology and Hepatology, Stony Brook University Hospital, 101 Nicolls Road HSC Level 17, Room 60, Stony Brook, NY 11794, USA
* Corresponding author.
E-mail address: Lionel.DSouza@stonybrook.edu

Gastrointest Endoscopy Clin N Am 29 (2019) 161–171
https://doi.org/10.1016/j.giec.2018.11.001
giendo.theclinics.com
1052-5157/19/© 2018 Elsevier Inc. All rights reserved.

and bacterial contamination of the biliary tree. Abnormalities in any part of this complex system can result in the stasis of bile with varied resultant clinical consequences.

With the increase in noninvasive imaging, whether for the evaluation of nonspecific abdominal pain or for other nongastrointestinal causes, there has been an increase in the detection of incidental biliary abnormalities, especially the finding of isolated biliary dilation. Although the primary goal in this clinical scenario is to identify those who might require biliary intervention for decompression, the increasing number of patients with clinically and biochemically asymptomatic biliary abnormalities leave the treating physician with the conundrum of whether to pursue invasive testing, or settle on watchful waiting. It is against this background that we begin to review the diagnostic approach to patients with unexplained biliary dilation.

BILIARY IMAGING TECHNIQUES

There are few data on the impact of EUS on the evaluation of isolated biliary dilation when other imaging tests such as transabdominal ultrasound (TUS) examination, computed tomography (CT) scans, and MRI or magnetic resonance cholangiopancreatography (MRCP) have failed to elucidate an etiology. The natural history of this clinical scenario has not been well-described, most likely because these nondiagnostic tests may reflect either a "normal" dilation of the bile duct in some instances, or the imaging test itself is limited in its ability to detect certain pathologies.

A normal bile duct can measure up to 6 to 8 mm in diameter, with 7 mm being the widely accepted upper limit of normal.[1–3] Unexplained dilation of the biliary tree is often seen in the setting of imaging performed as part of the workup for vague abdominal symptoms, or as a truly incidental finding on imaging performed for other reasons. As such, the clinical presentation can vary from the completely asymptomatic patient without any relevant biochemical derangements, to the patient with abdominal pain and/or elevated liver or pancreatic enzymes. A detailed history and physical examination along with noninvasive imaging tests to discern the etiology may not always result in a revelation of the exact cause. This may be partly due to the fact that the accuracy of most noninvasive imaging modalities is compromised by their inability to effectively evaluate the distal bile duct and periampullary region. Thus, further evaluation with EUS examination or endoscopic retrograde cholangiopancreatography (ERCP) may be indicated before accepting a nonobstructive cause in these patients.

TUS examination is often the first noninvasive imaging study ordered for the evaluation of either jaundice or nonspecific abdominal pain suspected to be of biliary origin. Although the presence of biliary dilation and the level of obstruction can be reliably demonstrated with TUS examination, the exact cause can be determined in only two-thirds of patients.[4,5] This is partly because overlying bowel gas and abdominal soft tissue often obscures the distal bile duct, ampulla, and pancreas. Although TUS examination is highly sensitive and specific for the detection of gallstones, the sensitivity for intraductal stones falls significantly to roughly 21% to 63% owing to various factors such as a limited acoustic window and a smaller duct diameter.[6–8] Hence, the diagnosis of choledocholithiasis is frequently delayed until clinical suspicion prompts the use of other imaging modalities. Similarly, TUS examination is insensitive for the detection of ampullary tumors owing to overlying bowel gas with an accuracy of approximately 15% in 1 series.[9,10]

The usefulness of the CT scan in the evaluation of a dilated bile duct depends on the cause. It is highly sensitive for the detection of pancreatic tumors, especially those greater than 2 cm.[11,12] However, for tumors smaller than 2 cm, the sensitivity can be as low as 77%.[13] The accuracy of CT scans for the detection of small ampullary tumors, especially those confined to the duodenal lumen, is quite low.[10,14] Alternatively, a CT scan (either contrast enhanced or nonenhanced) performs better than TUS examination in the detection of intraductal stones with a reported sensitivity of between 72% and 88%.[15]

With the rightful decrease in the use of the diagnostic ERCP, MR cholangiography has evolved into the noninvasive gold standard for the evaluation of the biliary tree. It has been shown to be as sensitive as ERCP in the diagnosis of distal biliary strictures owing to pancreatic cancer.[16] The differentiation of a benign from a malignant biliary stricture on MRI/MRCP can be challenging, and although there are radiologic rules of thumb that can be considered, these imaging pearls often lack specificity.[17,18] MRCP is the noninvasive test of choice for the detection of common bile duct (CBD) stones with a high sensitivity and specificity.[19,20] However, for stones 3 mm or less in size, the sensitivity of MRCP decreases substantially to less than 50%.[21]

In recent years, EUS examination has cemented its role as the superior imaging modality for evaluation of the pancreaticobiliary tree. It has proven to be highly accurate in the detection of stones in the extrahepatic ducts (**Fig. 1**). A metaanalysis consisting of 3075 patients showed that EUS examination has a sensitivity as high as of 94% and specificity of 95% in detecting CBD stones.[22,23] EUS examination also has shown to perform well in the evaluation of biliary strictures (**Fig. 2**) with a metaanalysis demonstrating a sensitivity of 78% and specificity of 84% in detecting malignant biliary strictures.[23] The efficacy of EUS examination in distal biliary strictures is further augmented with the addition of fine needle aspiration to provide a sensitivity of 84% to 91% and a specificity of 71% to 100%[24,25] (**Fig. 3**). When ampullary lesions are a concern, direct endoscopic visualization with a side-viewing endoscope can effectively evaluate the periampullary area and allow for biopsies, with the role of EUS examination more often being to evaluate for deeper invasion of lesions or staging of ampullary tumors.

NONPATHOLOGIC CAUSES OF BILIARY DILATION

In the absence of clinical symptoms or abnormal liver tests, the pretest probability of finding pathology on further invasive testing is considered to be low, and nonobstructive etiologies are often suggested in the appropriate clinical setting. The more widely

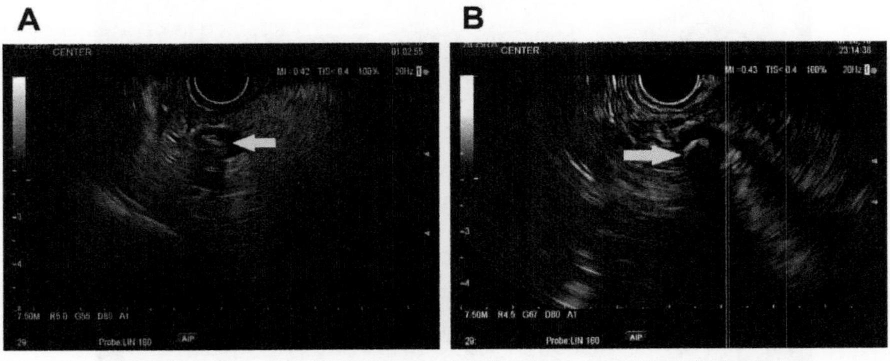

Fig. 1. (*A, B*). Endoscopic ultrasound images showing a cross-section of the distal common bile duct demonstrating a hyperechoic and shadowing intraductal structure consistent with a stone (*arrows*).

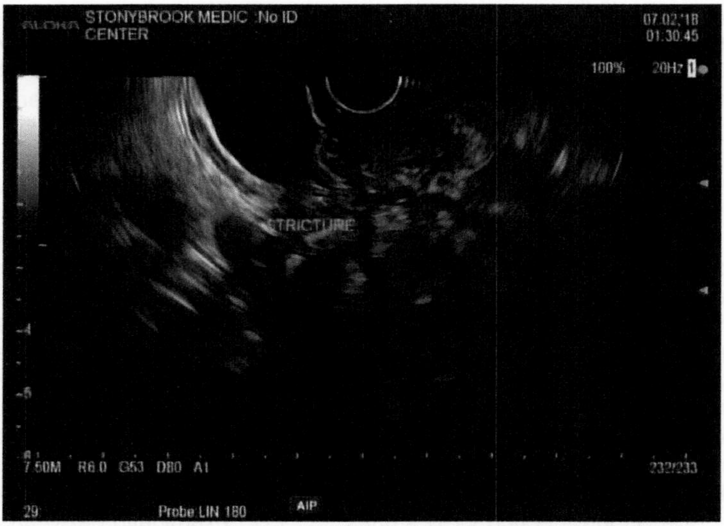

Fig. 2. Endoscopic ultrasound image demonstrating a stricture in the distal common bile duct.

quoted of these causes of biliary dilation include advanced age, chronic narcotic analgesic use, prior cholecystectomy, and previous biliary obstruction.

A prospective study of approximately 1000 patients showed that, although the bile duct does seem to dilate significantly with age, all patients in the study had bile ducts under the normal 7-mm cutoff.[26] Other studies have demonstrated similar findings with proposed upper limits in the elderly of 8.0 to 8.5 mm.[27–29] This scenario is especially true in the elderly with an intact gallbladder. This finding is, however, confounded

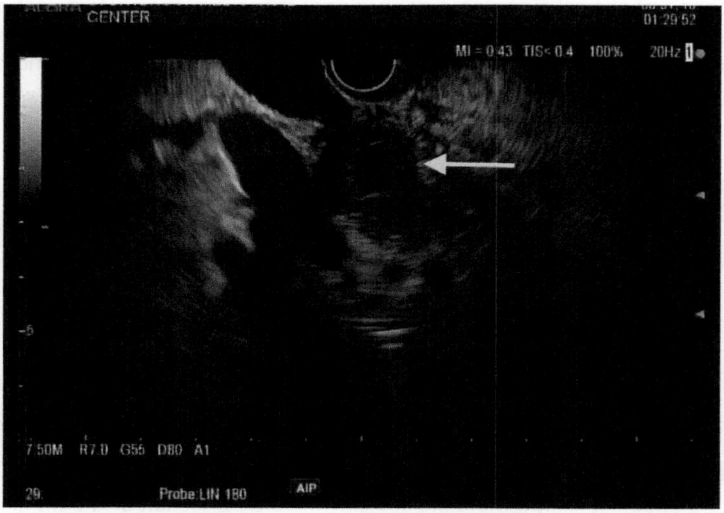

Fig. 3. Endoscopic ultrasound image showing a stricture of the distal common bile duct secondary to a mass in the head of the pancreas.

by the fact that certain obstructive etiologies such as malignancy are more common in the older patient and further investigation may be warranted when biliary dilation is significant (>8 mm), especially in the setting of symptoms or abnormal liver tests.

There has been much debate on the effect of the postcholecystectomy state on the size of the extrahepatic biliary tree. The gallbladder is believed to accommodate changes in pressure in the biliary tree, and thus, in its absence, can result in the transfer of these pressures to the bile duct causing dilation of the duct. Early studies suggested only a small change in the diameter of the bile duct after a cholecystectomy.[1] However, more recent retrospective studies have demonstrated significant increases in diameter, which has led to the suggestion that the upper limit of biliary diameter be increased to 10 mm in patients with prior cholecystectomy.[28–30] An alternative explanation in some patients may be that the biliary dilation may be secondary to a prior obstruction. The extrahepatic bile ducts are composed of mostly connective tissue with little or no smooth muscle. As such, prolonged distension of the bile duct can lead to permanent deformation, which may not normalize even after the obstruction is relieved.[1,31] In these 2 scenarios, further evaluation for the etiology of a dilated bile duct may not be required in the absence of biliary symptoms or abnormal liver tests.

An often underrecognized cause of isolated biliary dilation is the use of opiates. Opiates can cause an increase in the basal pressure and an increase in phasic contractions of the sphincter of Oddi leading to biliary dilation over time. One retrospective study showed an association, by TUS examination, of biliary dilation and addiction to opiates in asymptomatic patients with normal liver tests.[32] Another study evaluated 15 patients by EUS with a mean of 20 years of opiate addiction in the setting of abdominal pain and dilated extrahepatic ducts (10 of whom had normal liver tests). All 15 patients had biliary dilation without any evidence of other etiologies for obstruction.[33] Opiate use may also cause transient dilation of the biliary tree without elevations in liver enzymes, a phenomenon sometimes seen in imaging performed in the emergency room for unexplained abdominal pain where the patient may have already received intravenous narcotics before the imaging study. In the latter group of patients, repeat imaging often reveals resolution of the biliary dilation.

A rare cause of biliary dilation to consider is choledochal cysts. These cysts are congenital focal or segmental dilations of the biliary tree that may present in adulthood with abdominal pain or other vague abdominal symptoms. In addition, this finding can often be made incidentally on imaging performed for other reasons. Noninvasive imaging is often enough to make a definitive diagnosis; however, at times ERCP may be necessary to identify anomalous pancreaticobiliary anatomy and to rule out malignancy, which may develop in about 10% to 30% of adults with an increase in risk over time.[34]

THE IMPACT OF ENDOSCOPIC ULTRASOUND EXAMINATION IN ISOLATED BILIARY DILATION

Although the nonobstructive causes of unexplained biliary dilation discussed elsewhere in this article should be considered, the possibility of an occult pathology such as missed CBD stones or malignancy should be entertained and trigger further evaluation, particularly when clinical symptoms and/or biochemical abnormalities raise concern for these causes. There have been a few studies looking at the diagnostic impact of EUS examination in this clinical scenario (**Table 1**).

Studies have shown that TUS examination alone is not a sufficient test in the evaluation of a dilated biliary tree; on further investigation, a fair amount of pathology is often found. In a study by Kim and colleagues,[35] 77 asymptomatic patients with biliary

Table 1
Studies evaluating the impact of EUS on the evaluation of unexplained biliary dilation

	Patients with Normal Liver Tests	Positive Findings on EUS, n (%)	Patients with Abnormal Liver Tests	Positive Findings on EUS, n (%)
Malik et al,[42] 2007[a]	32	7 (21)	15	7 (46)
Rana et al,[44] 2013[a]	30	10 (33)	10	10 (100)
Sotoudehmanesh et al,[36] 2014	27	2 (7)	125	70 (56)
Bruno et al,[39] 2014[a]	57	12 (21)	N/A	N/A
Oppong et al,[45] 2014	40	7 (17)	N/A	N/A
Kwok et al,[40] 2009[a]	15	5 (33)	11	6 (55)
Steichen et al,[43] 2009	N/A	18%	N/A	51%

Abbreviations: EUS, endoscopic ultrasound; N/A, not applicable.
[a] Studies that included periampullary diverticulum and chronic pancreatitis as positive findings on EUS.

dilation (diagnosed by TUS examination alone) and normal liver tests were further investigated by either ERCP or CT scan, or repeat TUS examination. EUS examination was not performed in this study. Of the 49 patients who underwent ERCP, 20 patients had no lesions. However 29 of the 49 patients were found to have abnormalities that accounted for the biliary dilation, including periampullary diverticulum (n = 11), choledochal cyst (n = 4), anomalous pancreaticobiliary junction (n = 2), benign strictures (n = 10), and CBD mass (n = 2). Sotoudehmanesh and colleagues[36] performed a similar single-center prospective study of 152 patients with a dilated bile duct on TUS examination alone and subsequent evaluation with EUS. Only 32% and 45% of patients also underwent a CT scan and MRI/MRCP, respectively, after enrollment. In the subgroup of 27 patients who had normal liver tests, choledocholithiasis was found in 2 of the 27 patients. Five patients were thought to have had stones that had passed based on the clinical course. The remaining 20 of these 27 patients had nonpathologic findings—6 were normal, 6 had opium-induced dilation, and 8 had a prior cholecystectomy. In the other 125 patients with elevated liver tests, there were 32 cases of choledocholithiasis, 15 ampullary tumors, 14 distal cholangiocarcinomas and 9 pancreatic tumors. Thirty-five patients were thought to have passed a CBD stone, and the remainder were nonpathologic diagnoses. The high incidence of positive findings in the group of patients with elevated liver tests is most likely owing to the limited efficacy of TUS examination in identifying lesions in the distal bile duct and periampullary region.

The use of EUS examination as an additional diagnostic tool allows for not only the excellent visualization of the extrahepatic biliary tree, but also the systematic examination of the duodenal wall and the periampullary region. Although this is an invasive test, the procedure is well-tolerated and the complication rates have been shown to be low.[37,38] Although ERCP used to be considered the gold standard for the evaluation of biliary pathology, EUS examination has emerged as not only the safer, but also superior modality for evaluation of the pancreaticobiliary tree in this setting.

In cases of isolated biliary dilation without clinical symptoms or biochemical derangements, when an etiology is not identified on noninvasive imaging such as TUS examination, CT scan, or MRI, the clinical suspicion for biliary pathology is low.[39,40] In a study by Bruno and colleagues,[39] 57 patients with biliary dilation and normal liver enzymes were reviewed after the exclusion of those with a history of prior ERCP, biliary obstruction or jaundice. Forty-five patients (79%) did not have any abnormalities on EUS examination. Of the remaining 12, 6 patients had a periampullary diverticulum (with only 2 demonstrating indentation of the CBD), 2 had an ampullary adenoma, 2 had chronic pancreatitis, 1 had a 2-cm pancreatic head mass, and 1 had a CBD stone. During a mean follow-up period of 31 months, none of the patients with a negative EUS examination presented with relevant disease. The authors of this study raise an important point, valid for other similar studies, that there may be an overestimation of pathology because periampullary diverticula and chronic pancreatitis, in the absence of a consequent stricture, are not established causes of biliary obstruction and may be equally incidental findings.

In an abstract published in 2009 by Kwok and colleagues,[40] 30 patients with unexplained biliary dilation were evaluated by EUS examination. Four patients had a normal EUS examination without dilation, 15 patients revealed dilation but without specifically identified pathology, and 11 patients revealed abnormalities that consisted of choledocholithiasis, ampullary adenoma, cholangiocarcinoma, and chronic pancreatitis. In the 15 patients with unexplained dilation on EUS examination, there were no clinically significant events during the 16 month follow-up period.

Unlike patients with normal liver tests, the incidence of occult pathology may be higher in the presence of abnormal liver tests.[41] In a retrospective cohort of 47 patients with biliary dilation and no obvious pathology on prior imaging (including TUS examination, CT scan, or MRCP), 32 of 47 patients had normal liver enzymes representing the low suspicion group, whereas15 of 47 patients had elevated liver enzymes representing the moderate suspicion group.[42] The majority of patients (34 of 47) did not have any abnormalities on EUS examination to explain the dilation. In the low suspicion group, 2 of 32 patients were found to have significant pathology including a CBD stone and a periampullary diverticulum. Alternatively, in the moderate suspicion group, nearly one-half the patients (8 of 15 [53%]) had significant findings on EUS examination to explain their biliary dilation. The various pathologic lesions included 3 cases of CBD stones, 4 periampullary diverticula, and 1 ampullary tumor.

A second study published in abstract form by Steichen and colleagues[43] included 161 patients evaluated at a tertiary center for dilated bile duct where initial imaging failed to identify a cause. This study included patients with jaundice (21%) and patients with abnormal liver tests (43%) as separate categories, presumably with overlap. Of the patients with jaundice, 80% were found to achieve a diagnosis on EUS examination. The authors also reported that patients without jaundice or abnormal liver tests were less likely to have positive findings (18% vs 51%; $P<.0001$).

Rana and colleagues[44] retrospectively reviewed 40 patients referred to a single tertiary center for EUS examination for the evaluation of an unexplained dilation of the CBD. Of the 40 patients, 10 had elevated alkaline phosphatase levels. All of these 10 were found to have an abnormality on EUS examination, including 6 with stones, 2 with cholangiocarcinoma, and 2 with benign CBD strictures. Of the 30 with normal alkaline phosphatase levels, 20 had a normal EUS examination. The etiology in the other 10 patients with normal enzyme levels included 9 with choledocholithiasis and 1 with chronic pancreatitis. There was no difference in duct diameter between the groups with and without elevations in alkaline phosphatase, nor between the groups with and without pathology. The authors concluded that elevated liver tests portend a high pretest probability of pathologic findings, but that normal liver chemistries do not exclude the possibility of abnormalities in the biliary tree.

As these studies demonstrate, the presence of significant pathology in isolated asymptomatic biliary dilation is quite low, often revealing benign causes. Nonetheless, a healthy suspicion for malignant pathology should always be maintained and, in the appropriate clinical setting, less obvious nonobstructive etiologies should also be considered. A series by Oppong and colleagues[45] reviewed 83 patients with incidental CBD or/and pancreatic duct dilation with normal liver and pancreatic enzymes. Of these, 40 patients had isolated biliary dilation alone. Most of these patients (33 of the 40) did not have new findings on EUS examination. In fact, new findings on EUS examination were seen in only 7 of these 40 patients, including 3 with a CBD polyp, 3 with a stone, and 1 showing compression of the duct by the portal vein. Interestingly, all of the patients in this study with prior cholecystectomy fell into the larger group of 33 patients without new EUS findings.

SUMMARY

With the increased use of noninvasive imaging techniques to investigate abdominal complaints and other nongastrointestinal symptoms, there has been an increase in referrals to endosonographers for incidental findings such as isolated biliary dilation. Studies have demonstrated limitations in the ability of these noninvasive imaging modalities to distinguish clinically irrelevant variations in the biliary tree from pathologies with clinical consequence. Therefore, further diagnostic workup should be guided by the clinical presentation. Patients with symptoms localized to the biliary tree and/or abnormal liver tests have a higher pretest probability for significant pathology. The use of EUS examination as an additional investigative tool in these patients results in better evaluation of the distal CBD, the head of the pancreas, and the periampullary region. EUS examination in this group will often reveal significant findings that may lead to additional testing and/or intervention. In contrast, in asymptomatic patients with normal liver tests, the incidence of significant pathology is low. An otherwise normal EUS examination is reassuring in this group of patients and, if the patient

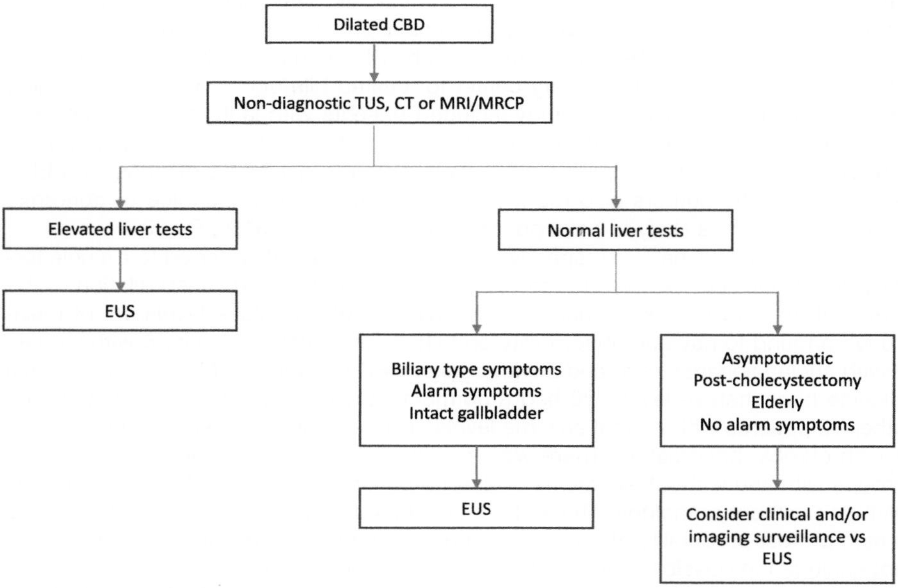

Fig. 4. Diagnostic approach to unexplained dilation of the extrahepatic bile duct. CBD, common bile duct; CT, computed tomography; EUS, endoscopic ultrasound; MRCP, magnetic resonance cholangiopancreatography; TUS, transabdominal ultrasound.

possesses an appropriate explanation for this isolated biliary dilation (eg, advanced age, chronic narcotic use, prior cholecystectomy, or prior treated biliary obstruction), it is reasonable to forego any further diagnostic workup and evaluation.

The evaluation of isolated dilation of the bile duct remains a challenge. Although the natural history of this condition may not be well-described, the data presented in this review suggest we may be able to stratify patients to those with and without a high likelihood of occult pathology. Thus, we propose an individually tailored approach (**Fig. 4**) based on current symptoms, the patient's history, liver, and pancreatic biochemistries, and an understanding of the expected diagnostic yield and risks of further investigation. Until more robust studies and long-term data become available, this process will help to minimize the chance of missed diagnoses while encouraging judicious use of health care resources.

REFERENCES

1. Coss A, Enns R. The investigation of unexplained biliary dilatation. Curr Gastroenterol Rep 2009;11(2):155–9.
2. Bowie JD. What is the upper limit of normal for the common bile duct on ultrasound: how much do you want it to be? Am J Gastroenterol 2000;95(4):897–900.
3. Niederau C, Müller J, Sonnenberg A, et al. Extrahepatic bile ducts in healthy subjects, in patients with cholelithiasis, and in postcholecystectomy patients: a prospective ultrasonic study. J Clin Ultrasound 1983;11(1):23–7.
4. Laing FC, Jeffrey RB, Wing VW, et al. Biliary dilatation: defining the level and cause by real-time US. Radiology 1986;160(1):39–42.
5. Cronan JJ. US diagnosis of choledocholithiasis: a reappraisal. Radiology 1986; 161(1):133–4.
6. Stott MA, Farrands PA, Guyer PB, et al. Ultrasound of the common bile duct in patients undergoing cholecystectomy. J Clin Ultrasound 1991;19(2):73–6.
7. Sugiyama M, Atomi Y. Endoscopic ultrasonography for diagnosing choledocholithiasis: a prospective comparative study with ultrasonography and computed tomography. Gastrointest Endosc 1997;45(2):143–6.
8. Majeed AW, Ross B, Johnson AG, et al. Common duct diameter as an independent predictor of choledocholithiasis: is it useful? Clin Radiol 1999;54(3):170–2.
9. Qiao QL, Zhao YG, Ye ML, et al. Carcinoma of the ampulla of Vater: factors influencing long-term survival of 127 patients with resection. World J Surg 2007;31(1): 137–43 [discussion: 144–6].
10. Skordilis P, Mouzas IA, Dimoulios PD, et al. Is endosonography an effective method for detection and local staging of the ampullary carcinoma? A prospective study. BMC Surg 2002;2:1.
11. Freeny PC, Marks WM, Ryan JA, et al. Pancreatic ductal adenocarcinoma: diagnosis and staging with dynamic CT. Radiology 1988;166(1 Pt 1):125–33.
12. Valls C, Andía E, Sanchez A, et al. Dual-phase helical CT of pancreatic adenocarcinoma: assessment of resectability before surgery. AJR Am J Roentgenol 2002; 178(4):821–6.
13. Bronstein YL, Loyer EM, Kaur H, et al. Detection of small pancreatic tumors with multiphasic helical CT. AJR Am J Roentgenol 2004;182(3):619–23.
14. Bakkevold KE, Arnesjø B, Kambestad B. Carcinoma of the pancreas and papilla of Vater: presenting symptoms, signs, and diagnosis related to stage and tumour site. A prospective multicentre trial in 472 patients. Norwegian Pancreatic Cancer Trial. Scand J Gastroenterol 1992;27(4):317–25.

15. Yeh BM, Liu PS, Soto JA, et al. MR imaging and CT of the biliary tract. Radiographics 2009;29(6):1669–88.
16. Adamek HE, Albert J, Breer H, et al. Pancreatic cancer detection with magnetic resonance cholangiopancreatography and endoscopic retrograde cholangiopancreatography: a prospective controlled study. Lancet 2000;356(9225):190–3.
17. Choi SH, Han JK, Lee JM, et al. Differentiating malignant from benign common bile duct stricture with multiphasic helical CT. Radiology 2005;236(1):178–83.
18. Park MS, Kim TK, Kim KW, et al. Differentiation of extrahepatic bile duct cholangiocarcinoma from benign stricture: findings at MRCP versus ERCP. Radiology 2004;233(1):234–40.
19. Hekimoglu K, Ustundag Y, Dusak A, et al. MRCP vs. ERCP in the evaluation of biliary pathologies: review of current literature. J Dig Dis 2008;9(3):162–9.
20. Romagnuolo J, Bardou M, Rahme E, et al. Magnetic resonance cholangiopancreatography: a meta-analysis of test performance in suspected biliary disease. Ann Intern Med 2003;139(7):547–57.
21. Nandalur KR, Hussain HK, Weadock WJ, et al. Possible biliary disease: diagnostic performance of high-spatial-resolution isotropic 3D T2-weighted MRCP. Radiology 2008;249(3):883–90.
22. Tse F, Liu L, Barkun AN, et al. EUS: a meta-analysis of test performance in suspected choledocholithiasis. Gastrointest Endosc 2008;67(2):235–44.
23. Garrow D, Miller S, Sinha D, et al. Endoscopic ultrasound: a meta-analysis of test performance in suspected biliary obstruction. Clin Gastroenterol Hepatol 2007;5(5):616–23.
24. Varadarajulu S, Tamhane A, Eloubeidi MA. Yield of EUS-guided FNA of pancreatic masses in the presence or the absence of chronic pancreatitis. Gastrointest Endosc 2005;62(5):728–36 [quiz: 751, 753].
25. Horwhat JD, Paulson EK, McGrath K, et al. A randomized comparison of EUS-guided FNA versus CT or US-guided FNA for the evaluation of pancreatic mass lesions. Gastrointest Endosc 2006;63(7):966–75.
26. Perret RS, Sloop GD, Borne JA. Common bile duct measurements in an elderly population. J Ultrasound Med 2000;19(11):727–30 [quiz: 731].
27. Bachar GN, Cohen M, Belenky A, et al. Effect of aging on the adult extrahepatic bile duct: a sonographic study. J Ultrasound Med 2003;22(9):879–82 [quiz: 883–5].
28. Senturk S, Miroglu TC, Bilici A, et al. Diameters of the common bile duct in adults and postcholecystectomy patients: a study with 64-slice CT. Eur J Radiol 2012;81(1):39–42.
29. Benjaminov F, Leichtman G, Naftali T, et al. Effects of age and cholecystectomy on common bile duct diameter as measured by endoscopic ultrasonography. Surg Endosc 2013;27(1):303–7.
30. Chawla S, Trick WE, Gilkey S, et al. Does cholecystectomy status influence the common bile duct diameter? A matched-pair analysis. Dig Dis Sci 2010;55(4):1155–60.
31. Mueller PR, Ferrucci JT, Simeone JF, et al. Observations on the distensibility of the common bile duct. Radiology 1982;142(2):467–72.
32. Farahmand H, PourGholami M, Fathollah MS. Chronic extrahepatic bile duct dilatation: sonographic screening in the patients with opioid addiction. Korean J Radiol 2007;8(3):212–5.
33. Sharma SS, Ram S, Maharshi S, et al. Pancreato-biliary endoscopic ultrasound in opium addicts presenting with abdominal pain. Endosc Ultrasound 2013;2(4):204–7.

34. Søreide K, Søreide JA. Bile duct cyst as precursor to biliary tract cancer. Ann Surg Oncol 2007;14(3):1200–11.
35. Kim JE, Lee JK, Lee KT, et al. The clinical significance of common bile-duct dilatation in patients without biliary symptoms or causative lesions on ultrasonography. Endoscopy 2001;33(6):495–500.
36. Sotoudehmanesh R, Nejati N, Farsinejad M, et al. Efficacy of Endoscopic Ultrasonography in Evaluation of Undetermined Etiology of Common Bile Duct Dilatation on Abdominal Ultrasonography. Middle East J Dig Dis 2016;8(4):267–72.
37. Amouyal P, Palazzo L, Amouyal G, et al. Endosonography: promising method for diagnosis of extrahepatic cholestasis. Lancet 1989;2(8673):1195–8.
38. Early DS, Acosta RD, Chandrasekhara V, et al. Adverse events associated with EUS and EUS with FNA. Gastrointest Endosc 2013;77(6):839–43.
39. Bruno M, Brizzi RF, Mezzabotta L, et al. Unexplained common bile duct dilatation with normal serum liver enzymes: diagnostic yield of endoscopic ultrasound and follow-up of this condition. J Clin Gastroenterol 2014;48(8):e67–70.
40. Kwok A, Lau J, Jones DB. Role of endoscopic ultrasound in evaluation of unexplained common bile duct dilation. Gastrointest Endosc 2009;69:AB250.
41. De Angelis C, Marietti M, Bruno M, et al. Endoscopic ultrasound in common bile duct dilatation with normal liver enzymes. World J Gastrointest Endosc 2015;7(8):799–805.
42. Malik S, Kaushik N, Khalid A, et al. EUS yield in evaluating biliary dilatation in patients with normal serum liver enzymes. Dig Dis Sci 2007;52(2):508–12.
43. Steichen JC, Lee JG, Chang KJ, et al. The utility of endoscopic ultrasound (EUS) in the evaluation of patients with bile duct dilation (BDD) of unclear etiology. Gastrointest Endosc 2009;69:AB244.
44. Rana SS, Bhasin DK, Sharma V, et al. Role of endoscopic ultrasound in evaluation of unexplained common bile duct dilatation on magnetic resonance cholangiopancreatography. Ann Gastroenterol 2013;26(1):66–70.
45. Oppong KW, Mitra V, Scott J, et al. Endoscopic ultrasound in patients with normal liver blood tests and unexplained dilatation of common bile duct and or pancreatic duct. Scand J Gastroenterol 2014;49(4):473–80.

Endoscopic Ultrasound–guided Liver Biopsy

David L. Diehl, MD

KEYWORDS

- Liver biopsy • Hepatic fibrosis • Cirrhosis • Abnormal liver tests • Core biopsy
- Fine-needle aspiration • Fine-needle biopsy

KEY POINTS

- Endoscopic ultrasound–guided liver biopsy (EUS-LB) is emerging as a cost-effective, safe, and well tolerated approach to liver biopsy.
- The ability of EUS-LB to target widely separated areas of liver allows more representative sampling.
- EUS-LB sampling with a 19G core needle using wet suction delivers liver cores of excellent length and minimal fragmentation, even in the setting of hepatic cirrhosis.
- In patients who need an upper endoscopy or diagnostic ultrasound as well as a liver biopsy, EUS-LB allows for efficient and cost-effective combination of services, which can lower overall costs for both procedures.

INTRODUCTION

For hepatologists, liver biopsy remains the gold standard for the assessment of chronic and subacute liver diseases in many cases. Timely application of this diagnostic test can lead to clarity in confusing or overlapping liver disorders.

The increasing awareness of the frequency of nonalcoholic steatohepatitis (NASH) and importance of this as a cause of cirrhosis and liver failure has brought renewed attention to accurate assessment of hepatic fibrosis. Great advances have been made in the noninvasive assessment of liver fibrosis, but often these cannot replace the need for biopsy.[1] Furthermore, noninvasive assessment of fibrosis can be misleading in some cases,[2] particularly with midrange amounts of fibrosis (so-called stages F2 and F3 fibrosis). With the increasing numbers of individuals with NASH and the anticipation of expanding pharmacologic therapies for this condition, it is likely that the need for liver biopsy for disease staging will increase.

Hepatologists have been largely getting out of the liver biopsy business, however, and farming these cases out to interventional radiology. The reasons for this are multiple: decrease in training and the ability to maintain liver biopsy case load,

Department of Gastroenterology and Nutrition, Geisinger Medical Center, 100 North Academy Avenue, 21-11, Danville, PA 17822, USA
E-mail address: dldiehl@geisinger.edu

Gastrointest Endoscopy Clin N Am 29 (2019) 173–186
https://doi.org/10.1016/j.giec.2018.11.002 **giendo.theclinics.com**
1052-5157/19/© 2018 Elsevier Inc. All rights reserved.

unavailability of image-guidance equipment in liver clinic or the endoscopy suite, and the time burden of postbiopsy recovery of patients undergoing liver biopsy.

The emergence of EUS-guided liver biopsy (EUS-LB) has allowed these procedures to come under the direct care of gastroenterologists and hepatologists, rather than leaking out to other departments.

METHODS OF LIVER BIOPSY

The first report of liver biopsy was by the well-known physician and scientist Paul Ehrlich in 1883. To accomplish a liver biopsy, a percutaneous (PC) site of puncture of the right lobe of the liver was identified by percussion of the liver span. The early proceduralists used a 14G or 16G needle to obtain a core biopsy specimen.

In recent years, image-guided target identification has become the standard approach, with this imaging accomplished with ultrasound or CT. Image guidance is important to avoid the adverse effects of gallbladder puncture or pneumothorax, rare complications of liver biopsy. With a specific apparatus that attaches to the ultrasound probe, real-time needle guidance can be accomplished, so that larger vessels can be identified and avoided. Real-time identification of vessels is not possible with CT-guided liver biopsy.

Transjugular (TJ) liver biopsy was first described in 1973[3] and remains an important approach to liver biopsy in patients with coagulopathy or those who require portal pressure measurements. Bleeding complications are rare, unless the biopsy needle inadvertently punctures the liver capsule, which can happen rarely in small cirrhotic livers.[4] Local complications at the site of vascular access (hematoma and pneumothorax) also can occur rarely.

The technique of EUS-LB was established in the past several years. Initially, a 19G trucut needle was used to accomplish the biopsy[5] (Quick-Core, Cook Medical, Bloomington, Indiana), but disappointing tissue yields led to abandonment of this approach. The discovery that a 19G EUS–fine-needle aspiration (FNA) needle could be used to accomplish EUS-LB with good tissue yields led to expansion in the use of EUS guidance for liver biosy.[6] There are currently several years of experience with the EUS-LB approach and a plethora of published experience demonstrating excellent tissue yields and procedural safety of this technique.[7,8]

TISSUE YIELDS OF ENDOSCOPIC ULTRASOUND–GUIDED LIVER BIOPSY COMPARED WITH OTHER METHODS OF LIVER BIOPSY

There are no prospective randomized trials of EUS-LB compared to TJ or PC liver biopsy. The author did a comparative study, however, of the 3 methods in a matched cohort of patients.[9] The biopsies of a group of 110 patients who had undergone EUS-LB were compared with biopsies of consecutive patients undergoing PC and TJ biopsy. Cirrhotic patients were excluded, because cirrhosis is known to decrease specimen lengths due to increased fragmentation. This study found that total specimen length and complete portal triad (CPT) count were comparable between the methods. Total specimen length and CPT were actually higher for EUS-LB than either TJ or PC when bilobar EUS biopsies were done (**Fig. 1**). This study, therefore, proved quantitative equivalency of EUS-LB to TJ or PC methods. For EUS-LB, a regular 19G EUS needle (not a core biopsy needle) was used for this study.

ADVANTAGES OF ENDOSCOPIC ULTRASOUND–GUIDED LIVER BIOPSY

There are several advantages of EUS-LB that have solidified its place as a method for liver biopsy. These include patients with a requirement for sedated liver biopsy, liver

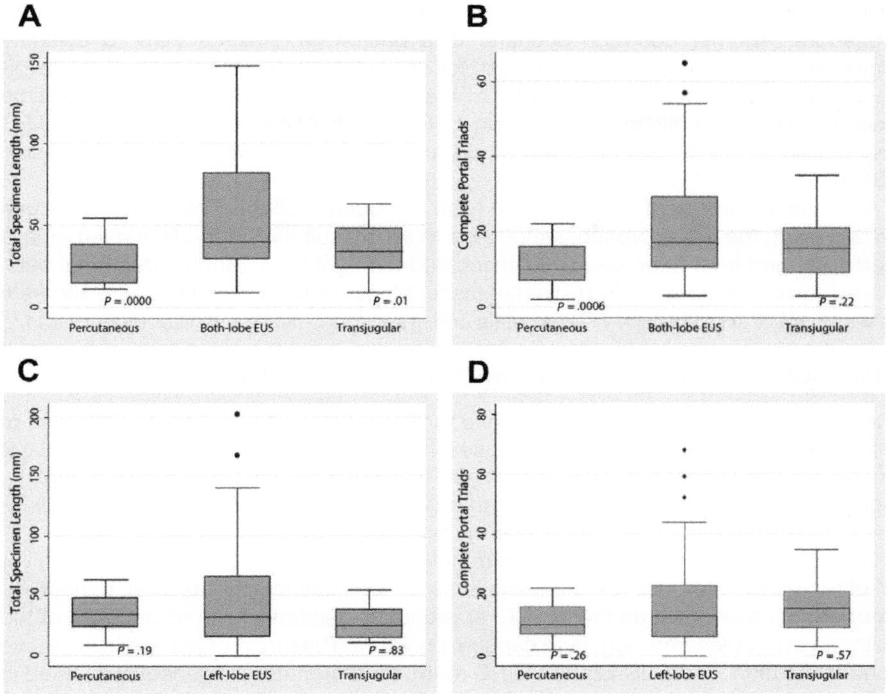

Fig. 1. (*A*) and (*B*) show total specimen length and number of CPTs, respectively, for the 3 methods of liver biopsy. Bilobar EUS-LB is superior to the PC method. (*C*) and (*D*) represent total specimen length and number of CPTs for left-lobe only EUS-LB, demonstrating equivalency of the methods for these measures.

biopsy in the pediatric patient, concomitant need for another endoscopic procedure along with liver biopsy, and requirement for bilobar liver biopsy.

Although PC or TJ liver biopsy is generally well tolerated, there is no question that EUS-LB is the most humane method of accomplishing liver biopsy. Some patients are extremely anxious before and during PC or TJ approaches, and because these procedures are generally done without sedation, only the brevity of the procedure (at least for PC) makes it tolerable. The author has noted patients who require a second liver biopsy to be very apprehensive about the second procedure, and EUS-LB can be offered to make it much more acceptable. For pediatric patients, these concerns are often even more pronounced. The additional small risk of sedation seems well worth the return in decreasing anxiety on the part of the pediatric patient and their parents.[10]

When there is a need for liver biopsy plus an endoscopic procedure, then EUS-LB is the most efficient and cost-effective way to accomplish this. The author frequently encounters situations requiring both procedures. In some cases, there is a need for esophagogastroduodenoscopy (EGD) to investigate dyspepsia, abdominal pain, gastroesophageal reflux disease, Barrett's esophagus evaluation, or surveillance or to rule out esophageal varices in suspected but not confirmed cirrhosis. It is also not uncommon for a patient to require an EUS as well as a liver biopsy. A common example is an EUS to rule out common bile duct pathology in cases of elevated liver tests. Absence of a common bile duct stone or biliary obstruction leads to liver biopsy, which would be done expeditiously rather than having the patient return for a second procedure. Another common scenario is a patient who needs EUS to evaluate abnormal CT imaging (a pancreatic cyst, for example) along with the need for liver biopsy. Again, the availability of EUS-LB at the same time is both cost saving and time saving. There are published data demonstrating safety of same-session EGD and PC liver biopsy.[11] The authors has not found any problems arising from same session EGD or EUS and EUS-LB.

A unique advantage of EUS-LB is the ease in procuring bilobar liver biopsy. This can be done with the PC approach, although is more difficult. For EUS-LB, the left lobe is readily imaged from the proximal stomach and the right lobe from the duodenal bulb. The ability to sample spatially distinct areas for biopsy may be useful for more accurate assessment of liver fibrosis, viral hepatitis activity, or post-transplant liver dysfunction.[12]

INDICATIONS AND CONTRAINDICATIONS FOR THE PROCEDURE

The indications for EUS-LB are like those for PC liver biopsy[13]: in brief, evaluation of liver diseases for which noninvasive assessment is inadequate. In addition, EUS-LB has expanded indications over PC. These include need for bilobar liver sampling, requirement for sedated liver biopsy, and patients who require an endoscopy or diagnostic EUS at the same time as a liver biopsy.

Contraindications for EUS-LB concern mainly coagulopathy from concomitant liver or other disease or use of anticoagulants or antiplatelet agents that cannot be stopped. In cases such as these, a TJ approach is generally favored because of the ability to avoid bleeding from liver capsule puncture. Presence of ascites is a relative contraindication, and EUS-LB (or the PC route, for that matter) is generally avoided in the presence of extensive intraperitoneal fluid and the TJ route favored. Small amounts of ascites are not considered a contraindication.

NEEDLE SELECTION

Historically, large needles (14G or 16G) were used for liver biopsy. These needles reliably delivered adequately long cores of tissue with a low amount of fragmentation. Use of these needles has largely given way, however, to spring-loaded Tru-Cut needles (**Fig. 2**), which are usually 18G at best, and often 20G Tru-Cut needles may be used. Therefore, use of a 19G EUS needle is more comparable to the currently used 18G needle than to the 14G to 16G needles of the past.

The largest EUS needle is 19G, and this has been the workhorse needle for EUS-LB. Recently, core-type needles have become available for EUS applications (Acquire, Boston Scientific, Marlborough, Massachusetts; SharkCore, Medtronic, Sunnyvale, California) (**Figs. 3** and **4**). The author has found that use of a 19G core biopsy needle for EUS-LB significantly increases specimen quality for every relevant metric, including total aggregate length, length of the longest piece, less fragmentation, and higher portal triad yields. The author considers a 19G core biopsy needle the preferred device for EUS-LB at present.

A 22G core needle is also available and is used by some endosonographers for EUS-LB. The core diameters, however, are approximately half that of the 19G needle. The author has shown that these narrower cores fragment extensively in the histology processing steps, leading to shorter specimens with increased fragmentation on the glass slide.[14] Due to this fragmentation, the author has found that the 22G core needle obtained an adequate specimen only 60% of the time compared with more than 90% with a 19G noncore EUS-FNA needle. The results of this study indicate that the 19G needle is preferred to a 22G core needle for EUS-LB.

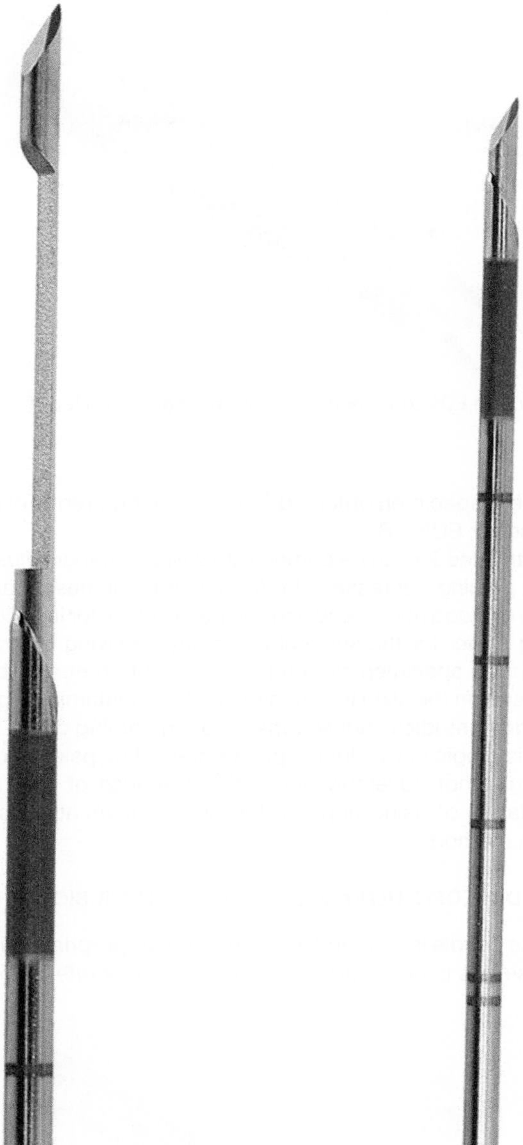

Fig. 2. Tip of the Tru-Cut biopsy needle (open and closed positions). (*Courtesy of* ProAct, Ltd., Corby, Northants, United Kingdom; with permission).

NEEDLE PREPARATION

Wet suction for EUS-FNA indicates the technique of removing the needle stylet and then flushing the needle lumen with fluid prior to attaching the vacuum syringe.[15] This technique was found to increase tissue yields of EUS-FNA of solid masses over dry suction. In a prospective crossover study, the author found that wet suction for EUS-LB was superior to dry suction in terms of less fragmentation of sample and

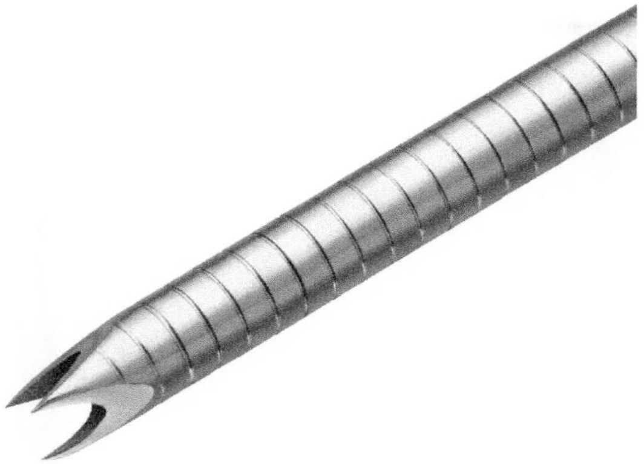

Fig. 3. Tip of the Acquire EUS core needle. (*Courtesy of* Boston Scientific, Marlborough, MA; with permission).

longer lengths of core specimen obtained.[16] The author currently exclusively uses the wet suction method for EUS-LB.

For wet suction, the needle can be primed with saline or heparin flush. The author has found that heparin priming decreases clot formation in the needle and, therefore, decreases production of blood noodles, which can be mistaken for liver cores. It also makes specimen handling easier for the surgical pathology receiving laboratory. In addition, decreased blood in the specimen makes pathologic interpretation by the pathologist easier, because tissue on the slide is enriched and less contaminating blood is present.

The author has done studies showing that heparin priming of the EUS needle does not interfere with histologic or cytologic appearances of biopsies and that immunohistochemical staining is not adversely affected.[17] Because of this, and the potential rheological advantages of using heparin, the author advocates using heparin flush for the wet suction method.

TECHNIQUE OF ENDOSCOPIC ULTRASOUND–GUIDED LIVER BIOPSY

After an appropriate needle is selected and prepared, appropriate targets are selected for biopsy. Because this is not a targeted biopsy of a discrete lesion, such as a liver

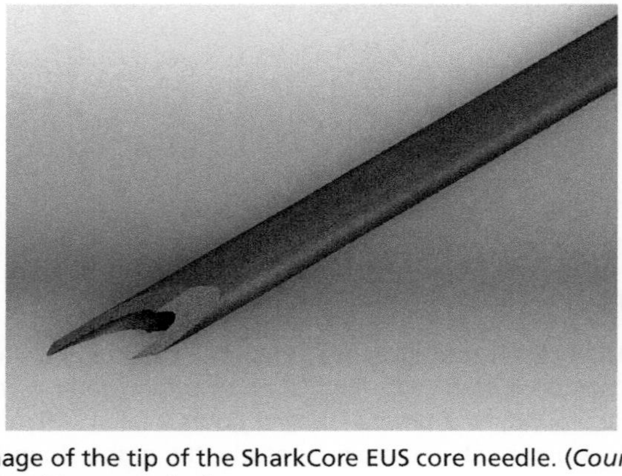

Fig. 4. Close-up image of the tip of the SharkCore EUS core needle. (*Courtesy of* Medtronic, Inc., Sunnyvale, CA; with permission).

metastasis, the process of target selection is different. In general, a long vessel-free trajectory is selected that allows uninterrupted needle passage to a depth of at least 3 cm (and potentially more) (**Fig. 5**). Care should be taken to confirm that if the left lobe of the liver is targeted, it is not confused with the spleen. In some cases of fatty liver, the echotexture of the liver can be surprisingly similar to the spleen.

After the needle is introduced through the duodenal bulb (right lobe) or gastric fundus (left lobe) and into the liver (**Fig. 6**), the suction syringe is turned on and several slow and deliberate needle passes with fanning are done. A single long pass often can deliver a long core of liver tissue, but the author tends to favor 3 needle passes to assure that specimen is obtained. After biopsy of the desired liver lobe, the suction syringe is turned off prior to removing the needle from the liver. The specimen is then chased from the needle lumen with either fluid flushing of the needle or reinsertion of the stylet.

Bilobar sampling decreases the chance of sampling error of the liver biopsy.[18–20] Another advantage of bilobar sampling is that if core yields from 1 lobe are less than adequate, increased yields from the other lobe can increase the overall amount of liver tissue and aid the pathologist. Bilobar sampling, however, is not strictly necessary if an adequate amount of tissue is obtained from one side. In patients who have had a Roux-en-Y gastric bypass, the left hepatic lobe is easily targeted, although it is generally not possible to obtain a biopsy from the right side of the liver.

SAMPLE HANDLING AFTER BIOPSY

Hepatologists who are used to doing PC liver biopsy may have been trained to put the obtained tissue core on a piece of gauze to assess adequacy of the biopsy. With specimens obtained by EUS-LB, this approach is not recommended due to the likelihood of introducing iatrogenic fragmentation of the specimen. The biopsy is extruded from the needle either with saline flush or with the stylet, directly into formalin. A tissue sieve

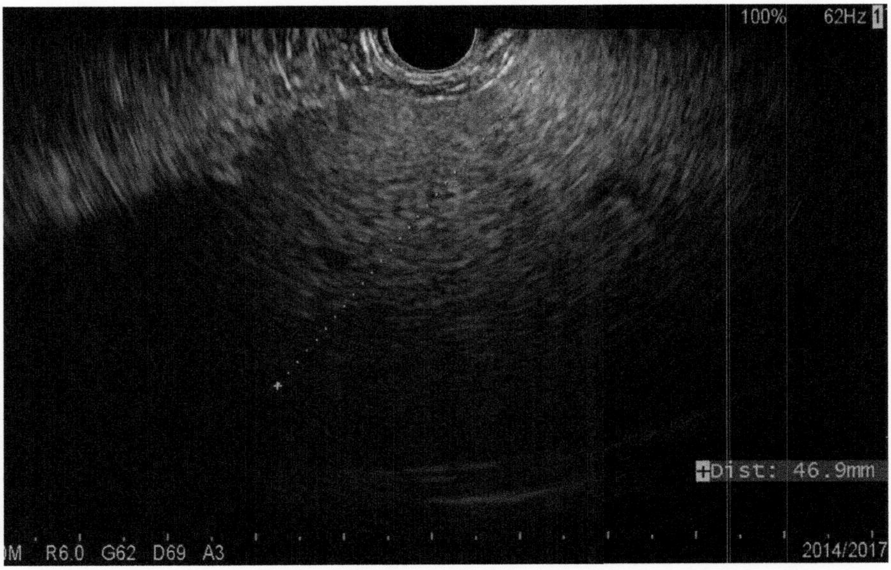

Fig. 5. Long needle trajectory of planned EUS-guided liver biopsy, right hepatic lobe (predicted trajectory indicated by dotted line).

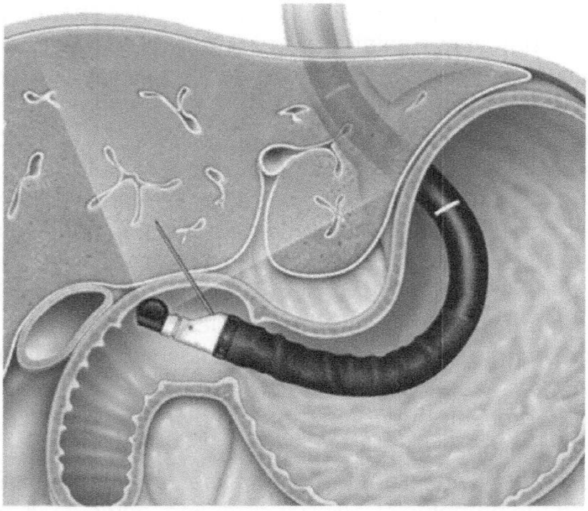

Fig. 6. Anatomic depiction of position of echoendoscope for right lobe EUS-LB. Transducer is positioned in the duodenal bulb. (*Courtesy of* Boston Scientific, Marlborough, MA; with permission).

can be used (**Fig. 7**) if there is a desire to wash away blood in the specimen (discussed previously).

The process of tissue fixation and embedding itself leads to unavoidable fragmentation. The risk of fragmentation is increased in fibrotic or cirrhotic tissue. The use of a 19G EUS core needle seems the best means possible of avoiding fragmentation and delivering longer tissue specimens, which are then easier for the pathologist to interpret (**Fig. 8**).

A large amount of blood is often obtained along with liver tissue during EUS-LB (**Fig. 9**). This does not present a safety concern, but the blood can make it hard at

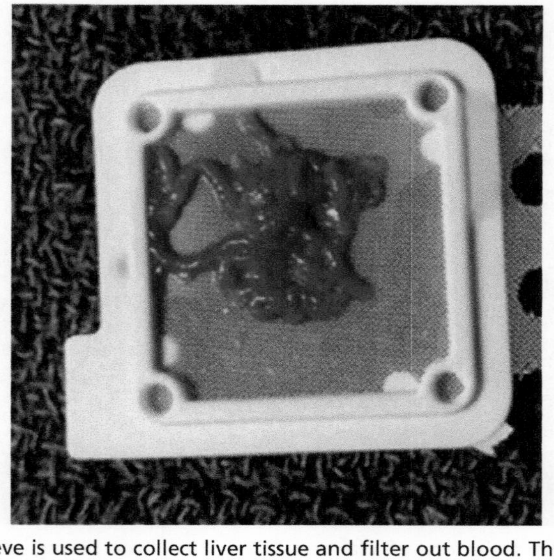

Fig. 7. A tissue sieve is used to collect liver tissue and filter out blood. This allows more accurate assessment of biopsy quantity immediately after EUS-LB.

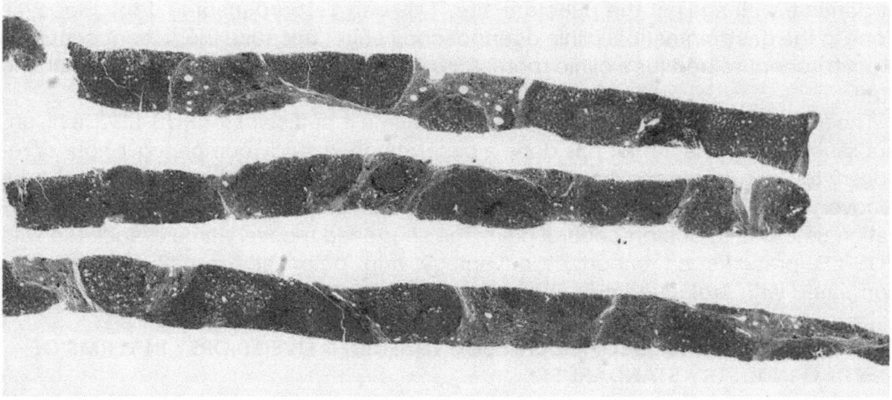

Fig. 8. Low-power photomicrograph of three long cores of cirrhotic liver. The newer 19G core biopsy needles allow these impressive lengths of biopsy without excessive tissue fragmentation, which is often seen with noncore needles (trichrome stain, original magnification ×10).

the time of the biopsy to determine if adequate liver tissue is obtained. In addition, the presence of blood makes the job of surgical pathology technicians harder, because they must separate the blood from the tissue prior to processing and embedding the liver tissue. The author has pioneered a procedural method involving heparin priming of the needle prior to biopsy, followed by tissue filtering and washing, to decrease these difficulties. The author has adapted a device to facilitate this process in the endoscopy suite and is developing a purpose-made tissue sieve device for general use, which should be available for use shortly.

POST–ENDOSCOPIC ULTRASOUND–GUIDED LIVER BIOPSY RECOVERY

Current guidelines for recovery time from PC liver biopsy are 2 hours to 4 hours, with the patient typically in a right decubitus position to offer tamponade of the

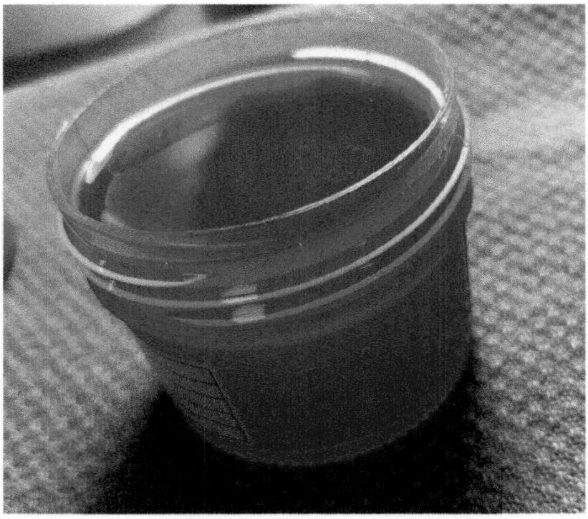

Fig. 9. Some EUS-LB samples have more blood in them, which can make assessment of adequacy of tissue acquisition harder.

abdominal wall against the puncture site. This can be burdensome if the biopsy is done in the gastrointestinal clinic or endoscopy suite, because the patient occupies a postprocedure bed (or a clinic room) for several hours while monitored by nursing staff.

The author has found that 1 hour of recovery time is sufficient for EUS-LB (Diehl, unpublished data). The author has done a case-matched study comparing 1 hour of recovery to 2 hours of recovery time after EUS-LB and found no advantage to 2-hour recovery in 90% of cases, with approximately 10% of patients requiring extra observation time due to postprocedural pain. The shortened recovery time associated with EUS-LB presents an important advantage and potential for real cost savings compared with prolonged outpatient procedure recovery.

TISSUE YIELDS OF ENDOSCOPIC ULTRASOUND–GUIDED LIVER BIOPSY IN TERMS OF MEETING INDUSTRY STANDARDS

Definitions of adequacy of a liver biopsy specimen has both quantitative and qualitative aspects. For some liver conditions (NASH, for example), more attention is paid to fibrosis and other features, whereas for others (primary biliary cirrhosis or autoimmune hepatitis, for example), a good assessment of the portal structures is critical. In the latter situations, having a higher number of CPTs is more important than in the former. In addition, expert liver pathologists are usually able to make diagnoses with smaller amounts of tissue compared with pathologists with less expertise, which can also change the weight of strict quantitative benchmarks.

There are several suggested metrics that have been suggested for quantitative adequacy of liver biopsies.[13,21,22] Most recommendations for total specimen length are from 15 mm to 20 mm, and adequacy of portal tracts has been quoted as from 6 to 10 complete portal tracts. EUS-LB does deliver cores of tissue that meet and exceed these benchmarks. The author finds that the use of the EUS core needle delivers longer specimens with more CPTs more consistently than a regular 19G EUS-FNA needle.[23]

COULD AN ENDOSCOPIC HEPATOLOGIST DO ENDOSCOPIC ULTRASOUND–GUIDED LIVER BIOPSY?

Learning EUS requires specialized additional training, usually in the context of a yearlong advanced endoscopy fellowship. This is understandable, given the wide range of organs and diseases addressed with EUS. But what if a physician only wants to do EUS-LB? Would it be possible to learn?

There are some examples of focused EUS procedures, in which a physician looks only at the organ system in question, without knowing how to perform an overall examination. Examples of this are transrectal endosonography, which may be performed by a colorectal surgeon, or esophageal or lung cancer staging, performed by a thoracic surgeon. In these examples, the operator does not necessarily need an in-depth understanding of EUS overall but only of the organ specifically examined. Short-format focused training programs exist for these indications.

A similar situation may apply to EUS-LB. With this procedure, attention is focused solely on the liver and how to safely accomplish biopsy. Most hepatologists are proficient at regular endoscopic procedures and could theoretically be taught how to pass the oblique-viewing echoendoscope, find the liver, and do the biopsy. In this way, the hepatologist could still be able to do the endoscopy in a patient who requires it and would not have to refer the liver biopsy to another practitioner, such as an interventional radiologist.

There are difficulties in bringing this possibility to reality, however. An important hurdle is for the hepatologist to get certified in doing an EUS procedure. At present, gastroenterology and gastrointestinal endoscopy societies do not make a distinction between a comprehensive EUS practice and a physician seeking to do EUS-LB only. According to current guidelines, this doctor would not likely have enough numbers of EUS procedures to certify. In addition, the ability to find and evaluate the common bile duct stone is important in a percentage of EUS-LB procedures, and this would entail more in-depth training for the hepatologist, which could be harder to accomplish.

For the present, at least, EUS-LB will likely remain in the purview of interventional endoscopists who perform EUS on a regular basis. As for other endoscopic procedures, adequate case volume is a key to establishing and maintaining competence. With expansion of EUS-LB, however, increased opportunities for training and certification in this procedure may be possible.

SUMMARY

As more clinical experience and published studies accumulate regarding EUS-LB, the niche for this diagnostic modality will continue to grow (**Boxes 1** and **2**). The development of the newer EUS core biopsy needles has been an important advance, and development of newer Tru-Cut needle technology may offer another way of obtaining excellent tissue cores of the liver. Development in technology to measure portal pressures via EUS in many cases will be complementary to EUS-LB and drive usage of both techniques. There remains a need for TJ approaches but likely only for patients with coagulopathy. There are multiple advantages to a sedated EUS-guided approach to liver biopsy for a wide range of stakeholders. Patients are likely to prefer a more comfortable and potentially safer procedure. There are advantages for health care workers, allowing higher procedural efficiency with decreased recovery time. And

Box 1
Endoscopic ultrasound–guided liver biopsy procedural checklist

Preprocedure

- Verify appropriate indication
- Verify no contraindications; confirm acceptable international normalized ratio and platelet count and patient not on anticoagulation or antiplatelet agents.
- Select needle (19G EUS needle, prefer EUS core biopsy needle, if available).
- Collect other supplies required for procedure: priming solution, formalin in specimen cups, and tissue filter, if desired.

Intraprocedure: target localization

- Target desired lobe of liver (or both, in some instances); proximal stomach for left lobe and duodenal bulb for right lobe
- For left lobe, confirm identify of liver and distinguish from spleen, which is seen from a similar location in the proximal stomach.
- Identify 2.5-cm to 5-cm trajectory for needle pass, which is free of vascular structures. Once adequate target is identified, open EUS needle and remove stylet.
- Prime needle with heparin flush or saline.
- Set vacuum in suction syringe (5–20 mL as desired), close stopcock, and attach to needle Luer connector.
- Introduce needle into channel of echoendoscope.

Intraprocedure: tissue acquisition

- Recheck adequate trajectory for needle.
- Lock endoscope knobs and have assistant hold the echoendoscope at the bite block.
- Introduce needle through gastric or duodenal wall with a quick, short stroke.
- Open stopcock.
- Steady and not overly fast needle pass into liver. Use as long a pass as possible, while avoiding vessels.
- One to three to-and-fro movements of needle with slight fanning motion of needle accomplished with elevator and/or large wheel.
- Before removing needle from liver, close stopcock on vacuum syringe.

Assessment of adequacy and tissue handling

- Express specimen from needle lumen by flushing with saline or heparin flush or by using the stylet.
- Flush specimen directly into formalin without other handling, and visually inspect contents to assess specimen adequacy.
- If using the tissue sieve method, flush tissue onto nylon mesh, then gently flush with saline to remove blood. Assess specimen adequacy by inspecting tissue on the sieve, then float specimen from sieve into the formalin jar.
- If inadequate tissue obtained, repeat biopsy from same liver lobe or the other one.

importantly, health care payers can benefit from potentially decreased costs and resource utilization.

The future role of EUS-LB looks bright and the author expects further growth and adoption of this approach as long as liver biopsy remains an important diagnostic modality.

Box 2
Indications and contraindications and situations where endoscopic ultrasound–guided liver biopsy may be preferred

Indication for EUS-LB

Any patient who requires a liver biopsy and can tolerate at least moderate sedation for an endoscopic procedure

Contraindications for EUS-LB

Coagulopathy with platelet count less than 50,000 or international normalized ratio greater than 1.5

Uninterruptible use of anticoagulants or antiplatelet agents

Large amount of ascites

Known cirrhosis or requirement for measurement of portal pressure

Specific situations where EUS-LB may be preferred to other means of liver biopsy

Requirement for sedated liver biopsy

Pediatric liver biopsy

Concomitant need for endoscopic procedure along with liver biopsy

Requirement for bilobar liver biopsy

REFERENCES

1. Caldwell S. Liver biopsy: the reports of its demise are greatly exaggerated. Clin Transl Gastroenterol 2016;7:e171.
2. Boursier J, Calès P. Clinical interpretation of Fibroscan® results: a real challenge. Liver Int 2010;30(10):1400–2.
3. Rösch J, Lakin PC, Antonovic R, et al. Transjugular approach to liver biopsy and transhepatic cholangiography. N Engl J Med 1973;289(5):227–31.
4. Lebrec D, Goldfarb G, Degott C, et al. Transvenous liver biopsy: an experience based on 1000 hepatic tissue samplings with this procedure. Gastroenterology 1982;83(2):338–40.
5. Dewitt J, McGreevy K, Cummings O, et al. Initial experience with EUS-guided Tru-cut biopsy of benign liver disease. Gastrointest Endosc 2009;69(3):535–42.
6. Stavropoulos SN, Im GY, Jlayer Z, et al. High yield of same-session EUS-guided liver biopsy by 19-gauge FNA needle in patients undergoing EUS to exclude biliary obstruction. Gastrointest Endosc 2012;75(2):310–8.
7. Diehl DL, Johal AS, Khara HS, et al. Endoscopic ultrasound-guided liver biopsy: a multicenter experience. Endosc Int Open 2015;3(3):E210–5.
8. Sey MS, Al-Haddad M, Imperiale TF, et al. EUS-guided liver biopsy for parenchymal disease: a comparison of diagnostic yield between two core biopsy needles. Gastrointest Endosc 2016;83(2):347–52.
9. Pineda JJ, Diehl DL, Miao CL, et al. EUS-guided liver biopsy provides diagnostic samples comparable with those via the percutaneous or transjugular route. Gastrointest Endosc 2016;83(2):360–5.
10. Johal AS, Khara HS, Maksimak MG, et al. Endoscopic ultrasound-guided liver biopsy in pediatric patients. Endosc Ultrasound 2014;3(3):191–4.
11. Stine JG, Liss G, Lewis JH. The safety of same-day endoscopy and percutaneous liver biopsy. Dig Dis Sci 2011;56(4):1201–6.
12. Larson SP, Bowers SP, Palekar NA, et al. Histopathologic variability between the right and left lobes of the liver in morbidly obese patients undergoing Roux-en-Y bypass. Clin Gastroenterol Hepatol 2007;5(11):1329–32.
13. Rockey DC, Caldwell SH, Goodman ZD, et al. American Association for the study of liver diseases. Liver biopsy. Hepatology 2009;49(3):1017–44.
14. Mok SR, Diehl DL, Johal AS, et al. Mo1245 19 versus 22-gauge fine needle biopsy for endoscopic ultrasound guided liver biopsy (EUS-LB): a prospective randomized trial. Gastrointest Endosc 2017;85(5):AB473–4.
15. Attam R, Arain MA, Bloechl SJ, et al. "Wet suction technique (WEST)": a novel way to enhance the quality of EUS-FNA aspirate. Results of a prospective, single-blind, randomized, controlled trial using a 22-gauge needle for EUS-FNA of solid lesions. Gastrointest Endosc 2015;81(6):1401–7.
16. Mok SR, Diehl DL, Johal AS, et al. A prospective pilot comparison of wet and dry heparinized suction for EUS-guided liver biopsy (with videos). Gastrointestinal endoscopy 2018;88(6):919–25.
17. Diehl DL, Mok SR, Khara HS, et al. Heparin priming of EUS-FNA needles does not adversely affect tissue cytology or immunohistochemical staining. Endosc Int Open 2018;6(3):E356.
18. Baunsgaard P, Sanchez GC, Lundborg CJ. The variation of pathological changes in the liver evaluated by double biopsies. Acta Pathol Microbiol Scand 1979;87: 51–7.
19. Abdi W, Millan JC, Mezey Y. Sampling variability on percutaneous liver biopsy. Arch Intern Med 1979;139:667–9.

20. Maharaj B, Maharaj RJ, Leary WP, et al. Sampling variability and its influence on the diagnostic yield of percutaneous needle biopsy of the liver. Lancet 1986;1: 523–5.
21. Bravo AA, Sheth SG, Chopra S. Liver biopsy. N Engl J Med 2001;344(7):495–500.
22. Shiha G, Sarin SK, Ibrahim AE, et al. Liver fibrosis: consensus recommendations of the Asian Pacific Association for the Study of the Liver (APASL). Hepatol Int 2009;3(2):323–33.
23. Ching-Campanioni R, Diehl DL, Confer B, et al. Mo1349 A prospective randomized trial of 19-Gauge (G) aspiration needle versus 19G core biopsy needle for endoscopic ultrasound-guided liver biopsy. Gastrointest Endosc 2018;87(6): AB457–8.

Advances in Endoscopic Imaging of the Biliary Tree

Saurabh Mukewar, MD*, David Carr-Locke, MD, FRCP, NYSGEF

KEYWORDS

• Biliary imaging • Cholangioscopy • Endomicroscopy • OCT

KEY POINTS

- Cholangioscopy has gained widespread popularity since the introduction of the digital single-operator cholangioscope.
- There has been improvement in techniques of direct peroral cholangioscopy.
- Newer indications for cholangioscopy are emerging.
- Image enhancement and newer imaging techniques are being developed.

INTRODUCTION

Endoscopic visualization of the biliary tree was first successfully performed more than 4 decades ago, with the first reported case in 1975.[1] There has been a refinement of cholangioscopy over the years, with improvement in endoscopes, accessories, and techniques. Wide application of this procedure was not possible, however, largely due to expensive and suboptimal devices. Use was limited to expert endoscopists for many years. More recently, with the introduction of a digital single-operator cholangioscope, this has changed. Cholangioscopy has gained popularity and is increasingly performed by endoscopists worldwide with high success rates. In addition, there have been developments in image enhancement and newer imaging techniques, such as intraductal ultrasound (IDUS), confocal laser endomicroscopy (CLE), and optical coherence tomography (OCT).

CHOLANGIOSCOPY SYSTEMS

Cholangioscopy can be performed via the percutaneous transhepatic or peroral routes. The percutaneous transhepatic approach can be associated with

Disclosure statement: S. Mukewar: Author discloses no conflict of interest. D. Carr-Locke: Royalties from US Endoscopy and Telemed Systems; Consultant for Boston Scientific Corporation and Mauna Kea Technologies; and Patent holder for Valentx and Ergogrip.

David H. Koch Medical Center, Department of Gastroenterology, Joan & Sanford I. Weill Medical, College of Cornell University, New York Presbyterian Hospital, 1278 York Avenue, 9th Floor, New York, NY 10065, USA
* Corresponding author.
E-mail address: saurabhmukewar@gmail.com

Gastrointest Endoscopy Clin N Am 29 (2019) 187–204
https://doi.org/10.1016/j.giec.2018.12.007
1052-5157/19/© 2018 Elsevier Inc. All rights reserved.

prolonged hospitalization and complications, such as bleeding, bile leak, and risk of metastases along the sinus tract or peritoneum.[2,3] It requires the creation of a mature, large-diameter track placed by interventional radiology, which may take several weeks to form. The oral route is generally preferred. Peroral cholangioscopy can be performed via either a direct approach (ie, direct advancement of an endoscope into the bile ducts) or an indirect approach (ie, mother-baby system with insertion of a cholangioscope through the instrumentation channel of a duodenoscope).

DIRECT PERORAL CHOLANGIOSCOPY

Direct peroral cholangioscopy (DPOC) involves advancement of an ultraslim forward-viewing endoscope through the patient's mouth directly into the bile ducts (**Fig. 1**). It requires prior endoscopic retrograde cholangiopancreatography (ERCP) with sphincterotomy or sphincteroplasty to facilitate advancement of the ultraslim endoscope across the papilla. The ultraslim endoscopes were originally designed for gastroscopy in pediatric patients or for traversing stenoses. The use of such endoscopes for performing cholangioscopy was first demonstrated in 1976.[4] All endoscopists must be aware that using gastroscopes for cholangioscopy carries a real risk of exerting excessive gas pressure (air or carbon dioxide) in the bile duct, with the possibility of gas embolism (**Fig. 2**). Air or carbon dioxide supply should, therefore, be disabled during cholangioscopy. The advantages of the direct method compared with indirect cholangioscopy include superior image quality (**Fig. 3**) and a larger channel for accessories. DPOC, however, is technically challenging. Looping of the endoscope in the stomach and the diameter of the endoscope often leads to difficulty in advancing the endoscope into the bile duct and maintaining stability. Several techniques and modifications have been suggested to overcome these challenges.

Freehand Technique

The freehand technique involves advancement of the slim endoscope directly into the papilla as for regular endoscopy. Once the endoscope is advanced in to the second part of duodenum, the tip is flexed to form a J-shaped configuration and the scope is then advanced into the bile duct.[5]

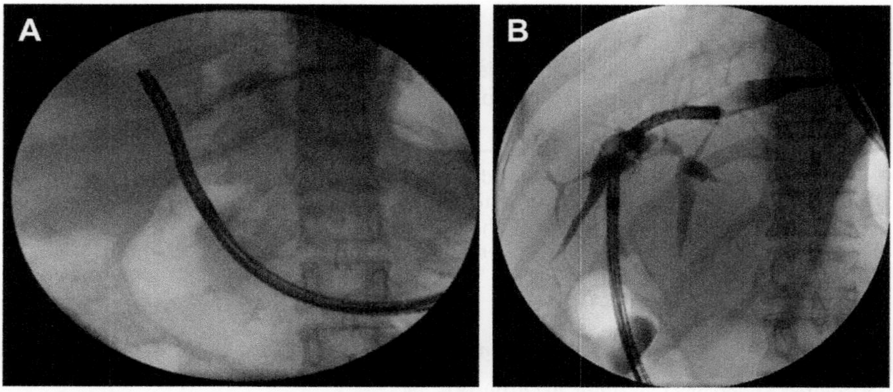

Fig. 1. Example of DPOC with small-caliber gastroscope (*A*) placed into the right hepatic duct and (*B*) placed into the left hepatic duct.

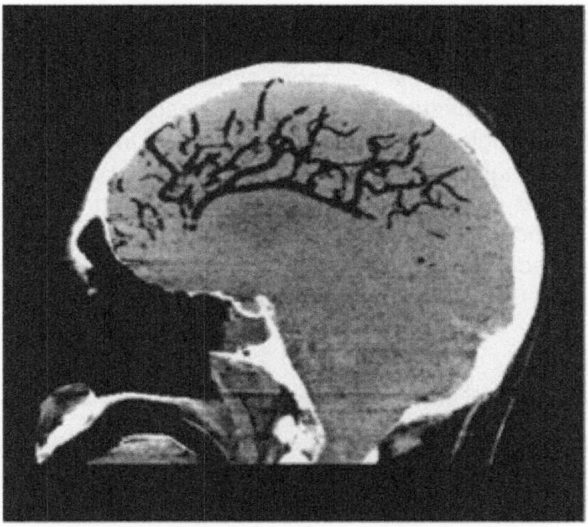

Fig. 2. CT scan of cerebral air embolus.

Tandem Technique

In the tandem technique, a guide wire is advanced into the bile ducts through a duodenoscope. The duodenoscope is then withdrawn and the slim endoscope is loaded over the guide wire into the bile ducts.[6] An overtube can be used to facilitate advancement of the endoscope to prevent looping of the endoscope in the stomach.[7]

Balloon Assisted Technique

An ultraslim endoscope preloaded with a balloon catheter over a guide wire is advanced into the duodenum, and biliary cannulation is performed with the guide wire. The balloon catheter is advanced into the bile ducts, inflated, and anchored. The endoscope is then advanced into the biliary tree with slight back traction of the

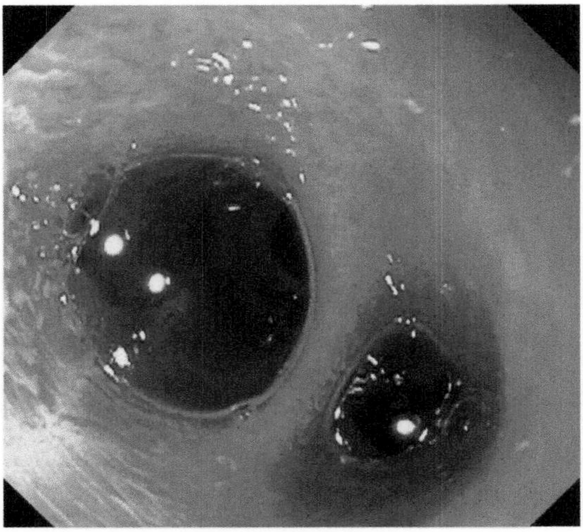

Fig. 3. Example of endoscopic image from DPOC.

inflated balloon catheter to assist in advancement of the endoscope.[8,9] Another balloon catheter type with a detachable exterior handle, allowing endoscope exchange, has been described but is no longer available (**Fig. 4**).

These techniques have limitations preventing widespread use of DPOCs. The freehand technique is challenging with high failure rates of intubating the bile duct. The guide wire or anchoring balloon assists in intubating the bile duct. Although the balloon anchors the device and provides stability while performing cholangioscopy, accessories cannot be advanced because the working channel is occupied by the anchoring balloon. To advance accessories, the balloon catheter needs to be removed, which makes the endoscope unstable during therapeutic applications, such as lithotripsy.

RECENT DEVELOPMENTS

Hybrid Balloon Catheter Anchoring Device

To overcome the limitation of an unstable endoscope after removal of balloon catheter anchoring devices, a new hybrid balloon catheter anchoring device has been described (**Fig. 5**).[10] In this anchoring device, the guide wire is tied to the distal end of the balloon catheter, which provides stability, especially while performing therapeutic procedures. Investigators have reported high technical success (>90%) with this catheter.[10]

Reusable Guiding Probe of Katz

The reusable guiding probe of Katz device is analogous to a papillotome, with a metal coil and an atraumatic tip (guide probe) (**Fig. 6**). The probe is advanced into the intrahepatic bile ducts via a duodenoscope. The duodenoscope is then removed and an ultraslim endoscope is advanced over the probe while the probe is kept under tension with a clamping device. This method prevents the looping of the ultraslim endoscope in the stomach due to stiffness of the probe. In a study of 17 patients, technical success of advancing cholangioscopes was 90% and for interventions was 85%.[11]

Double-bending Cholangioscope

In an attempt to overcome the difficulties of opposing vectors inherent in passing an endoscope in the axis of the upper gastrointestinal tract and then making an acute turn into the bile duct, a multibending cholangioscope was developed. In a recent study,

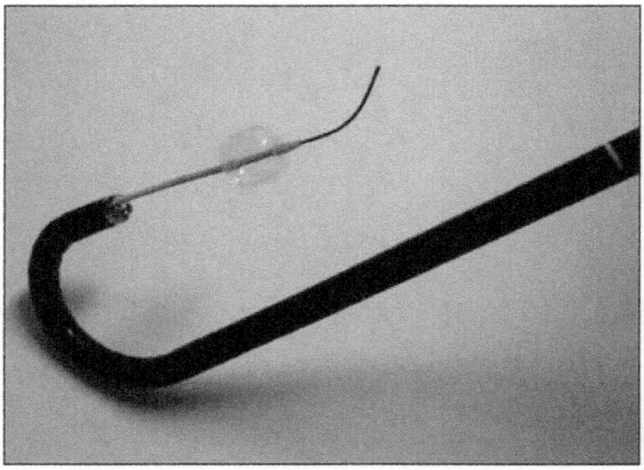

Fig. 4. Balloon assisted DPOC. (*Courtesy of* Dr Peter Kelsey, Boston, MA; with permission.)

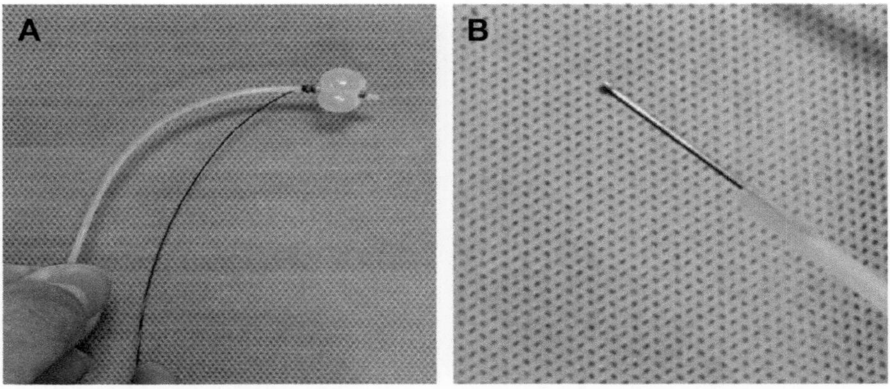

Fig. 5. Hybrid anchoring balloon for direct cholangioscopy. (*A*) A 0.021-inch guidewire tied to the balloon catheter at 2–3 mm from its distal end. (*B*) A specialized needle used to prevent deflation of the balloon after cutting the proximal handle portion of the balloon catheter. (*From* Li J, Guo SJ, Zhang JC, et al. A new hybrid anchoring balloon for direct peroral cholangioscopy using an ultraslim upper endoscope. Dig Endosc 2018;30(3):364–71, with permission.)

the second prototype version of this cholangioscope was evaluated.[12] It has 2 bending sections: a proximal section, which can be deflected in a single plane (90° up or 90° down), and a distal section, which can also be deflected in a single plane (160° up or 100° down). This endoscope was evaluated in a series of 41 patients undergoing cholangioscopy. In 7 patients, a freehand technique was attempted and failed in all. Using a guide wire or balloon assisted technique, a technical success of 88.2% was achieved in the remaining 34 cases and biliary interventions could be successfully performed in 88% of these cases.[13] The third prototype of this cholangioscope was developed with further modifications including a smaller distal end (4.9 mm compared with 5.2 mm of second prototype) and an ability defect the distal tip by 200° (compared with 160° with the second prototype) (**Fig. 7**).[14] In a study of 74 patients, the papilla was successfully entered in 97% cases, with an anchoring balloon needed in only 28%, and a majority of the bile ducts were cannulated by a freehand technique. This significantly reduced the procedure time in many cases. The targeted bile duct was entered in 84% of patients.[14]

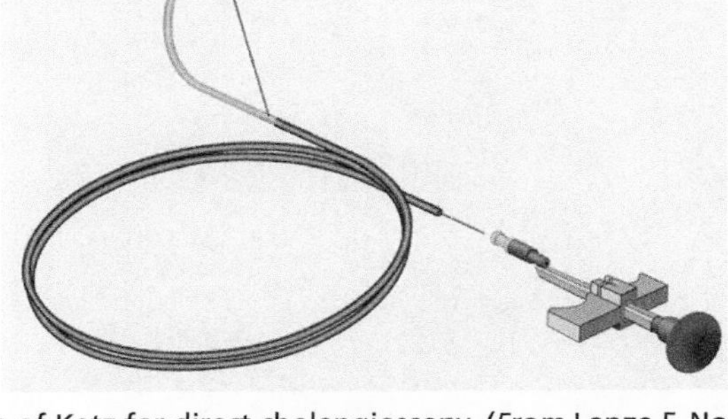

Fig. 6. Guide probe of Katz for direct cholangioscopy. (*From* Lenze F, Nowacki TM, Beyna T, et al. Direct peroral cholangioscopy with a new anchoring technique using the guide probe of Kautz - first clinical experiences. Endoscopy 2017;49(9):909–12, with permission.)

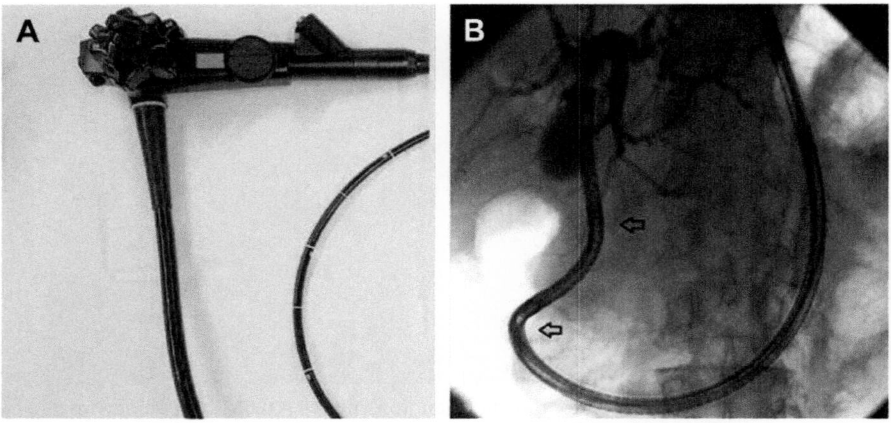

Fig. 7. Double-bending cholangioscope. (*A*) Photograph of the cholangioscope. (*B*) Radiographic image showing angulation of its two bending sections. (*From* Beyna T, Farnik H, Sarrazin C, et al. Direct retrograde cholangioscopy with a new prototype double-bending cholangioscope. Endoscopy 2016;48(10):929–33, with permission.)

INDIRECT CHOLANGIOSCOPY

Dual-operator System

In the dual-operator system, a baby cholangioscope is advanced into the bile duct through the working channel of a mother duodenoscope. In general, 2 operators are required to perform the procedure with 1 operating each endoscope (**Fig. 8**). Due to high cost, fragility of the instrument, and the need for 2 operators, dual operator system has fallen out of favor but, for decades, this was the only indirect system available. A video version of the baby endoscope is no longer available.

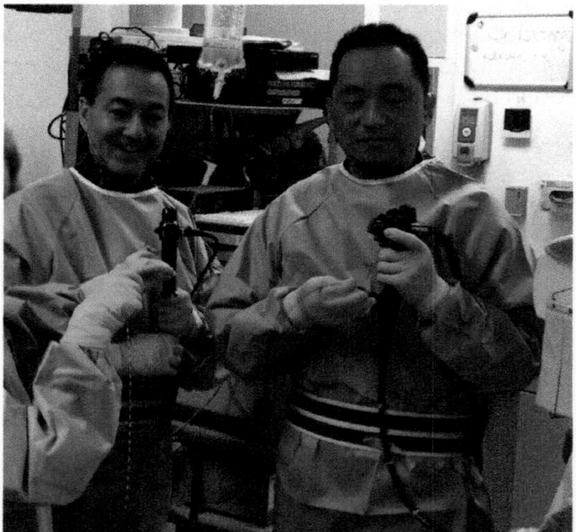

Fig. 8. Dual mother-baby cholangioscopy system (Hu Bing and John Martin demonstrating during the Cedars-Sinai International Symposium of Pancreaticobiliary Endoscopy).

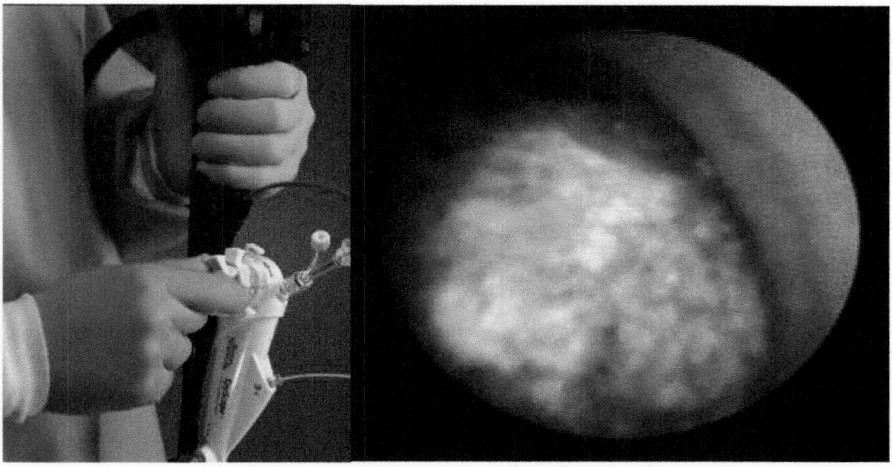

Fig. 9. Fiberoptic Spyglass (*A*) and bile duct image showing a stone (*B*). (*Courtesy of* Boston Scientific, Inc., Marlborough, MA.)

Single-operator System

Single operator cholangioscopy is performed with a single-operator cholangioscope initially made as a directable plastic sheath and a reusable optical combined light and image guide (Legacy SpyGlass, Boston Scientific, Marlborough, Massachusetts) (**Fig. 9**) now replaced by a completely disposable device with digital imaging (SpyGlass DS, Boston Scientific) (**Fig. 10**). The technique of insertion is similar to dual-operator cholangioscopy with advancement of the cholangioscope with or without a guide wire, except that the procedure can be performed by 1 operator controlling the carrier mother duodenoscope and the 3.3-mm diameter cholangioscope. The cholangioscope captures images digitally and has 4-way tip deflection and 2 channels, 1 for irrigation and 1 for suction, which also allows passing miniature instruments to achieve biopsy, endomicroscopy, laser lithotripsy, electrohydraulic lithotripsy, and snare or basket retrieval. In a recent study, it had superior visualization, image quality, and maneuverability than previous semidisposable, fiberoptic single-operator cholangioscopes.[15] Comparison between types of indirect cholangioscopy is illustrated in **Table 1**.

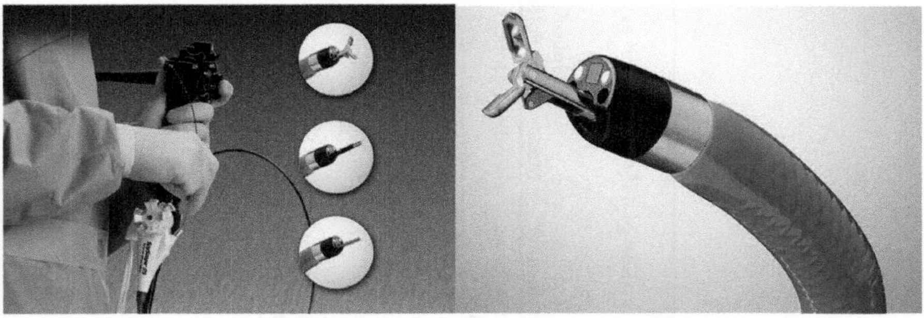

Fig. 10. Digital SpyGlass DS. (*Courtesy of* Boston Scientific, Inc., Marlborough, MA; with permission.)

Table 1
Comparison of different types of available indirect peroral cholangioscopes

Manufacturer	Model	Optical or Digital	Insertion Tube Diameter (mm)	Distal Diameter (mm)	Accessory Channel Diameter (mm)	Depth of Field (mm)	Angle of View (degrees)	Bending Section (degrees)	Working Length (mm)	Total Length (mm)	Single or Dual Operator
Pentax Tokyo, Japan	FCP-9P	Optical	3.1	3.1	1.2	1–50	90	90 up, 90 down	1900	2180	Dual
Olympus Shinjuku, Tokyo, Japan	CHF-BP30	Optical	3.4	3.1	1.2	1–50	90	160 up, 130 down	1870	2190	Dual
Boston Scientific Marlborough, MA	SpyGlass DS	Digital	3.6	3.5	1.2	??	120	30 up, 30 down 30 left 30 right	2140	2140	Single

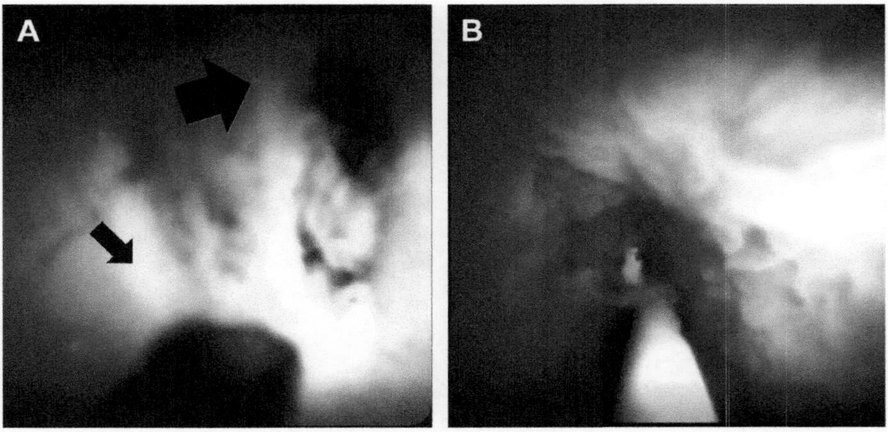

Fig. 11. SpyGlass DS image of bile duct stricture showing (*A*) stricture lumen (*large arrow*) and retained suture material (*small arrow*) and (*B*) same stricture being interrogated by a CLE probe. (*Courtesy of* Boston Scientific, Inc., Marlborough, MA.)

VISUALIZATION

Visualization during cholangioscopy can be achieved with water irrigation or CO_2 insufflation. CO_2 provides clearer images[16,17] than water but water is required for some of the therapeutic procedures, such as electrohydraulic or laser lithotripsy. The safety of CO_2 during cholangioscopy was demonstrated in a porcine model, where no barotrauma or change in vitals occurred after insufflation,[16] but care must always be taken to avoid high intraductal pressures and the risk of embolism.

INDICATIONS FOR CHOLANGIOSCOPY

Diagnostic

Diagnostic cholangioscopy is most often performed for evaluation of strictures (**Fig. 11**). A recent study also showed utility of cholangioscopy in precise mapping of the longitudinal extension of cholangiocarcinoma (**Fig. 12**) to the hepatic and papillary sides, which was not detected by ERCP in 20.0% and 11.6%, hepatic and papillary sides.[18] Cholangioscopy is also useful for evaluation of unexplained filling defects (**Fig. 13**), suspected biliary papillomatosis,[19] eosinophilic cholangitis,[20] suspected intraductal varices, and other abnormalities detected on CT, MRI, endoscopic ultrasound, and ERCP. Exact characteristics defining normal mucosa, inflammatory changes, and neoplasia are still being defined. Diagnostic sensitivity can be augmented during cholangioscopy by using various concomitant modalities, described later.

Therapeutic

Therapeutic cholangioscopy is performed for the removal of challenging stones by using intraductal electrohydraulic or laser lithotripsy (**Fig. 14**). A large, multicenter, retrospective study showed high success rates (>95%) for duct clearance with cholangioscopy-guided intraductal lithotripsy.[21] When compared with standard ERCP-directed therapy, cholangioscopy-guided laser lithotripsy shows higher duct clearance rates.[22] In another study, however, the success rate was similar to endoscopic papillary large balloon dilation.[23] In an interesting report, fluoroscopy/

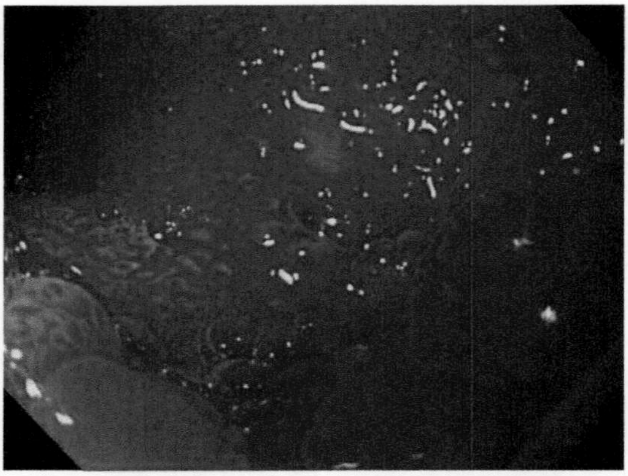

Fig. 12. Papillary mucosal changes proximal to an obstructing cholangiocarcinoma.

radiation-free ERCP for treating uncomplicated choledocholithiasis was performed with 100% technical success rate using cholangioscopy.[24]

In difficult strictures or with inability to advance a guide wire across a stricture, cholangioscopy-assisted guide wire placement can be achieved in up to 70% of cases[25,26] prior to tissue sampling and stent insertion.

In addition, cholangioscopy has also been used for photodynamic therapy for cholangiocarcinoma[27] and retrieval of proximally migrated stents[28,29] and a single case of intraductal polypectomy.[30]

NARROW BAND IMAGING OR EQUIVALENT LIGHT ENHANCEMENT MODES

During narrow band imaging (NBI), the illuminated white light is filtered to 2 colors—blue and green (wavelengths of 415 nm and 510 nm, respectively). The filtered light is absorbed by blood vessels resulting in an enhanced image of the vascular structures and the mucosal topography (**Fig. 15**). Multiple studies have consistently shown enhanced visualization with the use of NBI during cholangioscopy.[31–35] In a study of 12 patients—7 biliary cancers and 5 benign lesions—NBI was significantly better for visualization of surface structure and blood vessels compared with conventional white light cholangioscopy.[32] In a series of 38 patients with indeterminate biliary strictures, NBI enhanced the ability to differentiate benign from malignant lesions in 34 of the 38 cases by enhancing the surface structure.[35] In another study, percutaneous cholangioscopy was performed for evaluation of hepatobiliary malignancies in 36 patients.[33] In 13 patients, prior ERCP or magnetic resonance cholangiopancreatography (MRCP) could not accurately define the margin of the malignancy. Cholangioscopy with NBI improved the accuracy of detection of tumor margin in all 13 cases, which was later confirmed on surgical resection of the tumor.

CHROMOCHOLANGIOSCOPY

Chromoendoscopy is easily performed during endoscopy of the gastrointestinal tract for identification of dysplastic areas in Barrett esophagus,[36] inflammatory bowel disease,[37] and colon polyps[38] and in screening for gastric cancer.[39] Chromocholangioscopy enhances visualization, highlighting subtle changes in surface pattern of the bile ducts. Two studies evaluated the role of chromocholangioscopy with methylene blue. In a study of 45 cholangioscopy-guided biopsy specimens, variable methylene

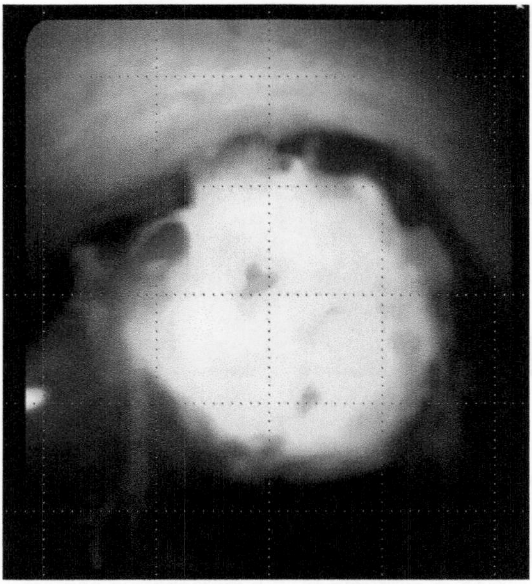

Fig. 13. Bile duct polyp.

blue uptake was seen depending on type of epithelium: 90% with normal epithelium, 69% with dysplastic epithelium, and none with malignant tissue.[40] In another study, 55 patients undergoing chromocholangioscopy, homogenous staining was observed in normal epithelium, heterogeneous dark staining was seen in inflammatory/dysplastic lesions and weak staining in benign strictures, such as primary sclerosing cholangitis (PSC) and post–liver transplant.[41] Mucin and exudates, however, can also stain with the dye, affecting accurate assessment of the biliary epithelium.[42] Thus, chromocholangioscopy can aid in enhancing the visualization of the biliary epithelium and improving characterization but has not become popular.

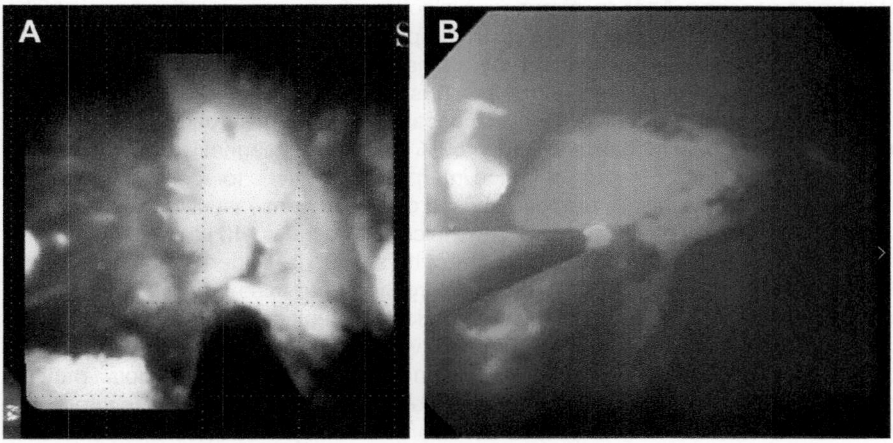

Fig. 14. (A) Electrohydraulic lithotripsy. (B) Laser lithotripsy.

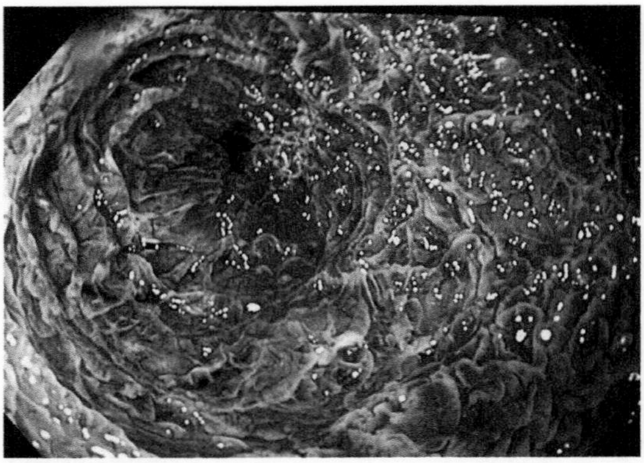

Fig. 15. NBI of the bile duct mucosa.

AUTOFLUORESCENCE IMAGING

Autofluorescence imaging (AFI) involves illumination of mucosa with a short and long wavelength light. The endogenous fluorophores in the tissue are stimulated and the fluorescent light emitted is captured by 2 hypersensitive cameras in red and green spectra. Normal tissue appears to emit green light and cancerous tissue dark green or black light.[43] In a study of 65 biliary lesions, AFI showed improvement in sensitivity from 88% to 100% over conventional cholangioscopy. The investigators describe better delineation of cancers with use of AFI. The specificity was reduced from 87.5% to 52.5%, however, due to false-positive results because granular non-neoplastic mucosa and bile appeared dark.[44] This technology is not widely available.

CONFOCAL LASER ENDOMICROSCOPY

CLE magnifies epithelial and subepithelial tissue 1000-fold to enable real-time microscopic examination of tissues (Cellvizio, Mauna Kea Technologies, Paris, France). During ERCP, CLE is performed with a probe (CholangioFlex miniprobe), designated as pCLE, either passed through a carrying catheter or through the instrument channel of a cholangioscope. After an intravenous injection of a fluorophore (fluorescein 10%), the targeted area is illuminated with a low-power laser (wavelength 488 nm), the emitted fluorescent light is captured by a small aperture in the probe, and real-time images are generated for evaluation. pCLE is particularly beneficial in patients with indeterminate biliary strictures (**Fig. 16**), because ERCP with brushings for cytology and biopsy have only modest sensitivity (50% to 70%) for diagnosis of cholangiocarcinoma in this setting.[45,46] A set of image interpretation criteria for identification of malignancy on CLE was initially proposed based on expert consensus, termed the Miami classification: thick white bands (>20 μm), thick dark bands (>40 μm), dark clumps or epithelial structures.[47] The presence of any of these criteria yielded a high sensitivity of 97% but low specificity of 33%. This was largely due to false-positive results in the setting of inflammation particularly from prior stent placement. Later, in another consensus meeting, the Paris classification was proposed to identify inflammatory conditions comprising 4 other criteria: vascular congestion, dark granular patterns with scales, increased interglandular space, and thickened reticular structure.[48] The thick dark bands are now known to be enlarged collagen bundles that have been changed by the neoplastic process.[49]

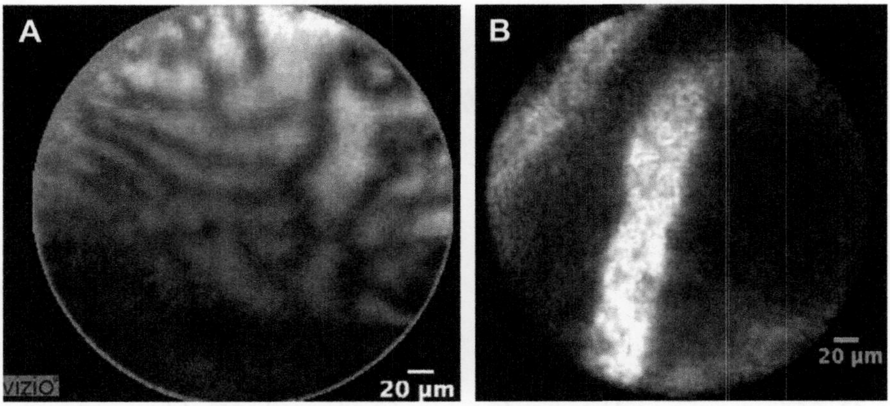

Fig. 16. pCLE of (*A*) normal bile duct and (*B*) cholangiocarcinoma.

Multicenter studies have evaluated the role of CLE for indeterminate biliary strictures. CLE had greater sensitivity for diagnosing biliary cancer compared with ERCP with tissue sampling (98% vs 45%).[50] The combination of CLE and ERCP with tissue sampling had greater accuracy than ERCP with tissue sampling alone. In another recent multicenter study, the sensitivity of CLE was 89% compared with conventional ERCP with tissue sampling (56%), and the combination of both had high accuracy of 88% for diagnosis of biliary cancer.[51] In a recent meta-analysis of CLE for biliary strictures, which included 8 studies with 280 patients, the pooled sensitivity for diagnosis of malignancy was 90% and specificity was 75%.[52] Thus, CLE is an established tool for diagnosis of malignancy in biliary strictures and in many centers is now part of a standard algorithm for diagnosis.[53]

INTRADUCTAL ULTRASONOGRAPHY

IDUS of the biliary tract can be performed using a high-frequency (12–30 MHz) ultrasound miniprobe that can be advanced into the accessory channel of the duodenoscope and into the bile duct. The image resolution of the bile ducts is superior to standard endoscopic ultrasound, due to proximity of the IDUS probe to the bile duct wall and the higher frequency of the probe at the expense of a more limited depth of penetration. In IDUS images, the bile duct wall appears to have 2 layers—the inner hypoechoic layer (which represents mucosa, muscularis propria, and fibrous layer of the subserosa) and the outer hyperechoic layer (which represents adipose layer of the subserosa, the serosa, and the interface echo between the serosa and surrounding organs).[54] IDUS findings can aid in differentiating PSC from immunoglobulin G4–related sclerosing cholangitis, with irregular margins, diverticulum-like outpouching, and disappearance of layers seen specifically in PSC.[55] Several studies have demonstrated the benefit of IDUS over cholangiography in evaluating patients with suspected choledocholithiasis.[56–58] In a series of 62 patients with suspected choledocholithiasis, the combination of ERC with IDUS was superior to ERC alone in diagnosing biliary stones/sludge (97% vs 87%).[56] In another study, IDUS had the highest sensitivity (95%) for detecting CBD stones compared with other modalities—ultrasound (20%), CT (40%), MRCP (80%), and ERCP (90%).[57]

IDUS is also better for evaluation of biliary strictures compared with standard modalities.[59,60] In a recent study of 193 patients with biliary obstruction, IDUS had a

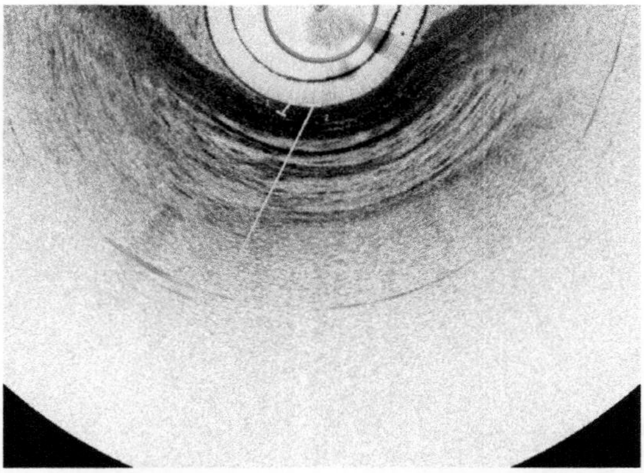

Fig. 17. OCT image of normal bile duct. (*Courtesy of* Dr Viren Joshi, MD, Advanced Digestive Institute, New Orleans, LA.)

sensitivity of 97% and specificity of 79% in identifying malignancy. Furthermore, IDUS has excellent performance in determining the local staging of cholangiocarcinoma, including longitudinal tumor extent and extension into adjacent blood vessels and organs.[61] IDUS is helpful in the management of patients with portal biliopathy, in differentiating biliary narrowing secondary to pericholedochal collaterals versus strictures.[62,63] IDUS was shown feasible and effective in performing ERCP without contrast cholangiography.[64] In another study, IDUS-guided endoscopic biliary drainage led to lower radiation exposure and slight increase in procedure time compared with endoscopic biliary drainage with conventional cholangiography.[65]

OPTICAL COHERENCE TOMOGRAPHY

OCT uses low intensity infrared light (wavelength 750–1300 nm), which is reflected or scattered from tissues to generate a cross-sectional tomographic image of the desired structure. OCT is analogous to ultrasound, except that it uses infrared light. For biliary imaging, the OCT probe is advanced into the bile duct through a biliary catheter (**Fig. 17**). The normal bile duct wall appears to have an inner hyporeflective layer corresponding to the epithelium, a hyperreflective layer corresponding to fibromuscular tissue, and a hyporeflective layer corresponding with the connective tissue.[66] In cases of biliary stricture, the second fibromuscular layer increases in size but the integrity of the 3 layers is maintained. In chronic inflammation of the bile duct wall, there is an increase in the thickness of the inner hyporeflective layer and the intermediate hyperreflective layer with backscattering of light.[67] With malignancy, the layers of the bile duct wall become disorganized and there are large nonreflective areas suggestive of tumor vessels. Recent experience with second-generation OCT also showed such characteristic patterns with PSC associated—benign and malignant strictures.[68] Arvanitakis and colleagues[69] evaluated the utility of OCT in 37 patients with biliary strictures. The sensitivity of OCT for diagnosis of malignancy ranged from 53% to 79% and specificity from 69% to 100%, depending on criteria used to define malignancy.[69]

SUMMARY

Endoscopic visualization of the biliary tree has undergone a major evolution over the past 4 decades. Where visualization began as 2-D fluoroscopic imaging, today endoscopists can routinely perform digital cholangioscopy and real-time optical endomicroscopy to further evaluate biliary tree abnormalities and, in many cases, guide direct endoscopic therapy.

REFERENCES

1. Takekoshi T, Takagi K. Retrograde pancreatocholangioscopy [in Japanese with English abstract]. Gastroenterol Endosc 1975;17:678–83.
2. Nimura Y, Shionoya S, Hayakawa N, et al. Value of percutaneous transhepatic cholangioscopy (PTCS). Surg Endosc 1988;2(4):213–9.
3. Oh HC, Lee SK, Lee TY, et al. Analysis of percutaneous transhepatic cholangioscopy-related complications and the risk factors for those complications. Endoscopy 2007;39(8):731–6.
4. Nakajima M, Akasaka Y, Fukumoto K, et al. Peroral cholangiopancreatosocopy (PCPS) under duodenoscopic guidance. Am J Gastroenterol 1976;66(3):241–7.
5. Brauer BC, Chen YK, Shah RJ. Single-step direct cholangioscopy by freehand intubation using standard endoscopes for diagnosis and therapy of biliary diseases. Am J Gastroenterol 2012;107(7):1030–5.
6. Larghi A, Waxman I. Endoscopic direct cholangioscopy by using an ultra-slim upper endoscope: a feasibility study. Gastrointest Endosc 2006;63(6):853–7.
7. Choi HJ, Moon JH, Ko BM, et al. Overtube-balloon-assisted direct peroral cholangioscopy by using an ultra-slim upper endoscope (with videos). Gastrointest Endosc 2009;69(4):935–40.
8. Moon JH, Ko BM, Choi HJ, et al. Intraductal balloon-guided direct peroral cholangioscopy with an ultraslim upper endoscope (with videos). Gastrointest Endosc 2009;70(2):297–302.
9. Lim P, Aggarwal V, Craig P. Role of balloon-assisted cholangioscopy in a multiethnic cohort to assess complex biliary disease (with videos). Gastrointest Endosc 2015;81(4):932–42.
10. Li J, Guo SJ, Zhang JC, et al. A new hybrid anchoring balloon for direct peroral cholangioscopy using an ultraslim upper endoscope. Dig Endosc 2018;30(3):364–71.
11. Lenze F, Nowacki TM, Beyna T, et al. Direct peroral cholangioscopy with a new anchoring technique using the guide probe of Kautz - first clinical experiences. Endoscopy 2017;49(9):909–12.
12. Itoi T, Sofuni A, Itokawa F, et al. Free-hand direct insertion ability into a simulated ex vivo model using a prototype multibending peroral direct cholangioscope (with videos). Gastrointest Endosc 2012;76(2):454–7.
13. Itoi T, Nageshwar Reddy D, Sofuni A, et al. Clinical evaluation of a prototype multibending peroral direct cholangioscope. Dig Endosc 2014;26(1):100–7.
14. Beyna T, Farnik H, Sarrazin C, et al. Direct retrograde cholangioscopy with a new prototype double-bending cholangioscope. Endoscopy 2016;48(10):929–33.
15. Shah RJ, Neuhaus H, Parsi M, et al. Randomized study of digital single-operator cholangioscope compared to fiberoptic single-operator cholangioscope in a novel cholangioscopy bench model. Endosc Int Open 2018;6(7):E851–6.
16. Mukewar S, Gorospe EC, Knipschield MA, et al. Effects of carbon dioxide insufflation during direct cholangioscopy on biliary pressures and vital parameters: a pilot study in porcine models. Gastrointest Endosc 2017;85(1):238–42.e1.
17. Ueki T, Mizuno M, Ota S, et al. Carbon dioxide insufflation is useful for obtaining clear images of the bile duct during peroral cholangioscopy (with video). Gastrointest Endosc 2010;71(6):1046–51.

18. Nishikawa T, Tsuyuguchi T, Sakai Y, et al. Preoperative assessment of longitudinal extension of cholangiocarcinoma with peroral video-cholangioscopy: a prospective study. Dig Endosc 2014;26(3):450–7.
19. Parsi MA. Biliary papillomatosis: diagnosis with direct peroral cholangioscopy. Gastrointest Endosc 2015;81(1):231–2.
20. Inamdar S, Trindade AJ, Sejpal DV. Bile duct mass determined to be eosinophilic cholangitis by digital cholangioscopy. Clin Gastroenterol Hepatol 2017;15(12): e173–4.
21. Brewer Gutierrez OI, Bekkali NLH, Raijman I, et al. Efficacy and safety of digital single-operator cholangioscopy for difficult biliary stones. Clin Gastroenterol Hepatol 2018;16(6):918–26.e1.
22. Buxbaum J, Sahakian A, Ko C, et al. Randomized trial of cholangioscopy-guided laser lithotripsy versus conventional therapy for large bile duct stones (with videos). Gastrointest Endosc 2018;87(4):1050–60.
23. Franzini T, Moura RN, Bonifacio P, et al. Complex biliary stones management: cholangioscopy versus papillary large balloon dilation - a randomized controlled trial. Endosc Int Open 2018;6(2):E131–8.
24. Barakat MT, Girotra M, Choudhary A, et al. A prospective evaluation of radiation-free direct solitary cholangioscopy for the management of choledocholithiasis. Gastrointest Endosc 2018;87(2):584–9.e1.
25. Woo YS, Lee JK, Noh DH, et al. SpyGlass cholangioscopy-assisted guidewire placement for post-LDLT biliary strictures: a case series. Surg Endosc 2016; 30(9):3897–903.
26. Bokemeyer A, Gross D, Bruckner M, et al. Digital single-operator cholangioscopy: a useful tool for selective guidewire placements across complex biliary strictures. Surg Endosc 2018. [Epub ahead of print].
27. Saumoy M, Kumta NA, Kahaleh M. Digital cholangioscopy for targeted photodynamic therapy of unresectable cholangiocarcinoma. Gastrointest Endosc 2016; 84(5):862.
28. Banerjee D, Perisetti A, Raghavapuram S, et al. Successful removal of proximally migrated biliary stent in a liver transplant patient by single-operator digital cholangioscopy. ACG Case Rep J 2018;5:e50.
29. Ogura T, Okuda A, Miyano A, et al. Successful digital cholangioscopy removal of a stent-retriever tip migrated into the periphery of the bile duct. Endoscopy 2018; 50(5):E113–4.
30. D'Souza LS, Korman A, Benias PC, et al. A novel technique for biliary polypectomy. Endoscopy 2017;49(10):E244–5.
31. Gupta R, Lakhtakia S, Santosh D, et al. Narrow band imaging cholangioscopy in hilar cholangiocarcinoma. Indian J Gastroenterol 2010;29(2):78–80.
32. Itoi T, Sofuni A, Itokawa F, et al. Peroral cholangioscopic diagnosis of biliary-tract diseases by using narrow-band imaging (with videos). Gastrointest Endosc 2007; 66(4):730–6.
33. Jang JW, Noh DH, Paik KH, et al. Effectiveness of cholangioscopy using narrow band imaging for hepatobiliary malignancies. Ann Surg Treat Res 2017;93(3): 125–9.
34. Mounzer R, Austin GL, Wani S, et al. Per-oral video cholangiopancreatoscopy with narrow-band imaging for the evaluation of indeterminate pancreaticobiliary disease. Gastrointest Endosc 2017;85(3):509–17.
35. Osanai M, Itoi T, Igarashi Y, et al. Peroral video cholangioscopy to evaluate indeterminate bile duct lesions and preoperative mucosal cancerous extension: a prospective multicenter study. Endoscopy 2013;45(8):635–42.

36. Kandiah K, Chedgy FJQ, Subramaniam S, et al. International development and validation of a classification system for the identification of Barrett's neoplasia using acetic acid chromoendoscopy: the Portsmouth acetic acid classification (PREDICT). Gut 2018;67(12):2085–91.
37. Flynn AD, Valentine JF. Chromoendoscopy for dysplasia surveillance in inflammatory bowel disease. Inflamm Bowel Dis 2018;24(7):1440–52.
38. Rex DK. Polyp detection at colonoscopy: endoscopist and technical factors. Best Pract Res Clin Gastroenterol 2017;31(4):425–33.
39. Kawahara Y, Takenaka R, Okada H, et al. Novel chromoendoscopic method using an acetic acid-indigocarmine mixture for diagnostic accuracy in delineating the margin of early gastric cancers. Dig Endosc 2009;21(1):14–9.
40. Maetani I, Ogawa S, Sato M, et al. Lack of methylene blue staining in superficial epithelia as a possible marker for superficial lateral spread of bile duct cancer. Diagn Ther Endosc 1996;3(1):29–34.
41. Hoffman A, Kiesslich R, Bittinger F, et al. Methylene blue-aided cholangioscopy in patients with biliary strictures: feasibility and outcome analysis. Endoscopy 2008; 40(7):563–71.
42. Brauer BC, Fukami N, Chen YK. Direct cholangioscopy with narrow-band imaging, chromoendoscopy, and argon plasma coagulation of intraductal papillary mucinous neoplasm of the bile duct (with videos). Gastrointest Endosc 2008; 67(3):574–6.
43. Uedo N, Iishi H, Tatsuta M, et al. A novel videoendoscopy system by using autofluorescence and reflectance imaging for diagnosis of esophagogastric cancers. Gastrointest Endosc 2005;62(4):521–8.
44. Itoi T, Yasushi S, Takeda K, et al. Improvement of choledochoscopy: chromoendocholedochoscopy, autofluorescence imaging, or narrow-band imaging. Dig Endosc 2007;19(Supp 1):S95–104.
45. Jailwala J, Fogel EL, Sherman S, et al. Triple-tissue sampling at ERCP in malignant biliary obstruction. Gastrointest Endosc 2000;51(4 Pt 1):383–90.
46. Navaneethan U, Hasan MK, Lourdusamy V, et al. Single-operator cholangioscopy and targeted biopsies in the diagnosis of indeterminate biliary strictures: a systematic review. Gastrointest Endosc 2015;82(4):608–14.e2.
47. Meining A, Shah RJ, Slivka A, et al. Classification of probe-based confocal laser endomicroscopy findings in pancreaticobiliary strictures. Endoscopy 2012;44(3): 251–7.
48. Caillol F, Filoche B, Gaidhane M, et al. Refined probe-based confocal laser endomicroscopy classification for biliary strictures: the Paris Classification. Dig Dis Sci 2013;58(6):1784–9.
49. Benias PC, Wells RG, Sackey-Aboagye B, et al. Structure and distribution of an unrecognized interstitium in human tissues. Sci Rep 2018;8(1):4947.
50. Meining A, Chen YK, Pleskow D, et al. Direct visualization of indeterminate pancreaticobiliary strictures with probe-based confocal laser endomicroscopy: a multicenter experience. Gastrointest Endosc 2011;74(5):961–8.
51. Slivka A, Gan I, Jamidar P, et al. Validation of the diagnostic accuracy of probe-based confocal laser endomicroscopy for the characterization of indeterminate biliary strictures: results of a prospective multicenter international study. Gastrointest Endosc 2015;81(2):282–90.
52. Liu Y, Lu Y, Sun B, et al. Probe-based confocal laser endomicroscopy for the diagnosis of undetermined biliary stenoses: a meta-analysis. Clin Res Hepatol Gastroenterol 2016;40(6):666–73.

53. Wang KK, Carr-Locke DL, Singh SK, et al. Use of probe-based confocal laser endomicroscopy (pCLE) in gastrointestinal applications. A consensus report based on clinical evidence. United European Gastroenterol J 2015;3(3):230–54.
54. Noda Y, Fujita N, Kobayashi G, et al. Comparison of echograms by a microscanner and histological findings of the common bile duct, in vitro study. Nihon Shokakibyo Gakkai Zasshi 1997;94(3):172–9 [in Japanese].
55. Naitoh I, Nakazawa T, Hayashi K, et al. Comparison of intraductal ultrasonography findings between primary sclerosing cholangitis and IgG4-related sclerosing cholangitis. J Gastroenterol Hepatol 2015;30(6):1104–9.
56. Das A, Isenberg G, Wong RC, et al. Wire-guided intraductal US: an adjunct to ERCP in the management of bile duct stones. Gastrointest Endosc 2001;54(1): 31–6.
57. Moon JH, Cho YD, Cha SW, et al. The detection of bile duct stones in suspected biliary pancreatitis: comparison of MRCP, ERCP, and intraductal US. Am J Gastroenterol 2005;100(5):1051–7.
58. Ueno N, Nishizono T, Tamada K, et al. Diagnosing extrahepatic bile duct stones using intraductal ultrasonography: a case series. Endoscopy 1997;29(5):356–60.
59. Chen L, Lu Y, Wu JC, et al. Diagnostic utility of endoscopic retrograde cholangiography/intraductal ultrasound (ERC/IDUS) in distinguishing malignant from benign bile duct obstruction. Dig Dis Sci 2016;61(2):610–7.
60. Vazquez-Sequeiros E, Baron TH, Clain JE, et al. Evaluation of indeterminate bile duct strictures by intraductal US. Gastrointest Endosc 2002;56(3):372–9.
61. Tamada K, Ueno N, Tomiyama T, et al. Characterization of biliary strictures using intraductal ultrasonography: comparison with percutaneous cholangioscopic biopsy. Gastrointest Endosc 1998;47(5):341–9.
62. Ramchandani M, Nageshwar Reddy D, Lakhtakia S, et al. Role of single-operator per-oral cholangioscopy and intraductal US in assessment of portal biliopathy (with videos). Gastrointest Endosc 2014;79(6):1015–9.
63. Bhatia V, Shasthry SM, Mukund A. Intraductal sonography in patients with portal cavernoma cholangiopathy. J Ultrasound Med 2016;35(3):651–9.
64. Lim SU, Park CH, Kee WJ, et al. Intraductal ultrasonography without radiocontrast cholangiogramin patients with extrahepatic biliary disease. Gut Liver 2015;9(4): 540–6.
65. Rew SJ, Lee DH, Park CH, et al. Comparison of intraductal ultrasonography-directed and cholangiography-directed endoscopic retrograde biliary drainage in patients with a biliary obstruction. Korean J Intern Med 2016;31(5):872–9.
66. Testoni PA, Mariani A, Mangiavillano B, et al. Main pancreatic duct, common bile duct and sphincter of Oddi structure visualized by optical coherence tomography: an ex vivo study compared with histology. Dig Liver Dis 2006;38(6):409–14.
67. Seitz U, Freund J, Jaeckle S, et al. First in vivo optical coherence tomography in the human bile duct. Endoscopy 2001;33(12):1018–21.
68. Tyberg A, Xu MM, Gaidhane M, et al. Second generation optical coherence tomography: preliminary experience in pancreatic and biliary strictures. Dig Liver Dis 2018;50(11):1214–7.
69. Arvanitakis M, Hookey L, Tessier G, et al. Intraductal optical coherence tomography during endoscopic retrograde cholangiopancreatography for investigation of biliary strictures. Endoscopy 2009;41(8):696–701.

Practical Management of Indeterminate Biliary Strictures

Aleksey Novikov, MD, Thomas E. Kowalski, MD,
David E. Loren, MD*

KEYWORDS

• Indeterminate biliary stricture • ERCP • EUS • PSC • Cholangiocarcinoma
• Cytology • FISH

KEY POINTS

- Indeterminate biliary strictures should be considered malignant unless proven otherwise.
- Clinical presentation, location of the stricture, and findings on cross-sectional imaging dictate the care of patients.
- The role of endoscopic ultrasound imaging has expanded for evaluation of the indeterminate biliary stricture compared with endoscopic retrograde cholangiopancreatography, particularly for distal strictures.
- Endoscopic ultrasound imaging with fine needle aspiration and endoscopic retrograde cholangiopancreatography with multimodal biopsies are often performed in a single session to maximize diagnostic efficiency.

INTRODUCTION

Indeterminate biliary strictures pose a particularly complex challenge, because patients and their physicians must weigh the malignant potential against benign etiologies in the face of the high risk of surgical resection. Many factors influence the level of concern for cancer, including the clinical presentation of the patient, results of serum tumor markers, anatomic location of strictures within the biliary tree, associated findings on imaging, and results of tissue sampling. In this article, we define indeterminate biliary stricture as the presence of biliary stricture on an imaging study without a defined tissue diagnosis. Unfortunately, there are no reliable serum tests

---

Disclosure Statement: A. Novikov: None. T. Kowalski: Consultant – Boston Scientific, Medtronics. D. Loren: Consultant - Boston Scientific, Olympus America.
Division of Gastroenterology and Hepatology, Thomas Jefferson University, 132 South 10th Street, 585 Main Building, Philadelphia, PA 19107, USA
* Corresponding author.
E-mail address: david.loren@jefferson.edu

Gastrointest Endoscopy Clin N Am 29 (2019) 205–214
https://doi.org/10.1016/j.giec.2018.12.003 giendo.theclinics.com
1052-5157/19/© 2018 Elsevier Inc. All rights reserved.

that can predict the presence of cancer or prognosticate when oncogenesis may occur. In observational studies, up to two-thirds of indeterminate biliary strictures are malignant, whereas up to one-fourth of all surgical resection specimens are benign.[1,2] Malignant biliary obstruction is most often due to cholangiocarcinoma or pancreatic adenocarcinoma, although less common etiologies must be considered. Expert evaluation of the indeterminate biliary stricture can minimize the morbidity associated with diagnostic procedures, avoid unnecessary surgery, and in some cases facilitate cure.

CLINICAL PRESENTATION

The most common clinical presentation of the indeterminate biliary stricture is painless jaundice; however, the spectrum ranges from an incidental radiologic finding in an asymptomatic individual to fulminant cholangitis. The clinical history plays a crucial role in evaluation because it provides clues to an underlying etiology. For example, malaise, fatigue, or weight loss may suggest malignancy, whereas a history of cholecystectomy increases the likelihood of a postoperative stricture. Particular attention should be given to signs and symptoms of chronic liver disease, as these may suggest an etiology (eg, primary sclerosing cholangitis [PSC] or portal cholangiopathy) and impact treatment options (eg, liver transplant vs resection for perihilar cholangiocarcinoma). Importantly, one must consider the clinical need for biliary intervention, because this consideration may direct diagnostic approaches to be performed during therapeutically indicated endoscopic retrograde cholangiopancreatography (ERCP) that otherwise may be appropriately deferred for less invasive diagnostic options such as endoscopic ultrasound (EUS) examination.

ETIOLOGY OF BILIARY STRICTURES

Obstruction of a bile duct may be due to lesions within the biliary lumen, from the bile duct itself, or from extrabiliary compression. Intraluminal obstruction, that is, obstruction not anatomically arising from the biliary mural layers, may be indistinguishable from other causes of biliary stricture on imaging alone. The atypical appearance of bile duct stones is most common whereas infrequent causes include hemobilia with obstructing clot, infectious etiologies (clonorchis, opisthorchis, and fasciola), and foreign bodies from a prior procedure or that migrated to the bile duct (eg, embolization coils, endoprostheses). An exophytic papillary malignancy may extend or even infarct into the lumen, causing an appearance of stricture on imaging.

Extraluminal etiologies include malignant compression from pancreatic or hepatocellular cancer, hepatic metastases, gallbladder cancer, and/or malignant adenopathy. Tissue confirmation of lymphatic metastasis may be diagnostic regarding the cell type of origin as well as render a patient inoperable (as in the case of gallbladder cancer and perihilar cholangiocarcinoma). Benign causes of extrabiliary obstruction include compression from a gallstone lodged in the cystic duct (Mirrizi syndrome), benign cysts (hepatic, pancreatic, choledochal cysts), and vascular structures in the case of portal cholangiopathy. One should be aware that on magnetic resonance cholangiopancreatography (MRCP) a flow void may occur secondary to the right hepatic artery crossing the common hepatic duct, which can mimic a biliary stricture.

Luminal strictures arising from the bile duct wall may be malignant, as in cholangiocarcinoma, or benign. The latter include autoimmune processes of PSC and IgG4-related sclerosing cholangitis, responses to infection, vascular injuries, and the sequelae of iatrogenic or other trauma (eg, long-standing choledocholithiasis).

PSC is a chronic, progressive cholestatic disease of unknown etiology that causes scarring and fibrosis in the intrahepatic and extrahepatic ducts with eventual progression to cirrhosis. A history of inflammatory bowel disease may be present in two-thirds of patients, whereas 5% of those with ulcerative colitis will develop PSC.[3] A dominant stricture is present in 45% of patients and should raise concern for cholangiocarcinoma complicating PSC. IgG4-related sclerosing cholangitis is an autoimmune cholangiopathy that is 70% prevalent in those with IgG4-related autoimmune pancreatitis, but may occur alone or in the setting of other extrabiliary IgG4-related diseases. This entity differs from PSC in that an elevated serum IgG4 level is present in 70% of patients, IgG4 infiltrates are seen on biopsy, and IgG4-related cholangitis is often responsive to steroid treatment. Elevated serum IgG4 levels are present in 10% of PSC patients, but there is no response to steroid treatment. Nonautoimmune causes of chronic pancreatitis may cause extrahepatic obstruction of the intrapancreatic portion of the common bile duct and estimates ranging between 3% and 46% of those with chronic pancreatitis.[4,5] AIDS cholangiopathy occurs when CD4 count falls below 100/mm^3 and is thought to be primarily due to opportunistic infections such as *Cryptosporidium*, *Microsporidium*, or cytomegalovirus.[6] Other inflammatory causes of biliary stricture such as hepatic pseudotumor, hepatic sarcoidosis, eosinophilic cholangitis, mast cell cholangitis, and histiocytosis X are extremely rare and better described elsewhere.[1,7–10]

Iatrogenic bile duct injury occurs in up to 0.5% of all open cholecystectomies and in up to 2.7% of all laparoscopic cholecystectomies owing to misidentification and subsequent ligation of the bile duct or owing to an inadvertent thermal injury.[11] Up to one-third of patients undergoing orthotropic liver transplantation experience biliary strictures either at the anastomosis or as a consequence of ischemic cholangiopathy, most commonly from hepatic artery thrombosis. Ischemic strictures may be single or multiple and affect both the intrahepatic and extrahepatic biliary trees.[12]

Malignant luminal strictures result from pancreatic cancer and cholangiocarcinoma, the latter of which is classified according to the anatomic location as extrahepatic, perihilar, or intrahepatic. PSC accompanied by a stricture is a common dilemma; up to 26% of all patients with PSC strictures will develop cancer, a 400-fold increase over the general population.[13] Establishing a diagnosis in this setting is particularly challenging owing to the low sensitivity and negative predictive value of cytologic brushings.[14] Primary biliary lymphoma carcinoid and neuroendocrine tumors have been reported, as have mural metastases from colon, hepatocellular, breast, renal cell, melanoma, and lung cancer.[15–17]

NONINVASIVE EVALUATION

Noninvasive imaging and serum blood tests are the first steps in assessing a patient with a biliary stricture. Absent PSC, the sensitivity of carcinoembryonic antigen and carbohydrate antigen 19-9 for cholangiocarcinoma is as low as 38% and 53% respectively, limiting their use in this setting. When PSC is present, the sensitivity of an elevated carbohydrate antigen 19-9 increases and should raise the index of suspicion for malignancy; however, one-third of patients will have benign findings.[18]

Transabdominal ultrasound examination may suggest the location of a biliary stricture, although detailed anatomic description is usually not possible because it is inferred by assessment of the description of dilated and normal-appearing biliary caliber (eg, normal common bile duct and dilated intrahepatics, suggest hilar obstruction). The sensitivity of ultrasound examination, even for common bile duct dilation, however, is as low as 85% and the identification of an etiology of obstruction is around

70% in expert hands.[19,20] Therefore, in these authors opinion, transabdominal ultrasound examination is reserved for clarification of findings on other modalities (eg, the assessment of a gallbladder mass as the suspected etiology of an indeterminate stricture) or to perform real-time vascular imaging in search of a vascular etiology of an indeterminate stricture.[21]

Computed tomography and MRCP provide comprehensive evaluation of the biliary tree as well as the adjacent organs and vessels. When compared with computed tomography, MRCP is more sensitive and specific for the diagnosis of strictures at the biliary hilum and in intrahepatic locations.[22–24] A metaanalysis showed MRCP to be comparable with ERCP in sensitivity for the diagnosis of biliary obstruction.[25,26] MRCP is more sensitive for biliary strictures, particularly intrahepatic duct strictures, because MRCP delineates completely occluded intrahepatic segments that are missed because they are not opacified by ERCP and because the increased intraluminal pressure associated with ERCP contrast injection may mask subtle caliber changes that can be noted on MRCP.

ENDOSCOPIC EVALUATION

Traditionally, ERCP has been the initial test for evaluation of extrahepatic, perihilar, and intrahepatic strictures because it allows for cytologic sampling, which may result in a tissue diagnosis upon which a treatment strategy can be based.[27,28] Cytology obtained during ERCP has an unacceptably low sensitivity of 15% to 60% for the detection of cancer,[29–31] although this rate can be improved to more than 60% when multiple methods of tissue acquisition are performed, such as the combination of brush cytology combined with fluoroscopically directed forceps biopsy and bile aspiration.[32]

With the advent of the single operator cholangioscope, direct visualization of strictures can be performed accompanied by directed biopsies with relative endoscopic efficiency. Limitations of earlier instruments included poor visualization within the duct and difficulty with passage of the biopsy forceps through the therapeutic channel. These challenges have been mitigated with subsequent iterations of the cholangioscope. The presence of abnormal tumor vessels is the strongest cholangioscopic predictor of cancer. Studies of single operator cholangioscope–directed biopsies have a sensitivity from 66% to 72%,[33,34] and single operator cholangioscope has recently been reported to decrease the cost of the evaluation of indeterminate strictures.[35] Despite the improved diagnostic yield associated with cholangioscopy and directed biopsies, one-third of malignant strictures still go undiagnosed.

Probe-based confocal laser endomicroscopy (pCLE) is an in vivo procedure for the analysis of the cellular structure of the biliary epithelium using confocal endomicroscopy that is performed during ERCP. pCLE has gained recognition as a technique that may aid in the assessment of the indeterminate biliary stricture with performance characteristics that exceed those of the pathology.[27,36] In a prospective, multicenter, international trial with 112 patients, pCLE combined with ERCP had a sensitivity of 89% compared with 53% for tissue sampling, although specificity was 72% for pCLE compared with 100% for tissue sampling.[37] A recent metaanalysis looking at 9 studies involving 447 patients with indeterminate biliary strictures found pCLE to have overall sensitivity of 87% for the detection of any malignancy.[38] The limitations of pCLE are that it is time consuming, uses the administration of a contrast agent (fluorescein), requires dedicated training in the interpretation of imaging, and suffers from suboptimal interobserver agreement.[39] These barriers may improve with further experience and refinement of the technology.

Optical coherence tomography (OCT) is an emerging technology that provides widefield in vivo cross-sectional imaging of the ductal wall at the microstructural level using low-intensity infrared light. This technology has a depth of penetration of 1 to 3 mm and lateral and axial resolution of 10 μm. Compared with pCLE, it allows for the imaging of a wide surface area of the bile duct, although studies on its clinical usefulness in biliary strictures are few.[40] The limited existing data have demonstrated sensitivities that exceed those of cytology with superior specificity compared with pCLE.[41,42] The role of biliary OCT in indeterminate strictures is under study.

EUS examination plays a central role in the evaluation of the indeterminate biliary stricture. When compared with ERCP, the complication rate of EUS examination is lower than that of ERCP. Through real-time imaging, the bile ducts can be visualized and sampled with the probe located in the stomach or duodenum, although the extrahepatic bile duct is more readily assessed than the hilum and more proximal ducts. Importantly, EUS examination can image periductal structures including lymph nodes and the gallbladder, which may be the cause of the biliary stricture and through sampling may not only be diagnostic, but provide tumor staging.[43,44] EUS examination typically images the common bile duct and associated structures better than structures at the hilum. In a large single-center retrospective trial, the sensitivity and specificity of distal stricture EUS-guided fine needle aspiration (FNA) for cholangiocarcinoma was significantly superior to EUS-guided FNA of proximal lesions (81% vs 59%).[45] EUS examination and ERCP can be safely combined for better results. In a study of patients with obstructive jaundice, combined EUS examination with or without FNA and ERCP yielded an overall sensitivity and specificity of 84.6% and 100%, respectively, with an acceptable complication rate of 10.5%, which is within the reported rate of adverse events for therapeutic ERCP.

MOLECULAR DIAGNOSTICS

To improve the diagnostic yield from tissue acquired during ERCP and EUS examination with FNA, molecular assays have been studied. The most clinically impactful test is fluorescent in situ hybridization (FISH), an assay that detects chromosomal abnormalities in DNA by the use of complimentary nuclear hybridizing fluorescent probes. FISH has been studied as an independent test, as well as in combination with other diagnostic modalities, and it is the incremental diagnostic yield of FISH testing that is most clinically valuable.[46,47] A retrospective study evaluating 281 patients over a 10-year period demonstrated a 66% sensitivity of FISH in combination with cytology. Importantly, the diagnostic yield was seen in patients with previously placed stents, a scenario that often confounds cytologic interpretation.[48] Moreover, FISH testing is beneficial in the management of patients with PSC in whom the discrimination of malignant strictures is confounded by cytologic atypia from inflammation, and can provide evidence of cancer, particularly when serial examinations are performed.[49]

Mutation profiling of free DNA on the supernatant from biliary brushings (PancraGEN, Interpace Diagnostics, Parsippany-Troy Hills, NJ) has recently been shown to improve the sensitivity and specificity of tissue sampling at ERCP. Notably, this modality does not require the brush itself and may be ordered after an initial cytology analysis. DNA is assessed for KRAS oncogene mutations, loss of heterozygosity, and tumor suppressor gene mutations at 10 genomic loci that are associated with malignant strictures. The additional usefulness of mutation profiling improves the sensitivity over cytology alone (44%) and is additive to cytology and FISH in the diagnosis of malignant biliary strictures with a sensitivity of 66% and 97% specificity.[50] The role of mutation profiling in PSC has yet to be determined.

Intraductal ultrasound (IDUS) uses a wire-guided probe for imaging from within the biliary lumen. This uncommonly performed technique has been demonstrated to improve the diagnostic accuracy of indeterminate strictures through high-resolution imaging of the biliary mural layers, identification of masses, sessile tumors, and adenopathy. In a large study of 264 patients who had IDUS and subsequent surgery for indeterminate biliary strictures, the sensitivity was found to be 93% and specificity 89.5%.[51] Additionally, there are data supporting that IDUS can better identify malignant strictures in the setting of PSC when compared with ERCP alone.[52,53] IDUS has not proliferated as a technology for indeterminate stricture because it has limited depth of penetration, and does not facilitate tissue acquisition the sine qua non for indeterminate stricture, whereas transluminal EUS can both image and sample target structures.

CLINICAL APPROACH TO THE PATIENT WITH INDETERMINATE BILIARY STRICTURE

The decision regarding how to approach a given patient must take into account the clinical presentation, location of the stricture, findings on cross-sectional imaging local expertise, and available technologies. In all patients serum testing is performed for a complete blood count, coagulation studies, hepatic function panel, carbohydrate antigen 19-9 and IgG4 levels. If IgG4-related cholangiopathy is suspected, a course of steroids may be given to assess response to treatment yet being sure to perform appropriate testing to exclude malignancy.

INDETERMINATE DISTAL BILIARY STRICTURE

For distal strictures that are more than 2 cm below the biliary hilum the initial test of choice is EUS with FNA, which can be performed independently or in conjunction with ERCP. EUS has a higher diagnostic yield than ERCP in this setting and can obviate the need for more invasive testing.[45,54] ERCP may be indicated based on clinical grounds (cholangitis or pruritus) or if EUS-guided needle aspiration of the biliary wall is performed, a stent is often placed to manage the biliary injury. There are recent data that suggest a biliary stent may not be necessary after EUS-FNA of the bile duct, it is our practice to place a biliary stent if the needle penetrated into biliary lumen.[55] When a mass or compressive lesion is identified on EUS this can be safely sampled without ERCP. ERCP may be performed in the same or a later session because a diagnosis has not been obtained at EUS examination and, if performed, cholangioscopy with biopsy, brush cytology, and fluoroscopic-guided biopsies are taken.

PERIHILAR OBSTRUCTION

Proximal biliary strictures involving the hilum are particularly problematic as the yield of EUS-guided sampling is lower and in fact may be contraindicated particularly for those who may be considered for liver transplantation. EUS examination is the initial test performed to assess the anatomy, identify the etiology of the stricture and identify nodes or adjacent structures that may be sampled. If a perihilar biliary based mass is identified, EUS with FNA will not be performed for candidates who may benefit from liver transplant. EUS-guided biopsy of the hilum has been associated with a high likelihood of peritoneal carcinomatous in up to 83% of patients and may prevent the patient from proceeding to transplant.[56] After EUS examination, ERCP should be performed with either pCLE or OCT if possible, cholangioscopy with biopsy if available, brush cytology, and fluoroscopic-guided biopsies. If PSC is suspected, sampling is performed for FISH. Should cytology be nondiagnostic, the preserved supernatant is sent for free DNA mutation profiling. Biliary decompression is uniformly performed to decrease the risk of cholangitis and has been shown to improve patient survival.[57]

INTRAHEPATIC BILIARY STRICTURE

Patients with intrahepatic strictures may present with minimal if any symptoms or with constitutional complaints of malaise and, less frequently, jaundice. When an intrahepatic biliary stricture is identified, one must consider the clinical history and noninvasive testing first with potential predisposing conditions including previous surgery or transplant, inflammatory bowel disease (PSC), IgG4-related disease, radiation, choledocholithiasis, infection, and known biliary anomalies. A high index of suspicion for cancer must be maintained particularly if a mass is seen on imaging, because malignancy is present in 50% to 70% of strictures.[58] For the suitable candidate without a predisposing condition, proceeding directly to surgery is appropriate, as a nondiagnostic evaluation does not adequately preclude the presence of cancer. For the majority of patients, evaluation is performed initially with ERCP (with pCLE or OCT if feasible) cholangioscopy with biopsy, brush cytology, FISH testing, and, if nondiagnostic, mutation profiling of supernatant DNA. Care is taken to decompress biliary segments proximal to the stricture to minimize the risk of cholangitis. If malignancy is suspected on any of the results, resection should be performed, even if cancer is not definitively confirmed. When surgery is not performed, a strategy of interval evaluation with blood tests and noninvasive imaging is performed at 3-months intervals, at which time repeat ERCP should be considered.

REFERENCES

1. Bowlus C, Olson K, Gershwin E. Evaluation of indeterminate biliary strictures. Nat Rev Gastroenterol Hepatol 2016;13:28–37.
2. Tummala P, Munigala S. Patients with obstructive jaundice and biliary stricture ± mass lesion on imaging prevalence of malignancy and potential role of EUS-FNA. J Clin Gastroenterol 2013;47(6):532–7.
3. Barkin JA, Levy C, Souto EO. Endoscopic management of primary sclerosing cholangitis. Ann Hepatol 2017;16(6):842–50.
4. Sarles H, Sahel J. Cholestasis and lesions of the biliary tract in chronic pancreatitis. Gut 1978;851–7. https://doi.org/10.1136/gut.19.9.851.
5. Abdallah AA, Krige JEJ, Bornman PC. Biliary tract obstruction in chronic pancreatitis. HPB (Oxford) 2007;9(6):421–8.
6. Ducreux M, Buffet C, Lamy P, et al. Diagnosis and prognosis of AIDS-related cholangitis. AIDS 1995;9(8):875–80.
7. Abdalian R, Heathcote EJ. Sclerosing cholangitis: a focus on secondary causes. Hepatology 2006. https://doi.org/10.1002/hep.21405.
8. Walter D, Hartmann S, Herrmann E, et al. Eosinophilic cholangitis is a potentially underdiagnosed etiology in indeterminate biliary stricture. World J Gastroenterol 2017. https://doi.org/10.3748/wjg.v23.i6.1044.
9. Kennedy PTF, Zakaria N, Modawi SB, et al. Natural history of hepatic sarcoidosis and its response to treatment. Eur J Gastroenterol Hepatol 2006. https://doi.org/10.1097/01.meg.0000223911.85739.38.
10. Baron TH, Koehler RE, Rodgers WH, et al. Mast cell cholangiopathy: another cause of sclerosing cholangitis. Gastroenterology 1995. https://doi.org/10.1016/0016-5085(95)90658-4.
11. N II, Davidoff AM, Pappas TN, et al. Mechanisms of major biliary injury during 1991:196–202.

12. Mourad MM, Algarni A, Liossis C, et al. Aetiology and risk factors of ischaemic cholangiopathy after liver transplantation. World J Gastroenterol 2014;20(20): 6159–69.
13. Lindor KD, Kowdley KV, Harrison ME. ACG clinical guideline: primary sclerosing cholangitis. Am J Gastroenterol 2015;110(5):646–59.
14. Levy MJ, Baron TH, Clayton AC, et al. Prospective evaluation of advanced molecular markers and imaging techniques in patients with indeterminate bile duct strictures. Am J Gastroenterol 2008;103(5):1263–73.
15. Cochrane J, Schlepp G. Metastatic breast cancer to the common bile duct presenting as obstructive jaundice. Case Rep Gastroenterol 2015;9(2):278–84.
16. Karakatsanis A, Vezakis A, Fragulidis G, et al. Obstructive jaundice due to ampullary metastasis of renal cell carcinoma. World J Surg Oncol 2013;11:262.
17. Marks JA, Rao AS, Loren D, et al. Malignant melanoma presenting as obstructive jaundice secondary to metastasis to the Ampulla of Vater. JOP 2010;11(2):173–5.
18. Sinakos E, Saenger AK, Keach J, et al. Many patients with primary sclerosing cholangitis and increased serum levels of carbohydrate antigen 19-9 do not have cholangiocarcinoma. Clin Gastroenterol Hepatol 2011;9(5):434–9.e1.
19. Skoczylas K, Pawełas A. Ultrasound imaging of the liver and bile ducts - expectations of a clinician. J Ultrason 2015;15(62):292–306.
20. Laing FC, Jeffrey RB. Choledocholithiasis and cystic duct obstruction: difficult ultrasonographic diagnosis. Radiology 1983;146(2):475–9. Available at: Radiologyfile:///Users/Alekseynovikov/Downloads/Radiology14626849098Pdf.
21. Abdelaziz O, Attia H. Doppler ultrasonography in living donor liver transplantation recipients: intra- and post-operative vascular complications. World J Gastroenterol 2016;22(27):6145–72.
22. Nesbit GM, Johnson CD, James EM, et al. Cholangiocarcinoma: diagnosis and evaluation of resectability by CT and sonography as procedures complementary to cholangiography. Am J Roentgenol 1988;151(5):933–8.
23. Saluja SS, Sharma R, Pal S, et al. Differentiation between benign and malignant hilar obstructions using laboratory and radiological investigations: a prospective study. HPB (Oxford) 2007;9(5):373–82.
24. Rösch T, Meining A, Frühmorgen S, et al. A prospective comparison of the diagnostic accuracy of ERCP, MRCP, CT, and EUS in biliary strictures. Gastrointest Endosc 2002;55(7):870–6.
25. Romagnuolo J, Bardou M, Rahme E, et al. Magnetic resonance cholangiopancreatography: a meta-analysis of test performance in suspected biliary disease background: magnetic resonance cholangiopancreatography 2003.
26. Kaltenthaler EC, Walters SJ, Chilcott J, et al. MRCP compared to diagnostic ERCP for diagnosis when biliary obstruction is suspected: a systematic review. BMC Med Imaging 2006;6:9.
27. American Society for Gastrointestinal Endoscopy (ASGE) Standards of Practice Committee., Anderson MA, Appalaneni V, Ben-Menachem T, et al. The role of endoscopy in the evaluation and treatment of patients with biliary neoplasia. Gastrointest Endosc 2013;77(2):167–74.
28. ASGE Standards of Practice Committee, Chathadi KV, Chandrasekhara V, Acosta RD, et al. The role of ERCP in benign diseases of the biliary tract. Gastrointest Endosc 2015;81(4):795–803.
29. Fogel EL, DeBellis M, McHenry L, et al. Effectiveness of a new long cytology brush in the evaluation of malignant biliary obstruction: a prospective study. Gastrointest Endosc 2006. https://doi.org/10.1016/j.gie.2005.08.039.

30. De Bellis M, Sherman S, Fogel EL, et al. Tissue sampling at ERCP in suspected malignant biliary strictures (Part 2). Gastrointest Endosc 2002. https://doi.org/10.1016/S0016-5107(02)70123-5.
31. Strongin A, Singh H, Eloubeidi MA, et al. Role of endoscopic ultrasonography in the evaluation of extrahepatic cholangiocarcinoma. Endosc Ultrasound 2013. https://doi.org/10.7178/eus.05.003.
32. Korc P, Sherman S. ERCP tissue sampling. Gastrointest Endosc 2016;84(4):557–71. https://doi.org/10.1016/j.gie.2016.04.039.
33. Laleman W, Verraes K, Van Steenbergen W, et al. Usefulness of the single-operator cholangioscopy system SpyGlass in biliary disease: a single-center prospective cohort study and aggregated review. Surg Endosc 2017;31(5):2223–32.
34. Navaneethan U, Konjeti R, Venkatesh PG, et al. Early precut sphincterotomy and the risk of endoscopic retrograde cholangiopancreatography related complications: an updated meta-analysis. World J Gastrointest Endosc 2014;6(5):200–8.
35. Deprez PH, Garces Duran R, Moreels T, et al. The economic impact of using single-operator cholangioscopy for the treatment of difficult bile duct stones and diagnosis of indeterminate bile duct strictures. Endoscopy 2018;50(2):109–18.
36. Karia K, Kahaleh M. A review of probe-based confocal laser endomicroscopy for pancreaticobiliary disease. Clin Endosc 2016. https://doi.org/10.5946/ce.2016.086.
37. Slivka A, Gan I, Jamidar P, et al. Validation of the diagnostic accuracy of probe-based confocal laser endomicroscopy for the characterization of indeterminate biliary strictures: results of a prospective multicenter international study. Gastrointest Endosc 2015. https://doi.org/10.1016/j.gie.2014.10.009.
38. Gao YD, Qu YW, Liu HF. Comparison of diagnostic efficacy between CLE, tissue sampling, and CLE combined with tissue sampling for undetermined pancreaticobiliary strictures: a meta-analysis. Scand J Gastroenterol 2018. https://doi.org/10.1080/00365521.2018.1448435.
39. Talreja JP, Sethi A, Jamidar PA, et al. Interpretation of probe-based confocal laser endomicroscopy of indeterminate biliary strictures: is there any interobserver agreement? Dig Dis Sci 2012. https://doi.org/10.1007/s10620-012-2338-6.
40. Mahmud MS, May GR, Kamal MM, et al. Imaging pancreatobiliary ductal system with optical coherence tomography: a review. World J Gastrointest Endosc 2013. https://doi.org/10.4253/wjge.v5.i11.540.
41. Arvanitakis M, Hookey L, Tessier G, et al. Intraductal optical coherence tomography during endoscopic retrograde cholangiopancreatography for investigation of biliary strictures. Endoscopy 2009. https://doi.org/10.1055/s-0029-1214950.
42. Tyberg A, Xu M-M, Gaidhane M, et al. Second generation optical coherence tomography: preliminary experience in pancreatic and biliary strictures. Dig Liver Dis 2018. https://doi.org/10.1016/j.dld.2018.05.019.
43. Topazian M. Endoscopic ultrasonography in the evaluation of indeterminate biliary strictures. Clin Endosc 2012. https://doi.org/10.5946/ce.2012.45.3.328.
44. Eloubeidi MA, Chen VK, Jhala NC, et al. Endoscopic ultrasound-guided fine needle aspiration biopsy of suspected cholangiocarcinoma. Clin Gastroenterol Hepatol 2004. https://doi.org/10.1053/S1542-3565(04)00005-9.
45. Mohamadnejad M, Dewitt JM, Sherman S, et al. Role of EUS for preoperative evaluation of cholangiocarcinoma: a large single-center experience. Gastrointest Endosc 2011. https://doi.org/10.1016/j.gie.2010.08.050.

46. Kipp BR, Stadheim LM, Halling SA, et al. A comparison of routine cytology and fluorescence in situ hybridization for the detection of malignant bile duct strictures. Am J Gastroenterol 2004;99(9):1675–81.
47. Smoczynski M, Jablonska A, Matyskiel A, et al. Routine brush cytology and fluorescence in situ hybridization for assessment of pancreatobiliary strictures. Gastrointest Endosc 2012;75(1):65–73.
48. Brooks C, Gausman V, Kokoy-Mondragon C, et al. Role of fluorescent in situ hybridization, cholangioscopic biopsies, and EUS-FNA in the evaluation of biliary strictures. Dig Dis Sci 2018. https://doi.org/10.1007/s10620-018-4906-x.
49. Quinn KP, Tabibian JH, Lindor KD. Clinical implications of serial versus isolated biliary fluorescence in situ hybridization (FISH) polysomy in primary sclerosing cholangitis. Scand J Gastroenterol 2017;52(4):377–81.
50. Kushnir VM, Mullady DK, Das K, et al. The diagnostic yield of malignancy comparing cytology, FISH, and molecular analysis of cell free cytology brush supernatant in patients with biliary strictures undergoing endoscopic retrograde cholangiography (ERC): a prospective study. J Clin Gastroenterol 2018. https://doi.org/10.1097/MCG.0000000000001118.
51. Meister T, Heinzow HS, Woestmeyer C, et al. Intraductal ultrasound substantiates diagnostics of bile duct strictures of uncertain etiology. World J Gastroenterol 2013;19(6):874–81.
52. Itoi T, Nageshwar Reddy D, Sofuni A, et al. Clinical evaluation of a prototype multibending peroral direct cholangioscope. Dig Endosc 2014;26(1):100–7.
53. Tischendorf JJW, Meier PN, Schneider A, et al. Transpapillary intraductal ultrasound in the evaluation of dominant bile duct stenoses in patients with primary sclerosing cholangitis. Scand J Gastroenterol 2007;42(8):1011–7.
54. Weilert F, Bhat YM, Binmoeller KF, et al. EUS-FNA is superior to ERCP-based tissue sampling in suspected malignant biliary obstruction: results of a prospective, single-blind, comparative study. Gastrointest Endosc 2014. https://doi.org/10.1016/j.gie.2013.12.031.
55. Onda S, Ogura T, Kurisu Y, et al. EUS-guided FNA for biliary disease as first-line modality to obtain histological evidence. Therap Adv Gastroenterol 2016;9(3):302–12.
56. Heimbach JK, Sanchez W, Rosen CB, et al. Trans-peritoneal fine needle aspiration biopsy of hilar cholangiocarcinoma is associated with disease dissemination. HPB (Oxford) 2011;13(5):356–60.
57. Cassani LS, Chouhan J, Chan C, et al. Biliary decompression in perihilar cholangiocarcinoma improves survival: a single-center retrospective analysis. Dig Dis Sci 2018. https://doi.org/10.1007/s10620-018-5277-z.
58. Yeo D, Perini MV, Muralidharan V, et al. Focal intrahepatic strictures: a review of diagnosis and management. HPB (Oxford) 2012;14(7):425–34.

Stenting for Benign and Malignant Biliary Strictures

Jason G. Bill, MD[a], Daniel K. Mullady, MD[b,*]

KEYWORDS

- Biliary stenting • Biliary obstruction • Malignant biliary obstruction
- Benign biliary stricture

KEY POINTS

- Endoscopic retrograde cholangio-pancreatography (ERCP) plays a major role in managing benign and malignant biliary obstruction.
- In the setting of malignant biliary obstruction, ERCP is indicated to palliate symptoms (eg, pruritus) and to provide biliary decompression in those who are not immediate surgical candidates.
- The choice of stent (plastic vs metal) depends on the patient's underlying diagnosis and long-term treatment plan.
- The endoscopic approach in stenting of benign biliary strictures varies based on the underlying etiology.

INTRODUCTION

Endoscopic retrograde cholangiopancreatography (ERCP) is commonly performed for biliary obstruction resulting from both malignant and benign etiologies. A therapeutic endoscopist must have a thorough understanding of the etiologies, demographics, risk factors and diagnostic techniques to develop a tailored approach to each clinical scenario. Benign biliary strictures have a wide range of etiologies, most of which result in obstruction due to underlying inflammation, ischemia, and fibrosis. Malignant biliary obstruction is most commonly seen in pancreatic adenocarcinoma and cholangiocarcinoma, and the approach to stenting may differ pending on presentation, location of the mass, and treatment goals. This review covers the approach to patients with benign and malignant biliary obstruction with a focus on technical and procedural aspects of biliary stenting.

Disclosure Statement: D. Mullady is a consultant for Boston Scientific. J. Bill has no disclosures to report.
[a] Washington University School of Medicine in St. Louis, 660 South Euclid Avenue, Campus Box 8124, St Louis, MO 63110, USA; [b] Interventional Endoscopy, Washington University School of Medicine in St. Louis, 660 South Euclid Avenue, Campus Box 8124, St Louis, MO 63110, USA
* Corresponding author.
E-mail address: mulladyd@wustl.edu

Gastrointest Endoscopy Clin N Am 29 (2019) 215–235
https://doi.org/10.1016/j.giec.2018.12.001 giendo.theclinics.com
1052-5157/19/© 2018 Elsevier Inc. All rights reserved.

GENERAL PRINCIPLES OF ENDOSCOPIC MANAGEMENT

Indications for Stenting

Stenting should be used for benign etiologies indications for ERCP including obtaining tissue to exclude the presence of malignancy, treatment of jaundice and associated symptoms, and to remediate the stricture. In the setting of malignant etiologies, stenting is performed to palliate jaundice and associated symptoms, most notably pruritus, and to decrease bilirubin to allow for the administration of chemotherapy and/or radiation therapy.

Endoscopic Tools

The endoscopic tools used during ERCP for biliary stenting including guidewires, sphincterotomes, dilators, and various types of stents. The endoscopist should be familiar with the available tools and especially familiar with tools available at his or her medical center. The American Society of Gastrointestinal Endoscopy has multiple technology review articles pertaining to the types of sphincterotomes, guidewires, and stents available for use.[1–3]

Guidewires

Guidewires are important in ERCP to gain access to the duct of interest, traverse strictures, and to serve as a scaffold over which devices and stents can be advanced and positioned. 0.035 in guidewires are most common; however, tight strictures may require smaller diameter (0.025 in, 0.021 in, or 0.018 in), a hydrophilic coating, or an angulated tip. Ultimately there is little in the way of comparative data, and wire usage is determined by individual preference and local availability. For tight distal biliary strictures or difficult-to-traverse hilar strictures, generally small-diameter, hydrophilic, and angled tipped wires are preferred.

Biliary stents

There are many biliary plastic (PS) and self-expandable metallic stents (SEMS) from various manufacturers, and discussion of each available stent is outside of the scope of this article. However, there are a few important principles regarding stent design and size. Plastic biliary stents are composed of polyethylene, polyurethane, or Teflon, with diameters from 5 Fr to 12 Fr and lengths from 1 to 18 cm. There are additional features that vary between stents, such as flanges versus pigtail fixation, center versus duodenal bend, and side holes.

Self-expandable metal stents (SEMS) have been developed primarily for use in the setting of malignant biliary obstruction. Three types of SEMS are available: fully covered (fcSEMS), partially covered (pcSEMS), and uncovered (uSEMS). uSEMS and pcSEMS are reserved for malignant strictures only and should not be used in the absence of confirmed malignancy. fcSEMS are used for malignant obstruction, but they are also being increasingly used for benign biliary strictures, largely limited to the extrahepatic bile duct, although there are reports of bilateral fcSEMS used for perihilar strictures. Although tissue ingrowth seems to be less common with fcSEMS, stent migration is more common than with uSEMS. The major advantage of SEMS over PS is longer patency and therefore reduced need for routine stent exchanges and unplanned intervention because of stent occlusion.[4]

Another caveat that must be considered prior to placement of SEMS is related to the effect on a patient's operative plan and resectability. Regarding biliary strictures in the setting of pancreatic adenocarcinoma, a retrospective review including 241 patients demonstrated that placement of SEMS was deemed safe and did not interfere or pose any technical difficulty for definitive surgical resection.[5] Therefore, in patients with a resectable malignant distal bile duct stricture, a short intrapancreatic or covered SEMS may be used and would not impede pancreatic resection. In the setting of perihilar obstruction, the use of metal stents should only be performed at tertiary care centers in direct communication with a hepatobiliary surgeon. Inappropriate use of use of transpapillary metal stents should be avoided, as this may increase the surgical complexity of resection by opacifying undrained segments, compromising tissue acquisition, or making local resection impossible.

Preprocedural evaluation As ERCP has become primarily a therapeutic rather than diagnostic procedure, a thorough preprocedural evaluation is important to develop a plan for biliary stenting. One of the most important aspects in the preprocedure evaluation is obtaining high-quality cross-sectional imaging that will allow the endoscopist to localize and define the stricture and assess for atrophic segments that should be avoided during ERCP since stenting atrophic segments will not lead to appreciable improvement in liver chemistries and increase the risk for postprocedural cholangitis. Furthermore, in the setting of malignancy, imaging will allow for preprocedure planning with regard to future resectability of a malignant biliary stricture, plans for neoadjuvant chemotherapy, and possible portal vein embolization. These are important considerations that will affect the location of stent placement and type of stent used.

Classification of stricture

The most commonly used system that provides a systematic preoperative assessment of local spread or location of the stricture is the Bismuth-Corlette Classification (**Fig. 1**, **Table 1**). Multiple other classifications have been developed but will not be mentioned because of the focused nature of this article.

MALIGNANT BILIARY OBSTRUCTION

It is estimated in 2018 that a total of 55,000 new cases of pancreatic cancer and over 50,000 liver, gallbladder, and other biliary tract malignancies will be diagnosed in the

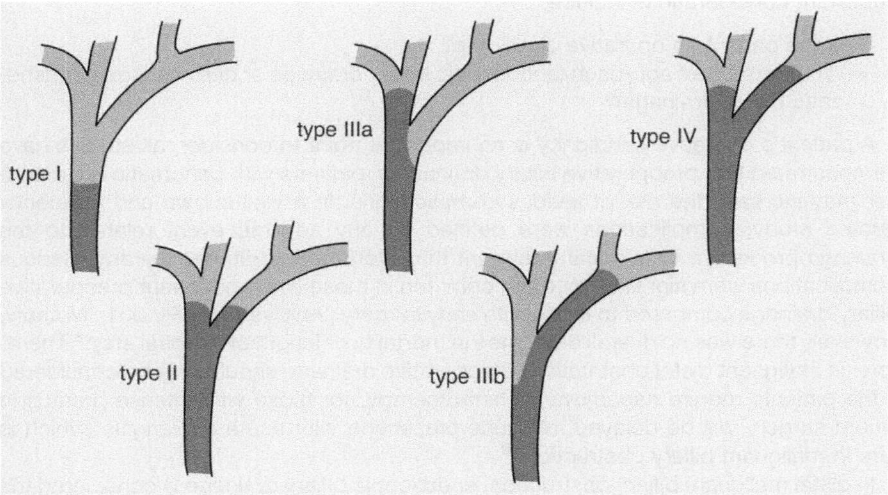

Fig. 1. Bismuth-Corlette classification. (*From* Khan SA, Davidson BR, Goldin RD, et al. Guidelines for the diagnosis and treatment of cholangiocarcinoma: an update. Gut 2012;61(12):1657–69; with permission.)

Table 1
Bismuth-Corlette classification of hilar strictures

Type	Definition
I	Involving the common hepatic duct
II	Tumor involves the common hepatic duct at the confluence of the right and left hepatic ducts
IIIa	Tumor involves the confluence and extends into the right hepatic duct
IIIb	Tumor involves the confluence and extends into the left hepatic duct
IV	Tumor involves both the right and left hepatic ducts

From Siddiqui AA, Mehendiratta V, Loren D, et al. Self-expanding metal stents (SEMS) for preoperative biliary decompression in patients with resectable and borderline-resectable pancreatic cancer: outcomes in 241 patients. Dig Dis Sci 2013;58(6):1744–50; with permission.

United states.[6] Pancreatic cancer is estimated to be the second leading cause of cancer death in the United States by 2030,[7] and only 15% to 20% of cases are deemed potential operative candidates. Given the increasing prevalence and generally poor prognosis, biliary drainage is often required for therapeutic and palliative indications.

From a technical standpoint, malignant strictures of the biliary system can be classified based on the location of obstruction: distal lesions (those involving the common bile duct) versus perihilar lesions. With some caveats, the general approach to stenting in malignant distal biliary obstruction is similar across all etiologies. Perihilar strictures, on the other hand, are approached differently when choosing the optimal endoscopic technique. Given the differing approaches, this section will be divided into how one should approach malignant distal biliary obstruction and how one should approach perihilar malignancies.

TECHNIQUE AND APPROACH IN MALIGNANT DISTAL BILIARY OBSTRUCTION

Patient Selection

Important considerations include:

- Is the patient an operative candidate?
- What is the best approach (endoscopic biliary drainage or percutaneous transhepatic biliary drainage)?

A patient's operative candidacy is an important point to consider, as studies have demonstrated that preoperative biliary drainage in patients with pancreatic head cancer may increase the risk of serious complications. In a well-known and frequently quoted study, complications were defined by any adverse event related to the drainage procedure or surgical treatment that prompted additional therapy. Serious complications were significantly more common in those who underwent preoperative biliary drainage compared to those with early surgery (39% vs 74%; *P*<.001). Notably, however, there was no overall difference in mortality or length of hospital stay.[8] Therefore, in malignant distal obstruction, preoperative drainage should only be considered if the patients require neoadjuvant chemotherapy, for those with intense pruritus in whom surgery will be delayed, or those presenting with acute cholangitis (which is rare in malignant biliary obstruction).[9]

In distal malignant biliary obstruction, endoscopic biliary drainage is considered the treatment of choice compared with percutaneous techniques. This is because of an overall lower rate of adverse events, less repeat procedures, and the lack of external drainage catheters.[10]

Endoscopic Technique

Cholangiography should be obtained to define the location and severity of the stricture. Although controversial, the authors generally suggest sphincterotomy prior to stent placement.

Injection of contrast proximal to (upstream from) the stricture will ensure that the endoscopist obtains an adequate cholangiogram that will guide further decision making not only regarding the location of stent placement and type of stent but also guide the endoscopist as to which, if any, segments to avoid. Injection of contrast into atrophic segments places the patient at an increased risk for cholangitis and should therefore be avoided. Whether a sphincterotomy is performed prior to stent placement remains controversial, as initial studies demonstrated a decreased risk in post-ERCP pancreatitis.[11] This, however, has not been replicated in a recent analysis including only those with unresectable pancreatic adenocarcinoma before placement of SEMS.[12] Despite this, unless the patient is on therapeutic anticoagulation or is unable to hold antiplatelet agents, the authors generally perform sphincterotomy prior to stent placement given early data demonstrating a decrease in rates of post-ERCP pancreatitis, to facilitate placement of multiple transpapillary stents, and to allow ease of obtaining deep biliary cannulation during subsequent procedures.

OUTCOMES OF BILIARY STENTING IN MALIGNANT DISTAL BILIARY OBSTRUCTION

PS and SEMS have similar short-term efficacy and are appropriate options for initial management in most patients in whom the treatment plan is not well-established. Although 1-month patency rates are similar, large randomized trials demonstrate a significant benefit in stent patency in SEMS versus PS.[13] The biliary stents available and considerations in patients with malignant distal biliary obstruction are reviewed in **Table 2**.

Results from cost-effective analyses have suggested that if anticipated survival is greater than 4 months or if the cost of SEMS is less than 50% of the cost of the ERCP, then SEMS may be favored. As chemotherapy regimens improve, it is often difficult to truly determine a patient's mortality risk during initial ERCP, so the decision is not always straightforward. The most recent prospective trial evaluated 54 patients who were undergoing neoadjuvant chemotherapy for pancreatic adenocarcinoma, 16 with fcSEMS, 17 with uSEMS, and 21 with PS. The PS group had extra in-hospital costs because of stent occlusion, and therefore, no stent was superior in cost-effectiveness. Furthermore, the fcSEMS resulted in fewer days of neoadjuvant treatment delay and a longer time to stent occlusion.[14] Therefore, the authors tend to favor the use of fcSEMS

Table 2
Stent choice in distal malignant biliary obstruction

Stent Type	Patient Selection
Plastic biliary stents	• If the patient is an operative candidate • If survival is expected to be <4 mo[9]
fcSEMS	• Can be placed in those who are operative candidates • Can be cost effective if the patient's survival is expected to be more than 4 mo[9] • Stent of choice in those planning to receive neoadjuvant chemotherapy prior to surgical resection[14]
uSEMS	• Short (intrapancreatic) stents can be placed in those planning to receive neoadjuvant chemotherapy prior to surgical resection • Nonoperative candidates with poor expected survival

in the setting of malignant distal biliary obstruction when overall survival is unclear, especially when the patient is to receive neoadjuvant chemotherapy.

Stent-Related Cholecystitis

Data from multiple retrospective studies have demonstrated that placement of fcSEMS across the cystic duct takeoff may result in an increased risk of acute cholecystitis when compared with placement of uSEMS or PS.[15–19] However, data from randomized controlled trials have failed to demonstrate similar results, demonstrating no difference in rates of acute cholecystitis with placement of fcSEMS.[20,21] Apparent risk factors for the development of cholecystitis include tumor involving the cystic duct ostium and the presence of cholelithiasis prior to stent placement.[17] Based on the current data, the authors tend to favor the use of fcSEMS in those where the stent can be placed below the cystic duct ostium, or in those who are post-cholecystectomy.

APPROACH TO PERIHILAR MALIGNANT BILIARY OBSTRUCTION

About 20% of malignant biliary obstructions are caused by malignancies involving the hilum, most commonly cholangiocarcinoma (Klatskin tumor). Other lesions include hepatocellular carcinoma, gallbladder cancer, and metastatic disease (most commonly colorectal cancer). Although the goals of endoscopic management are similar, to make a diagnosis and to restore the flow of bile, there are specific considerations pertaining to perihilar strictures that will be discussed in this section.

Patient Selection

Physicians should determine whether the patient is an operative candidate, and the best approach to take with the patient.

Studies have demonstrated that preoperative cholangitis may be a risk factor for postoperative liver failure, which again emphasizes the importance of preventing complications in the perioperative period.[22] Specifically, biliary drainage should only be performed for those who require neoadjuvant chemotherapy, with cholangitis, or those with intense pruritus.[9]

In general, because of high safety, efficacy, ability to sample tissue, and the avoidance of external drains, endoscopic intervention is the preferred and most common approach. However, observational data have shown that select patients may benefit from up front percutaneous transhepatic biliary drainage (PTBD). In a retrospective cohort study of 288 patients with potentially resectable perihilar cholangiocarcinoma, 38% of those with Bismuth 3 or 4 hilar lesions required additional preoperative drainage with PTBD after initial attempt at ERCP.[23] The led the authors to recommend first-line PTBD over ERCP in this select group of patients (Bismuth II-IV). Eagerly awaited are results from a multicenter randomized controlled trial comparing PTBD and ERCP for palliation of malignant hilar obstruction, which hopefully will provide evidence basis for the optimal approach to biliary drainage in these patients.[24]

Preprocedural Evaluation

For any perihilar stricture, a thorough preprocedural evaluation should be performed including cross-sectional imaging with MRI/MRCP or contrast-enhanced computed tomography (CT). The goal of imaging is to provide a road map for the endoscopist and assist in developing a preprocedural plan to target specific segments, while avoiding atrophic segments or segments that will be resected or embolized. Imaging also allows the multidisciplinary team to assess for resectability, which may obviate the need for preoperative biliary drainage or direct the endoscopist to the appropriate side of the liver to stent. Furthermore, if radical liver surgery is being considered, the size of individual liver segments can be assessed, and portal vein embolization (PVE) can be performed in order to induce hypertrophy of the future liver remnant. In general, draining 50% of the liver volume is associated with better outcomes and improved survival. Stenting an atrophic sector resulted in drainage of less than 30% of the total liver volume and was shown to be clinically not beneficial and resulted in more post-procedural cholangitis.[25,26]

Endoscopic Techniques

Avoid injection of contrast into atrophic segments, those that may be resected, or those that may need to be targeted for portal vein embolization

The injection of contrast into segments that either will not drain well or those where access is not deemed to be beneficial may increase the risk for postprocedural cholangitis and thereby increase the risk of postoperative liver failure.[22] To avoid this, the best strategy is to obtain high-quality cross-sectional imaging in the preprocedural period. This will allow the endoscopist to target specific segments and inject contrast after wire access to the desired segment has been achieved. A limited amount of contrast should be injected in all patients with complex hilar strictures to avoid filling undesirable segments.

Bilateral drainage is preferred

For those undergoing endoscopic biliary drainage, considerations regarding stent placement include use of plastic versus SEMS, unilateral versus bilateral stenting, and side-by-side versus Y- configuration when placing SEMS. Regarding unilateral versus bilateral stenting, a metanalysis of 36 studies concluded that bilateral metal stenting seems to have a lower overall number of complications and higher odds of lowering the bilirubin, but did not alter the 30-day mortality.[27] Given improved clinical outcomes with bilateral stenting, the authors' approach is to place bilateral stents in order to optimize biliary drainage unless one of the liver lobes appears atrophic.

When using the side-by-side method for placement of SEMS, the authors cannulate both the right and left systems and maintain wire access to both sides prior to stent placement. SEMS are then inserted and deployed sequentially (when using traditional SEMS) or simultaneously (when using 6F stent introducers) (**Fig. 2**). Regarding the stent in stent technique, wire access to both sides is obtained. The first SEMS is then placed, typically in the more angulated left hepatic duct. Another wire is then placed through the lumen of the first SEMS and advanced through the interstices alongside of the wire that was initially placed. The first wire is then removed, and a second SEMs is inserted over the wire through the interstices of the first SEMS into the contralateral ductal system, resulting in a Y-shaped configuration[28] (**Fig. 3**). When this method was first described, a fenestration was made through the interstices of the initially placed SEMS to facilitate placement of the second stent.[29] Currently, stents with an open cell design have been developed to assist with bilateral stent within stent insertion techniques.[30] Both side-by-side and stent-in-stent technique are clinically feasible and safe in patients with hilar obstruction, and success is likely dependent on individual patient factors. Side-by-side configuration may be limited in settings where there is minimal ductal dilatation to facilitate placement. The largest prospective study comparing side-by-side versus stent-in-stent technique involved 52 consecutive patients demonstrating similar technical success between the 2 groups, with a longer cumulative duration of stent patency in the side-by-side group. Of note however, there was a significant increase in adverse events in the side-by-side group (44% vs 13%, $P = .016$).[31]

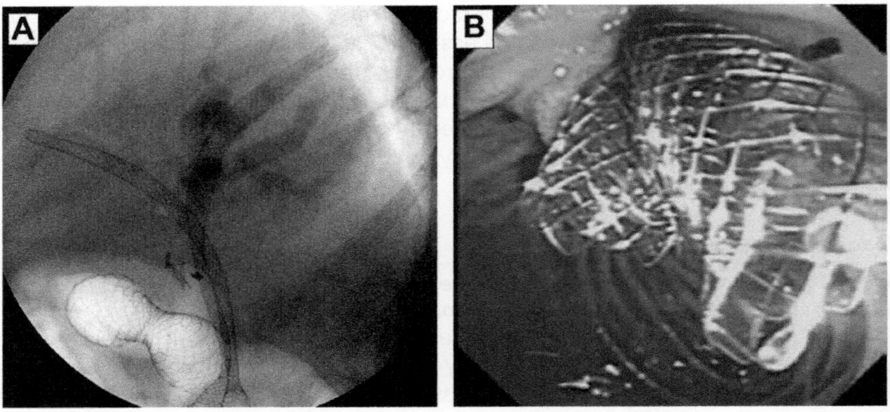

Fig. 2. (*A*) Side-by-side SEMS in a patient with unresectable hilar cholangiocarcinoma. Note also the duodenal stent that was placed for concurrent malignant gastric outlet obstruction. (*B*) intraduodenal double-barrel appearance of side-by-side SEMS. This allows for selective cannulation into each side of the liver should reintervention be required.

Antibiotics are recommended only if there is failure or suspicion of failure to drain the targeted biliary system or any undrained segment.[32]

Transpapillary versus suprapapillary stenting

The sphincter of Oddi is important, as it may act as a mechanical barrier preventing backflow into the biliary system. Therefore, it has been theorized that placement of stents above the biliary orifice in malignant hilar obstruction may result in lower rates of cholangitis and lower rates of stent occlusion. In a large retrospective study involving 172 patients, placement of SEMS above the papilla provided similar success rates, stent patency, and stent occlusion rates.[33] Although deemed noninferior in this study, reintervention is frequently required and may be more difficult when stents are placed above the sphincter. Therefore, this technique remains controversial and currently has not gained widespread use.

RECURRENT BILIARY OBSTRUCTION

PS and SEMS are proven therapies for symptom relief and palliation. As 5-year survival rates continue to increase for pancreatic, liver, and biliary malignancies, performing ERCP for stent occlusion is likely to become more frequent. Stent patency for SEMS in the setting of perihilar tumors ranges from 150 to 557 days, with stent occlusion occurring 22% to 50% patients.[34] Risk factors for recurrent obstruction include stenting in the setting of gallbladder carcinoma, left-sided stent placement, and cholangitis prior to SEMS placement. Stent occlusion is typically caused by tissue ingrowth, sludge, debris, or tumor extension.

If the patient has had prior plastic stenting, stents are exchanged for a fcSEMS or uSEMS. If the patient has had a prior uSEMS, the authors would generally place a fcSEMS within the previous stent. Other methods to manage stent occlusion include repeated balloon sweeps or balloon sweeps followed by placement of plastic stents through the lumen of the prior placed uSEMS.

A novel approach using radiofrequency ablation to treat biliary stent occlusion in malignant biliary obstruction appears to be safe and effective, however has yet to be evaluated in larger randomized controlled trials.[35–37] The RFA catheter (Habib EndoHPB;

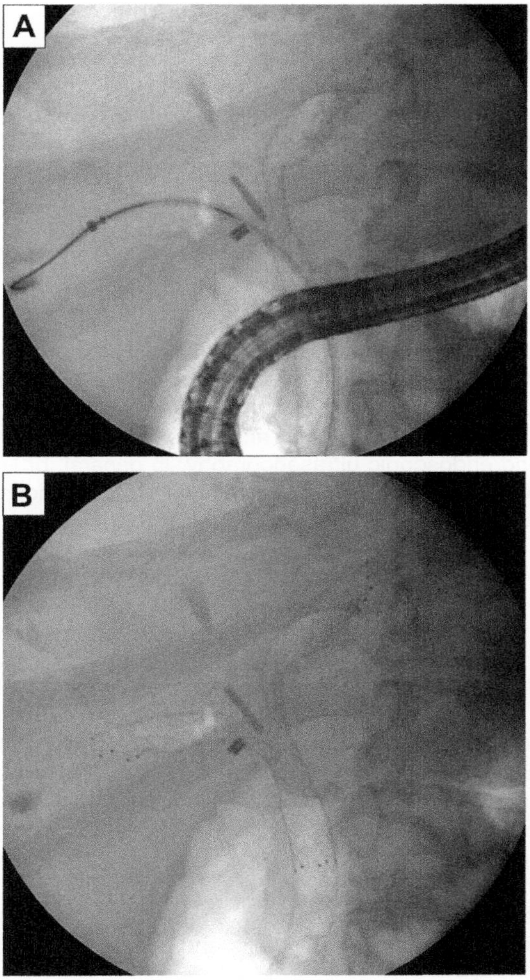

Fig. 3. Y-configuration SEMS for unresectable perihilar cholangiocarcinoma. (*A*) After placing the first stent, wire access has been gained through the interstices of the first stent to the contralateral liver followed by another stent over the wire. (*B*) Final fluoroscopic appearance after deployment of the second stent.

Emcision Ltd, London, United Kingdom) is a single-use, disposable device that can be advanced over a 0.035 in guidewire and is used for endoluminal delivery of RFA.[38] A recent meta-analysis, involving a total of 505 patients, demonstrated a mean difference in stent patency of 51 days, favoring those patients who received RFA. Furthermore, a survival analysis demonstrated improved survival in patients treated with RFA (hazard ratio, 1.395; 95% confidence interval [CI], 1.145–1.7; $P<.001$).[37] The authors admit that data in this analysis were limited to small observational studies, prompting the need for larger randomized trials to draw definitive conclusions. Other questions remain, as it is unclear whether RFA would be more effective when used with plastic versus metal biliary stents or if RFA should be performed with initial stent placement or used after a metal stent has been clogged in the setting of tumor ingrowth.

APPROACH TO STENTING FOR BENIGN BILIARY STRICTURES

Benign biliary strictures have diverse etiologies resulting in biliary obstruction primarily because of local inflammation or ischemia resulting in scaring/fibrosis. Common etiologies of benign biliary strictures are listed in **Table 3**. Although each condition requires special consideration, many of the same principles can be applied. The goals of endoscopic therapy in benign biliary strictures are to exclude malignancy and provide effective biliary decompression to prevent further complications such as secondary sclerosing cholangitis.

ENDOSCOPIC TECHNIQUE AND APPROACH

Ruling out Malignancy

Although outside of the scope of this article, there are many studies comparing diagnostic strategies utilized to effectively rule out malignancy in the setting of biliary strictures. The endoscopist needs to have a thorough understanding of the available diagnostic modalities. These include tissue acquisition (brushings, cytology, biopsies), cholangioscopy, and endoscopic ultrasonography. In general, brush cytology has a lower sensitivity (30%–57% vs 43%–81%) than that of forceps biopsy, with both having similar specificity (90%–100%).[39,40] Endoscopic ultrasonography enables detailed visualization of the ampulla, extrahepatic bile duct and hilum, pancreas, and surrounding structures. Fine needle aspiration (FNA) of surrounding nodes can have a sensitivity of up to 89%.[41–43] In general, particularly in patients who are candidates for resection or transplantation, FNA of the tumor should be avoided because of the risk of seeding the needle tract or peritoneum.[44] Cholangioscopy enables direct visualization of bile duct strictures and sight-directed targeted biopsy of abnormal-appearing tissue. It has been shown to increase the sensitivity from 78.1 to 93.4 and NPV from 68.6 to 100 and has an overall sensitivity similar to that of brushings and cytology of 60%.[45,46] Probe-based CLE is a technique that allows detailed high-resolution images of biliary epithelium, and while studies have demonstrated higher sensitivity of CLE over tissue acquisition methods, its poor interobserver reliability, high false positivity rate (specificity of 67%), and overall lack of availability and expertise make it less utilized.[47–49]

Of note, stent placement prior to tissue acquisition may lead to granulation tissue or inflammation and can affect pathology results and diagnostic accuracy. Thus, early

Table 3
Etiologies of benign biliary strictures

Inflammatory	• Chronic pancreatitis • Primary sclerosing cholangitis • Immunoglobulin G (IgG)4 cholangiopathy
Postoperative	• After cholecystectomy • After liver transplantation
Other	• Trauma • Radiation • Mirizzi syndrome • Infectious • Human immunodeficiency virus cholangiopathy • Portal biliopathy • Tuberculosis • Recurrent pyogenic cholangitis • Choledochal cysts

referral to a tertiary care center with expertise in these ancillary techniques is extremely important.

Cholangiography

A cholangiogram is obtained to further define the stricture characteristics, estimate the diameter of the ducts, and to aid in diagnosis. Notably long strictures (those >14 mm) or those with an irregular appearance are more suspicious for malignancy.[50]

Stricture Dilation

Dilation of benign strictures by balloon or passage dilators is generally performed prior to stent placement. The size of the dilating balloon is determined by the size of the bile duct distal to the stricture. The balloon is advanced over the wire and inflated under fluoroscopic guidance for 30 to 60 seconds. Dilation soon (within 30 days) after a biliary anastomosis carries an increased risk of dehiscence and bile leak.[51,52] Therefore, the authors generally forego prestenting dilation in these situations.

Stent Choice

Plastic stents remain the standard of care for management of benign biliary strictures despite recent data demonstrating equal effectiveness of fcSEMS in certain clinical scenarios.[53] When using PS, 1 or 2 10 Fr PS will initially be placed side by side across the stricture. Every 3 to 4 months, the ERCP is repeated with additional dilation and placement of an increasing number of stents. Stenting is continued until the stricture has been remediated.[54–58] The decision to discontinue stenting has been based on either the disappearance of the stricture using fluoroscopy, the ease at which a balloon biliary catheter is passed, or timing (after a fixed 12-month interval).[54,56,59] In a retrospective analysis, stricture recurrence was predicted if, following endoscopic therapy, the diameter of the stricture was less than 75% compared with the surrounding bile duct.[60] There are few data comparing specific endpoints to endoscopic therapy and therefore, the decision is based mostly on endoscopist preference and experience.

The use of fcSEMS has gained popularity in the setting of benign biliary strictures. uSEMS or pcSEMS should not be used for benign biliary strictures because of their lack of removability. fcSEMS have the advantage of longer patency time compared with PS, therefore potentially decreasing the overall number of ERCPs required to remediate the stricture. In a randomized controlled trial of 102 patients, fcSEMS were found to be noninferior in regards to success rates compared with PS (87.7% vs 87.3%; $P = .007$) but demonstrated a significantly faster rate of stricture resolution (225 days in the plastic stent group vs 181 days in the fcSEMS group).[57] Importantly, however, there is a significant rate (approximately 9%) of stent migration with the use of fcSEMS, which varies greatly depending on etiology.[61,62] The final concern in the setting of long indwell times is the possibility of developing a stricture at the proximal or distal portion of the SEMS. In 1 retrospective study of 37 patients, de novo strictures after stent removal occurred in 8.1% of patients.[63] Currently the only fcSEMS approved in the United States for benign disease is the Wallflex stent (Boston Scientific), but its indication is limited to biliary obstruction because of chronic pancreatitis. However, there is extensive experience and data for off-label use of both the Wallflex stent and the Viabil stent (Gore Medical) for benign biliary strictures. Despite the widespread experience and data regarding safety and efficacy, the authors recommend a thorough documented discussion with the patient when using these stents off-label for managing benign biliary obstruction.

MANAGEMENT BASED ON ETIOLOGY

Chronic Pancreatitis

An estimated 10% to 30% of patients with underlying chronic pancreatitis develop distal biliary strictures, making it the most common etiology of benign biliary obstruction.[64]

Indications for biliary drainage include cholangitis, jaundice, and persistent cholestasis (greater than 1 month).

Endoscopic technique

Placement of biliary stents in the setting of a bile duct stricture secondary to chronic pancreatitis remains similar to other benign etiologies of the distal common bile duct. After cannulation, a cholangiogram should be obtained with contrast injected proximal to the stricture. A biliary sphincterotomy is then performed to assist with stent insertion and to assist in future reinterventions and placement of multiple stents. Balloon dilation can be performed but is not a requirement to facilitate stent placement. In general, multiple 10 Fr stents should be placed, and ERCP is repeated every 3 months. The stricture is then re-evaluated with repeat cholangiogram. Treatment is deemed successful when contrast is seen freely flowing into the duodenum and when there is no longer a waist seen with balloon dilation. Historically, PS stents have been placed, and it has been recommended to perform placement of 10 Fr stents in sequential fashion every 3 months until fluoroscopic resolution or after 12 to 18 months. More recent trials, however, have demonstrated comparable efficacy with placing fcSEMS.[65]

Outcomes of endoscopic intervention

CBD strictures in the setting of chronic pancreatitis seem to be more resistant to endoscopic therapy than other benign etiologies, especially in the setting of chronic calcific pancreatitis.[66] Higher success rates with endoscopic therapy have been seen with 2 approaches: placement of multiple PS and more recently with the use of fcSEMS.

Plastic stents

Long-term outcomes are suboptimal (12%-44%) with the use of single PS, and use should only be considered for biliary decompression as a bridge to surgery.[67–70] Similar to other benign etiologies, placement of multiple PS has demonstrated improved outcomes but requires frequent endoscopic intervention. With this approach, success rates have ranged from 44% to 92%.[56]

Self-expandable metal stents

A randomized controlled trial published in 2015 demonstrated comparative efficacy of fcSEMS versus PS when looking at rates of recurrent strictures (88% in both groups).[65] The fcSEMS group also required fewer repeat procedures. In another large multinational study, stricture resolution occurred in 79.7% of patients with a median indwell period of 11.3 months.[61] This has led some to recommend up-front placement of fcSEMS for biliary obstruction secondary to chronic pancreatitis.

Postoperative Strictures

Postoperative strictures can generally be categorized as postcholecystectomy and post-transplant biliary strictures. Post-transplant strictures can be further broken down into early (<30 days) versus late strictures and anastomotic versus nonanastomotic.

Endoscopic technique

Endoscopic therapy is accepted as first-line therapy for all kinds of postoperative biliary strictures. Similar principles of endoscopic therapy apply. Importantly, knowing which type of biliary reconstruction was performed will be important during preprocedural planning. The most common post-transplant anastomosis is a duct-to-duct anastomosis, but hepaticojejunostomy is sometimes performed, particularly in patients with primary sclerosing cholangitis (PSC). Knowing postoperative anatomy is extremely important, particularly because a hepaticojejunostomy requires use of a pediatric colonoscope or enteroscope and may not be reachable via a peroral approach.

Cholangiography

In general, cholangiography is important to delineate the location, length, and characteristics of the stricture. Anastomotic strictures are generally focal, short, and localized compared with nonanastomotic strictures.[71,72] Nonanastomotic strictures are generally caused by underlying ischemia and therefore are more numerous and diffuse, often involving the hilum and intrahepatic bile ducts.[73] Obtaining thorough cholangiography in suspected postcholecystectomy biliary injury is extremely important in ruling out other diagnoses, identifying a transected bile duct or bile leak, and delineating the location of the suspected injury.

Dilation

In post-transplant strictures, balloon dilation alone without stent placement generally is not performed, as studies have demonstrated recurrence of strictures, with long-term success rates of only 30% to 40%.[52,74] Care should be taken in the early post-operative phase, as those patients may be at a higher risk of anastomotic injury. In general, the authors recommend performance of dilation prior to stent placement. There are no data comparing balloon dilation and stenting versus balloon dilation alone when discussing postcholecystectomy bile duct strictures.

Stent choice

As in other benign biliary strictures, the sequential placement of 10 Fr plastic biliary stents has been the gold standard, but newer data have demonstrated effectiveness of fcSEMS.[57,75]

Outcomes of Endoscopic Therapy

Post-transplant

Outcomes of stenting for anastomotic strictures are altered based on timing and location of stricture formation. Early outcomes (<30 days) are caused by local postoperative edema/inflammation and have an excellent response to endoscopic therapy. Most resolve within 3 months of initial therapy.[72,76] Success rates of endoscopic treatment of late anastomotic strictures is similar but requires a more prolonged course of therapy. Success rates range from 80% to 90%.[77–79] Given the nature of nonanastomotic strictures, endoscopic therapy is less effective. Rates of long-term response are poorly defined but have ranged from 50% to 75%, with at least 25% of patients eventually undergoing repeat transplantation.[80]

Postcholecystectomy

ERCP has been demonstrated to be a safe and effective long-term approach, as success rates are cited up to 90% at 12 months, with a recurrence rate of 20% to 30%.[80] Most studies pertain to sequential placement of multiple PS, although there are increasing data with the use of fcSEMS.[61]

Primary Sclerosing Cholangitis

PSC is a cholestatic liver disease characterized by immune-mediated inflammation leading to ductal fibrosis and stricture formation of both the intrahepatic and extrahepatic bile ducts. Endoscopic management is generally indicated in the presence of jaundice, pruritus, and imaging findings of a dominant stricture, which occurs in 40% to 50% of patients with PSC. Dominant strictures are defined as a stenosis less than 1.5 mm in diameter in the CBD and less than 1 mm in the hepatic ducts and usually are associated with upstream dilation of the biliary tree.[81]

Endoscopic technique

ERCP is reserved for patients with symptomatic jaundice in the presence of a dominant biliary stricture. Although improvement in serum alkaline phosphatase to normal or below 1.5 times the upper limit of normal has been shown to decrease the risk of cholangiocarcinoma,[82] the authors do not perform ERCP in the setting of isolated alkaline phosphatase elevation.

Cholangiography

Cholangiography can be obtained via ERCP, percutaneous transhepatic cholangiography (PTC), or MRCP. Given the noninvasive nature of MRCP along with an extremely high sensitivity and specificity, ERCP should be reserved in those patients who cannot undergo MRI or for therapeutic purposes in the setting of a dominant stricture.[83,84] When performing ERCP in a patient with PSC, a minimal amount of contrast should be injected in order to minimize post-ERCP cholangitis.

Sphincterotomy

It is unclear if endoscopic biliary sphincterotomy provides benefit or harm in the setting of PSC. The authors generally will perform biliary sphincterotomy to assist in stent placement and to provide easier access for repeated biliary interventions. Some would advocate a small sphincterotomy rather than complete because of the theoretic risk of ascending cholangitis.[85] There are no data to support this hypothesis.

Balloon dilation

Balloon dilation alone of dominant strictures is accepted as first-line therapy in the setting of PSC, as studies have demonstrated improvement in symptoms (pruritus, jaundice, pain), liver chemistries, and longer liver transplantation-free survival.[86–89] The authors generally recommend dilation of dominant strictures with balloon dilators starting with a 4 mm or 6 mm balloon and sequentially increasing depending on the duct diameter above and below the stricture.

Balloon dilation versus stenting

Stenting is generally not performed for PSC-related strictures because of studies demonstrating a high rate of early stent occlusion. This is thought to be related to the extensive inflammatory cellular debris that develops in patients with PSC.[90] If stenting is performed, it is generally recommended to have short-term interval follow-up, defined by removal in 1 to 2 weeks following insertion.[88] This approach, however, has recently been questioned. In a recent multicenter trial of patients with PSC and a dominant stricture, short-term stents were not superior to balloon dilation and were associated with a significantly higher occurrence of adverse events.[91] Furthermore, a recent multicenter randomized trial of patients with PSC and a dominant stricture demonstrated a lack of superiority to stenting versus balloon dilation alone, along with an increased risk of post-ERCP pancreatitis and cholangitis.[91] Therefore, the authors' approach is to perform balloon dilation alone as the initial treatment of dominant strictures. They reserve stenting for PSC-related strictures in rare instances of refractory strictures or early recurrence of strictures and avoid long-term stenting in these situations whenever possible.

Antibiotic prophylaxis

PSC patients have multifocal strictures; therefore, complete drainage may not be feasible during ERCP. Current guidelines from the American Society of Gastrointestinal Endoscopy recommend routine antimicrobial prophylaxis for PSC patients who are undergoing ERCP.[92]

Outcomes of Endoscopic Interventions

Although there are few high-quality studies evaluating the efficacy of ERCP in the setting of PSC, it appears clear from multiple large retrospective studies that ERCP tends to prolonged survival. In a large study using the Mayo Risk Score to predict outcomes, the 5-year survival was significantly improved in those with dominant strictures who underwent ERCP therapy (83% vs 65%; $P = .027$).[93] These findings were replicated in another large retrospective study that again reported higher 3-year and 4-year survival in those who underwent ERCP.[94]

It should be noted that performing ERCP in patients with PSC carries significant risk of complications that range from 7.3% to 20%.[93,94] The most common complication is post-ERCP pancreatitis followed by cholangitis, sepsis, ductal perforation, bleeding, and liver abscesses.[81] This emphasizes the importance of limited contrast injection and careful patient selection.

SUMMARY

The approach to stenting biliary strictures depends on several variables including benign versus malignant etiology and extrahepatic versus perihilar location. Benign biliary strictures have been managed traditionally with serial PS placement, generally every 3 months, until fluoroscopic resolution or for 12 to 18 months. More recently, benign extrahepatic biliary strictures have been successfully remediated using fcSEMS with data for their safety and efficacy. However, using fcSEMS for benign strictures generally remains off-label. For malignant biliary strictures, an important decision is PS versus SEMS. SEMS have longer patency. However, reintervention is usually more challenging through indwelling SEMS, and SEMS may interfere with subsequent surgical resection, particularly for perihilar strictures. The endoscopist should understand the advantages and disadvantages to various stents and the available data regarding stenting malignant and benign biliary strictures. Whenever possible, the endoscopist should work in a multidisciplinary fashion with surgery, interventional radiology, and oncology to individualize treatment based on a particular patient's disease, treatment, and prognosis, and to optimize clinical outcomes.

REFERENCES

1. Somogyi L, Chuttani R, Croffie J, et al. Guidewires for use in GI endoscopy. Gastrointest Endosc 2007;65(4):571–6.
2. ASGE Technology Committee, Kethu SR, Adler DG, Conway JD, et al. ERCP cannulation and sphincterotomy devices. Gastrointest Endosc 2010;71(3):435–45.
3. ASGE Technology Assessment Committee, Pfau PR, Pleskow DK, Banerjee S, et al. Pancreatic and biliary stents. Gastrointest Endosc 2013;77(3):319–27.
4. Siiki A, Helminen M, Sand J, et al. Covered self-expanding metal stents may be preferable to plastic stents in the treatment of chronic pancreatitis-related biliary strictures: a systematic review comparing 2 methods of stent therapy in benign biliary strictures. J Clin Gastroenterol 2014;48(7):635–43.
5. Siddiqui AA, Mehendiratta V, Loren D, et al. Self-expanding metal stents (SEMS) for preoperative biliary decompression in patients with resectable and borderline-

resectable pancreatic cancer: outcomes in 241 patients. Dig Dis Sci 2013;58(6): 1744–50.
6. Siegel RL, Miller KD, Jemal A. Cancer statistics, 2016. CA Cancer J Clin 2016; 66(1):7–30.
7. Bekkali NLH, Oppong KW. Pancreatic ductal adenocarcinoma epidemiology and risk assessment: Could we prevent? Possibility for an early diagnosis. Endosc Ultrasound 2017;6(Suppl 3):S58–61.
8. van der Gaag NA, Rauws EA, van Eijck CH, et al. Preoperative biliary drainage for cancer of the head of the pancreas. N Engl J Med 2010;362(2):129–37.
9. Dumonceau JM, Tringali A, Blero D, et al. Biliary stenting: indications, choice of stents and results: European Society of Gastrointestinal Endoscopy (ESGE) clinical guideline. Endoscopy 2012;44(3):277–98.
10. Inamdar S, Slattery E, Bhalla R, et al. Comparison of adverse events for endoscopic vs percutaneous biliary drainage in the treatment of malignant biliary tract obstruction in an inpatient national cohort. JAMA Oncol 2016;2(1):112–7.
11. Zhou H, Li L, Zhu F, et al. Endoscopic sphincterotomy associated cholangitis in patients receiving proximal biliary self-expanding metal stents. Hepatobiliary Pancreat Dis Int 2012;11(6):643–9.
12. Hayashi T, Kawakami H, Osanai M, et al. No benefit of endoscopic sphincterotomy before biliary placement of self-expandable metal stents for unresectable pancreatic cancer. Clin Gastroenterol Hepatol 2015;13(6):1151–8.e2.
13. Kaassis M, Boyer J, Dumas R, et al. Plastic or metal stents for malignant stricture of the common bile duct? Results of a randomized prospective study. Gastrointest Endosc 2003;57(2):178–82.
14. Gardner TB, Spangler CC, Byanova KL, et al. Cost-effectiveness and clinical efficacy of biliary stents in patients undergoing neoadjuvant therapy for pancreatic adenocarcinoma in a randomized controlled trial. Gastrointest Endosc 2016; 84(3):460–6.
15. Fumex F, Coumaros D, Napoleon B, et al. Similar performance but higher cholecystitis rate with covered biliary stents: results from a prospective multicenter evaluation. Endoscopy 2006;38(8):787–92.
16. Ornellas LC, Stefanidis G, Chuttani R, et al. Covered Wallstents for palliation of malignant biliary obstruction: primary stent placement versus reintervention. Gastrointest Endosc 2009;70(4):676–83.
17. Suk KT, Kim HS, Kim JW, et al. Risk factors for cholecystitis after metal stent placement in malignant biliary obstruction. Gastrointest Endosc 2006;64(4): 522–9.
18. Yoon WJ, Lee JK, Lee KH, et al. A comparison of covered and uncovered Wallstents for the management of distal malignant biliary obstruction. Gastrointest Endosc 2006;63(7):996–1000.
19. Jang S, Stevens T, Parsi M, et al. Association of covered metallic stents with cholecystitis and stent migration in malignant biliary stricture. Gastrointest Endosc 2018;87(4):1061–70.
20. Telford JJ, Carr-Locke DL, Baron TH, et al. A randomized trial comparing uncovered and partially covered self-expandable metal stents in the palliation of distal malignant biliary obstruction. Gastrointest Endosc 2010;72(5):907–14.
21. Yang MJ, Kim JH, Yoo BM, et al. Partially covered versus uncovered self-expandable nitinol stents with anti-migration properties for the palliation of malignant distal biliary obstruction: a randomized controlled trial. Scand J Gastroenterol 2015;50(12):1490–9.

22. Olthof PB, Wiggers JK, Groot Koerkamp B, et al. Postoperative liver failure risk score: identifying patients with resectable perihilar cholangiocarcinoma who can benefit from portal vein embolization. J Am Coll Surg 2017;225(3):387–94.
23. Wiggers JK, Groot Koerkamp B, Coelen RJ, et al. Preoperative biliary drainage in perihilar cholangiocarcinoma: identifying patients who require percutaneous drainage after failed endoscopic drainage. Endoscopy 2015;47(12):1124–31.
24. Al-Kawas F, Aslanian H, Baillie J, et al. Percutaneous transhepatic vs. endoscopic retrograde biliary drainage for suspected malignant hilar obstruction: study protocol for a randomized controlled trial. Trials 2018;19(1):108.
25. Chang WH, Kortan P, Haber GB. Outcome in patients with bifurcation tumors who undergo unilateral versus bilateral hepatic duct drainage. Gastrointest Endosc 1998;47(5):354–62.
26. Vienne A, Hobeika E, Gouya H, et al. Prediction of drainage effectiveness during endoscopic stenting of malignant hilar strictures: the role of liver volume assessment. Gastrointest Endosc 2010;72(4):728–35.
27. Puli SR, Kalva N, Pamulaparthy SR, et al. Bilateral and unilateral stenting for malignant hilar obstruction: a systematic review and meta-analysis. Indian J Gastroenterol 2013;32(6):355–62.
28. Law R, Baron TH. Bilateral metal stents for hilar biliary obstruction using a 6 Fr delivery system: outcomes following bilateral and side-by-side stent deployment. Dig Dis Sci 2013;58(9):2667–72.
29. Silverman W, Slivka A. New technique for bilateral metal mesh stent insertion to treat hilar cholangiocarcinoma. Gastrointest Endosc 1996;43(1):61–3.
30. Chahal P, Baron TH. Expandable metal stents for endoscopic bilateral stent-within-stent placement for malignant hilar biliary obstruction. Gastrointest Endosc 2010;71(1):195–9.
31. Naitoh I, Hayashi K, Nakazawa T, et al. Side-by-side versus stent-in-stent deployment in bilateral endoscopic metal stenting for malignant hilar biliary obstruction. Dig Dis Sci 2012;57(12):3279–85.
32. Almadi MA, Barkun JS, Barkun AN. Stenting in malignant biliary obstruction. Gastrointest Endosc Clin N Am 2015;25(4):691–711.
33. Cosgrove N, Siddiqui AA, Adler DG, et al. A comparison of bilateral side-by-side metal stents deployed above and across the sphincter of oddi in the management of malignant hilar biliary obstruction. J Clin Gastroenterol 2017;51(6):528–33.
34. Miura S, Kanno A, Masamune A, et al. Risk factors for recurrent biliary obstruction following placement of self-expandable metallic stents in patients with malignant perihilar biliary stricture. Endoscopy 2016;48(6):536–45.
35. Steel AW, Postgate AJ, Khorsandi S, et al. Endoscopically applied radiofrequency ablation appears to be safe in the treatment of malignant biliary obstruction. Gastrointest Endosc 2011;73(1):149–53.
36. Xia N, Gong J, Lu J, et al. Percutaneous intraductal radiofrequency ablation for treatment of biliary stent occlusion: a preliminary result. World J Gastroenterol 2017;23(10):1851–6.
37. Sofi AA, Khan MA, Das A, et al. Radiofrequency ablation combined with biliary stent placement versus stent placement alone for malignant biliary strictures: a systematic review and meta-analysis. Gastrointest Endosc 2018;87(4):944–51.e1.
38. McCarty TR, Rustagi T. New indications for endoscopic radiofrequency ablation. Clin Gastroenterol Hepatol 2018;16(7):1007–17.

39. De Bellis M, Sherman S, Fogel EL, et al. Tissue sampling at ERCP in suspected malignant biliary strictures (Part 1). Gastrointest Endosc 2002;56(4):552–61.
40. Glasbrenner B, Ardan M, Boeck W, et al. Prospective evaluation of brush cytology of biliary strictures during endoscopic retrograde cholangiopancreatography. Endoscopy 1999;31(9):712–7.
41. Eloubeidi MA, Chen VK, Jhala NC, et al. Endoscopic ultrasound-guided fine needle aspiration biopsy of suspected cholangiocarcinoma. Clin Gastroenterol Hepatol 2004;2(3):209–13.
42. Garrow D, Miller S, Sinha D, et al. Endoscopic ultrasound: a meta-analysis of test performance in suspected biliary obstruction. Clin Gastroenterol Hepatol 2007; 5(5):616–23.
43. Lee JH, Salem R, Aslanian H, et al. Endoscopic ultrasound and fine-needle aspiration of unexplained bile duct strictures. Am J Gastroenterol 2004;99(6): 1069–73.
44. Lundstedt C, Stridbeck H, Andersson R, et al. Tumor seeding occurring after fine-needle biopsy of abdominal malignancies. Acta Radiol 1991;32(6):518–20.
45. Navaneethan U, Hasan MK, Lourdusamy V, et al. Single-operator cholangioscopy and targeted biopsies in the diagnosis of indeterminate biliary strictures: a systematic review. Gastrointest Endosc 2015;82(4):608–14.e2.
46. Fukuda Y, Tsuyuguchi T, Sakai Y, et al. Diagnostic utility of peroral cholangioscopy for various bile-duct lesions. Gastrointest Endosc 2005;62(3):374–82.
47. Kahaleh M, Giovannini M, Jamidar P, et al. Probe-based confocal laser endomicroscopy for indeterminate biliary strictures: refinement of the image interpretation classification. Gastroenterol Res Pract 2015;2015:675210.
48. Talreja JP, Sethi A, Jamidar PA, et al. Interpretation of probe-based confocal laser endomicroscopy of indeterminate biliary strictures: is there any interobserver agreement? Dig Dis Sci 2012;57(12):3299–302.
49. Wallace MB, Fockens P. Probe-based confocal laser endomicroscopy. Gastroenterology 2009;136(5):1509–13.
50. Bain VG, Abraham N, Jhangri GS, et al. Prospective study of biliary strictures to determine the predictors of malignancy. Can J Gastroenterol 2000;14(5): 397–402.
51. Thuluvath PJ, Pfau PR, Kimmey MB, et al. Biliary complications after liver transplantation: the role of endoscopy. Endoscopy 2005;37(9):857–63.
52. Zoepf T, Maldonado-Lopez EJ, Hilgard P, et al. Balloon dilatation vs. balloon dilatation plus bile duct endoprostheses for treatment of anastomotic biliary strictures after liver transplantation. Liver Transpl 2006;12(1):88–94.
53. Dumonceau JM, Tringali A, Papanikolaou IS, et al. Endoscopic biliary stenting: indications, choice of stents, and results: European Society of Gastrointestinal Endoscopy (ESGE) Clinical Guideline - Updated October 2017. Endoscopy 2018;50(9):910–30.
54. Costamagna G, Pandolfi M, Mutignani M, et al. Long-term results of endoscopic management of postoperative bile duct strictures with increasing numbers of stents. Gastrointest Endosc 2001;54(2):162–8.
55. Costamagna G, Tringali A, Mutignani M, et al. Endotherapy of postoperative biliary strictures with multiple stents: results after more than 10 years of follow-up. Gastrointest Endosc 2010;72(3):551–7.
56. Draganov P, Hoffman B, Marsh W, et al. Long-term outcome in patients with benign biliary strictures treated endoscopically with multiple stents. Gastrointest Endosc 2002;55(6):680–6.

57. Cote GA, Slivka A, Tarnasky P, et al. Effect of covered metallic stents compared with plastic stents on benign biliary stricture resolution: a randomized clinical trial. JAMA 2016;315(12):1250–7.
58. Khan MA, Baron TH, Kamal F, et al. Efficacy of self-expandable metal stents in management of benign biliary strictures and comparison with multiple plastic stents: a meta-analysis. Endoscopy 2017;49(7):682–94.
59. Kuzela L, Oltman M, Sutka J, et al. Prospective follow-up of patients with bile duct strictures secondary to laparoscopic cholecystectomy, treated endoscopically with multiple stents. Hepatogastroenterology 2005;52(65):1357–61.
60. Parlak E, Dişibeyaz S, Ödemiş B, et al. Endoscopic treatment of patients with bile duct stricture after cholecystectomy: factors predicting recurrence in the long term. Dig Dis Sci 2015;60(6):1778–86.
61. Deviere J, Nageshwar Reddy D, Püspök A, et al. Successful management of benign biliary strictures with fully covered self-expanding metal stents. Gastroenterology 2014;147(2):385–95 [quiz: e15].
62. Zheng X, Wu J, Sun B, et al. Clinical outcome of endoscopic covered metal stenting for resolution of benign biliary stricture: Systematic review and meta-analysis. Dig Endosc 2017;29(2):198–210.
63. Kasher JA, Corasanti JG, Tarnasky PR, et al. A multicenter analysis of safety and outcome of removal of a fully covered self-expandable metal stent during ERCP. Gastrointest Endosc 2011;73(6):1292–7.
64. Costamagna G,, Boskoski I. Current treatment of benign biliary strictures. Ann Gastroenterol 2013;26(1):37–40.
65. Haapamaki C, Kylänpää L, Udd M, et al. Randomized multicenter study of multiple plastic stents vs. covered self-expandable metallic stent in the treatment of biliary stricture in chronic pancreatitis. Endoscopy 2015;47(7):605–10.
66. Kahaleh M, Behm B, Clarke BW, et al. Temporary placement of covered self-expandable metal stents in benign biliary strictures: a new paradigm? (with video). Gastrointest Endosc 2008;67(3):446–54.
67. Deviere J, Devaere S, Baize M, et al. Endoscopic biliary drainage in chronic pancreatitis. Gastrointest Endosc 1990;36(2):96–100.
68. Smits ME, Rauws EA, van Gulik TM, et al. Long-term results of endoscopic stenting and surgical drainage for biliary stricture due to chronic pancreatitis. Br J Surg 1996;83(6):764–8.
69. Vitale GC, Reed DN Jr, Nguyen CT, et al. Endoscopic treatment of distal bile duct stricture from chronic pancreatitis. Surg Endosc 2000;14(3):227–31.
70. Familiari P, Boškoski I, Bove V, et al. ERCP for biliary strictures associated with chronic pancreatitis. Gastrointest Endosc Clin N Am 2013;23(4):833–45.
71. Thethy S, Thomson BNj, Pleass H, et al. Management of biliary tract complications after orthotopic liver transplantation. Clin Transplant 2004;18(6): 647–53.
72. Verdonk RC, Buis CI, Porte RJ, et al. Anastomotic biliary strictures after liver transplantation: causes and consequences. Liver Transpl 2006;12(5):726–35.
73. Ito K, Siegelman ES, Stolpen AH, et al. MR imaging of complications after liver transplantation. AJR Am J Roentgenol 2000;175(4):1145–9.
74. Schwartz DA, Petersen BT, Poterucha JJ, et al. Endoscopic therapy of anastomotic bile duct strictures occurring after liver transplantation. Gastrointest Endosc 2000;51(2):169–74.
75. Tal AO, Finkelmeier F, Filmann N, et al. Multiple plastic stents versus covered metal stent for treatment of anastomotic biliary strictures after liver

transplantation: a prospective, randomized, multicenter trial. Gastrointest Endosc 2017;86(6):1038–45.
76. Pasha SF, Harrison ME, Das A, et al. Endoscopic treatment of anastomotic biliary strictures after deceased donor liver transplantation: outcomes after maximal stent therapy. Gastrointest Endosc 2007;66(1):44–51.
77. Graziadei IW, Schwaighofer H, Koch R, et al. Long-term outcome of endoscopic treatment of biliary strictures after liver transplantation. Liver Transpl 2006;12(5): 718–25.
78. Morelli J, Mulcahy HE, Willner IR, et al. Long-term outcomes for patients with post-liver transplant anastomotic biliary strictures treated by endoscopic stent placement. Gastrointest Endosc 2003;58(3):374–9.
79. Tabibian JH, Asham EH, Han S, et al. Endoscopic treatment of postorthotopic liver transplantation anastomotic biliary strictures with maximal stent therapy (with video). Gastrointest Endosc 2010;71(3):505–12.
80. Rustagi T, Jamidar PA. Endoscopic management of benign biliary strictures. Curr Gastroenterol Rep 2015;17(1):422.
81. Thosani N, Banerjee S. Endoscopic retrograde cholangiopancreatography for primary sclerosing cholangitis. Clin Liver Dis 2014;18(4):899–911.
82. Lindstrom L, Hultcrantz R, Boberg KM, et al. Association between reduced levels of alkaline phosphatase and survival times of patients with primary sclerosing cholangitis. Clin Gastroenterol Hepatol 2013;11(7):841–6.
83. Dave M, Elmunzer BJ, Dwamena BA, et al. Primary sclerosing cholangitis: meta-analysis of diagnostic performance of MR cholangiopancreatography. Radiology 2010;256(2):387–96.
84. Barkin JA, Levy C, Souto EO. Endoscopic management of primary sclerosing cholangitis. Ann Hepatol 2017;16(6):842–50.
85. Gotthardt D, Stiehl A. Endoscopic retrograde cholangiopancreatography in diagnosis and treatment of primary sclerosing cholangitis. Clin Liver Dis 2010;14(2): 349–58.
86. Johnson GK, Saeian K, Geenen JE. Primary sclerosing cholangitis treated by endoscopic biliary dilation: review and long-term follow-up evaluation. Curr Gastroenterol Rep 2006;8(2):147–55.
87. Lee JG, Schutz SM, England RE, et al. Endoscopic therapy of sclerosing cholangitis. Hepatology 1995;21(3):661–7.
88. Aabakken L, Karlsen TH, Albert J, et al. Role of endoscopy in primary sclerosing cholangitis: European Society of Gastrointestinal Endoscopy (ESGE) and European Association for the Study of the Liver (EASL) clinical guideline. Endoscopy 2017;49(6):588–608.
89. Gotthardt DN, Rudolph G, Klöters-Plachky P, et al. Endoscopic dilation of dominant stenoses in primary sclerosing cholangitis: outcome after long-term treatment. Gastrointest Endosc 2010;71(3):527–34.
90. van Milligen de Wit AW, van Bracht J, Rauws EA, et al. Endoscopic stent therapy for dominant extrahepatic bile duct strictures in primary sclerosing cholangitis. Gastrointest Endosc 1996;44(3):293–9.
91. Ponsioen CY, Arnelo U, Bergquist A, et al. No superiority of stents vs balloon dilatation for dominant strictures in patients with primary sclerosing cholangitis. Gastroenterology 2018;155(3):752–9.e5.
92. ASGE Standards of Practice Committee, Banerjee S, Shen B, Baron TH, et al. Antibiotic prophylaxis for GI endoscopy. Gastrointest Endosc 2008;67(6):791–8.

93. Baluyut AR, Sherman S, Lehman GA, et al. Impact of endoscopic therapy on the survival of patients with primary sclerosing cholangitis. Gastrointest Endosc 2001;53(3):308–12.
94. Gluck M, Cantone NR, Brandabur JJ, et al. A twenty-year experience with endoscopic therapy for symptomatic primary sclerosing cholangitis. J Clin Gastroenterol 2008;42(9):1032–9.

Endoscopic Management of Biliary Issues in the Liver Transplant Patient

James F. Crismale, MD, Jawad Ahmad, MD, FRCP*

KEYWORDS

• Biliary stricture • Bile leak • Liver transplantation • ERCP

KEY POINTS

- Biliary complications are common after liver transplantation and can lead to significant morbidity.
- Most of the common biliary complications after liver transplantation are recognized clinically and several risk factors have been identified.
- The therapeutic endoscopist plays a critical role in the management of biliary complications following liver transplantation with success rates of more than 90% in most situations, avoiding the need for interventional radiologic or surgical approaches.

INTRODUCTION

Biliary complications are known as the "Achilles heel" of liver transplantation (LT) and still remain a problem despite improved surgical technique and experience. Biliary strictures, anastomotic and nonanastomotic, and bile leaks may complicate deceased donor (DDLT) and living donor LT (LDLT), with both being more common after LDLT. Both may lead to significant morbidity, and in some cases, reduced graft and patient survival. Endoscopic retrograde cholangiopancreatography (ERCP) is the cornerstone of management of biliary complications following LT, and generally obviates percutaneous and surgical approaches. Herein, we discuss the pathophysiology, risk factors, diagnosis, and management of biliary complications following LT.

BILIARY STRICTURES

Anastomotic Strictures

Biliary strictures may occur in approximately 12.8% of patients following LT, although incidence ranges from 2% to 14%.[1,2] Anastomotic strictures are the most common,

Disclosure Statement: The authors have no financial conflicts of interest related to the contents of this article to disclose.
Recanati/Miller Transplantation Institute, Icahn School of Medicine at Mount Sinai, One Gustave L. Levy Place, New York, NY 10029, USA
* Corresponding author. Recanati/Miller Transplantation Institute, Icahn School of Medicine at Mount Sinai, One Gustave L. Levy Place, Box 1104, New York, NY 10029.
E-mail address: jawad.ahmad@mountsinai.org

Gastrointest Endoscopy Clin N Am 29 (2019) 237–256
https://doi.org/10.1016/j.giec.2018.11.003
giendo.theclinics.com
1052-5157/19/© 2018 Elsevier Inc. All rights reserved.

accounting for 80% of strictures.[3] These are defined as strictures occurring within 5 mm of the duct-to-duct anastomosis, and they typically occur within the first 6 months following LT (range, 2.5–9 months).[4] Risk factors for anastomotic strictures are numerous, and include those attributable to the donor and/or to surgical technique. Donor risk factors include advanced donor age, high donor body mass index, donation after cardiac death, prolonged cold ischemia time, and macrovesicular graft steatosis greater than 25%.[5–9] Surgical risk factors include surgical technique, tight anastomosis, disruption of the bile duct blood supply via excessive dissection or use of cautery, and size mismatch between the donor and recipient.[10] In the early post-transplant period (<1 month), technical issues related to surgical technique predominate, whereas later, anastomotic strictures occur related to relative ischemia at the site of anastomosis. Bile leaks at the anastomosis also predispose to subsequent stricture formation via local inflammation and fibrosis.[11] There are currently few data to suggest that one particular method of duct-to-duct anastomosis is beneficial over another (eg, end-to-end vs end-to-side or side-to-side). Furthermore, the available data suggest equivalent outcomes when using continuous versus interrupted suturing technique.[6]

Post-LT biliary strictures (anastomotic or nonanastomotic) may be suspected in the setting of elevated cholestatic liver enzymes and/or worsening jaundice and pruritus. Abdominal pain may be present, although in the absence of overt cholangitis, pain may not be a predominating symptom. If a biliary stricture is suspected, noninvasive imaging with ultrasound or magnetic resonance cholangiopancreatography (MRCP) may be helpful. Compared with a nontransplant population, ultrasound is somewhat less sensitive for detecting biliary dilatation and strictures in the post-LT setting, with an estimated sensitivity ranging from 40% to 70%; thus, a normal ultrasound should not rule out further investigation.[12] Ultrasound should be performed with Doppler evaluation of the hepatic artery to help identify pathology, such as hepatic artery thrombosis (HAT) or stenosis, which may be contributing to the formation of a biliary stricture. Compared with ultrasound, MRCP retains good sensitivity and specificity for identifying biliary obstruction in the post-LT setting (93% and 97.6%, respectively).[13,14] Pre-endoscopic MRCP may be helpful to provide a "road-map" for the endoscopist.

Endoscopic therapy of anastomotic strictures may involve balloon dilation with or without placement of plastic or metal biliary stents. Multiple sequential procedures are often necessary for successful treatment. A prerequisite for any endoscopic therapy is the ability to pass a guidewire past the area of stricture. If this cannot be accomplished because of angulation or another anatomic variant, then initial interventional radiology-guided percutaneous access with passage of a guidewire transhepatically into the bile duct is necessary, after which endoscopic intervention may be accomplished via a rendezvous technique.[4] In select cases, peroral cholangioscopy may be used to assist in obtaining direct visualization of the stricture when cannulation is difficult.[4,15] At the index procedure, sphincterotomy is typically performed to allow for easier bile drainage and for placement of multiple stents, if necessary.

Balloon dilation alone is initially successful in up to 89% of cases; however, the recurrence rate is high at 62%.[16] Given this, the current standard of care includes plastic biliary stent placement in addition to balloon dilation to help prevent reformation of the stricture (**Fig. 1**). Typically, the balloon is dilated to 4 to 10 mm, depending on the size of the donor duct and the time since transplantation.[17] Following dilation, a 7F to 10F plastic biliary stent is placed to assist in biliary drainage.[18] ERCP is repeated in approximately 2 to 3 months, whereupon the previously placed stent is removed, the stricture is again dilated, and one or more plastic stents are replaced across the stricture. This helps to increase the diameter of the anastomotic stenosis and minimizes the risk of stent occlusion by sludge and other debris with the subsequent development of cholangitis.[18] Typically, between two and four stents are used during subsequent procedures, although some authors promote a method of "maximal stent therapy," where up to six to eight plastic stents are inserted during any given session.[17,19,20] The mean number of ERCPs required for resolution of anastomotic strictures using this technique range from three to five, with long-term success rates ranging from 68% to 100%, and recurrence rates ranging from 0% to 37%.[10,18] The mean time to resolution ranges from 4 to 24 months.[4,10]

A variation on this technique is sequential stent addition, without interval dilation and stent exchange. In sequential stent addition, previously placed stents are not removed

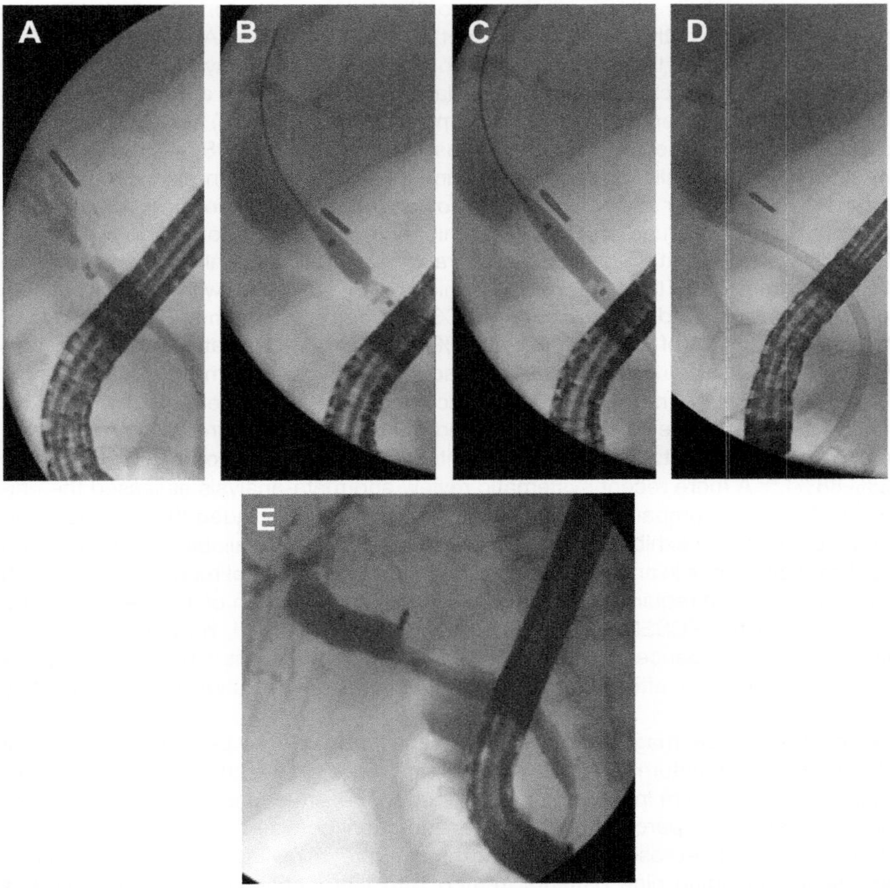

Fig. 1. Anastomotic stricture at the duct-to-duct anastomosis 5 months after orthotopic liver transplantation. The patient presented with rising liver biochemical tests and itching with MRCP concerning for a stricture. (*A*) Tight stricture at the anastomosis with prestenotic dilation of the donor duct. A wire has been passed through the stricture (*B*) and a 6-mm dilating balloon is being inflated across the stricture with a waist that then expands (*C*). A plastic stent has then been deployed across the stricture (*D*). After another ERCP and balloon dilation, two stents were inserted and a year later the stricture is markedly improved (*E*) and the patient had normal liver biochemical tests. (© 2018 Jawad Ahmad, MD, New York.)

during subsequent ERCP; instead, the bile duct is cannulated and additional stents are placed alongside previously placed biliary stents to serially dilate the stricture. In a recent prospective study comparing sequential stent addition with standard technique (interval dilation and stent exchange), outcomes were similar, with resolution of the stricture in 96% in both groups, with statistically similar rates of adverse events, including cholangitis, stent migration, bleeding, and pancreatitis. The authors of this study emphasize that this technique results in reduced procedure and fluoroscopy time, and lower device costs compared with standard interval dilation and stent exchange.[21]

Another modification to sequential balloon dilation and stent placement includes "rapid sequence" endoscopic management, where rather than repeat procedures every 2 to 3 months, ERCP is repeated at 2-week intervals, with stent removal and placement. One study examining the use of this technique reported a high success rate with resolution of the anastomotic stricture in 87% of cases. Additionally, they reported a faster time to resolution of approximately 107.6 days (although this is compared with historical data; this particular study did not have a control group).[22]

The use of fully-covered self-expanding metal stents (FCSEMS) has been proposed as an alternative to the use of multiple plastic stents (MPS). FCSEMS have a larger diameter (10 mm), equivalent to the combined diameter of seven plastic stents, and because of this wider diameter, have a lower predisposition to stent occlusion.[10] The main downside to use of FCSEMS is a higher migration rate compared with plastic stents, which occurs at a rate of 16%.[23] A randomized clinical trial comparing the use of SEMS with MPS to treat a variety of benign biliary strictures (with 65% of patients post-LT) demonstrated noninferiority of FCSEMS compared with MPS, with rates of stricture resolution of 92.6% and 85.4%, respectively.[24] Patients treated with FCSEMS in this study required fewer endoscopic procedures compared with patients treated with MPS. In a meta-analysis that included 200 patients treated with FCSEMS, a higher rate of stricture resolution was noted with stent duration greater than 3 months compared with patients who received stenting for less than 3 months (80%–95% vs 53%–88%).[23] A more recent systematic review and meta-analysis assessed the efficacy of FCSEMS compared with MPS. Although this only included three randomized controlled trials and exhibited significant heterogeneity, the available data suggest no significant difference in anastomotic stricture resolution or rate of recurrence, although fewer ERCPs were required to achieve resolution (with a mean of 1.69 fewer ERCPs per patient in the FCSEMS group).[25] The authors concluded, however, that there was insufficient evidence to suggest FCSEMS over MPS at this time. When used as secondary treatment after failure of MPS, the rate of resolution is approximately 77%.[10]

A novel technique, magnetic compression anastomosis, may be used in the case of refractory biliary strictures to avoid surgical revision. In this technique, two small circular magnets (2.4 mm in diameter) are placed at the site of anastomosis, one endoscopically and one percutaneously. The attraction between the magnets creates compression and necrosis at the site of the stricture, allowing recanalization. In one case series including nine patients treated with this technique, recanalization was observed in 77% of patients at a median recanalization time of 8.1 days. No recurrence was noted in the patients that responded, although follow-up was short-term at 4.8 months.[26]

Anastomotic strictures recur in 0% to 37% of patients treated with MPS at a mean time ranging from 1.5 to 24 months after therapy; in those treated with SEMS, it is approximately 23%.[10,25] The risk of recurrence seems highest among patients with a high intraoperative transfusion requirement, those who undergo a short duration of stenting (<12 months), and among patients with strictures that are identified more than 6 weeks after transplant.[10] Management of refractory anastomotic strictures may include the use of FCSEMS or magnetic compression anastomosis as described previously. Surgical revision of the anastomosis (eg, from a choledochocholedochostomy to Roux-en-Y hepaticojejunostomy [RYHJ]) or percutaneous drainage may be necessary as salvage therapy in up to 10% to 20% of patients.[25]

Nonanastomotic Strictures

By definition, nonanastomotic strictures (NAS) occur more than 5 mm from the site of the anastomosis. Cholangiocytes, more so than hepatocytes, are especially susceptible to ischemia. Such injury may result from macrovascular complications, including HAT or stenosis, or may result from damage to the microvasculature in the setting of ischemia/reperfusion injury, ABO blood group incompatibility, or chronic rejection. Strictures form when ischemic damage to the bile duct leads to fibrosis.[27] Thus, when NAS is suspected, in addition to imaging the biliary tree with ultrasound and/or MRCP, a careful evaluation of the hepatic artery via Doppler ultrasonography and/or computed tomography or magnetic resonance angiography is essential.[28]

Clinically, NAS may present with abnormal liver chemistries with or without clinically overt cholangitis. Damage to cholangiocytes may lead to sloughing of biliary epithelium leading to biliary cast formation. These casts may serve as a nidus for the development of cholangitis, which occurs in approximately 48% of patients with NAS.[29] The incidence of NAS varies from 5% to 25% post-DDLT; this wide variation in incidence results largely from inconsistent inclusion criteria in the literature.[11] In one of the largest studies of NAS, the median time to presentation was 4.1 months, and more than 50% of cases occurred within the first year following transplantation.[30] The cholangiographic appearance of NAS may be similar to that of primary sclerosing cholangitis (PSC); although recurrence of PSC post-LT should be considered in the differential diagnosis among patients who were transplanted for PSC, appearance of multiple biliary strictures within the first year following transplantation is more often related to biliary ischemia.[31]

HAT is the most common macrovascular complication associated with the formation of NAS. In cases of early HAT (within 3 weeks of LT), bile duct necrosis leads to stricture formation and cast deposition within the bile ducts; concomitant hepatic dysfunction necessitates retransplantation in 53% to 74% of patients.[32,33] In contrast, late HAT may present more insidiously, with NAS leading to jaundice, clinical cholangitis, or deranged liver enzymes.[33] It is important, therefore, to obtain imaging of the hepatic artery when patients present after transplantation with elevated liver enzymes. Risk factors for the development of late HAT include previous abdominal surgery, previous HAT, recipient age less than 50 years, and a small donor size.[33]

NAS unrelated to HAT often occur in the setting of other microvascular injury or immunologic injury, including following prolonged ischemia time, the use of deceased after cardiac death (DCD) donors, ABO incompatibility, and chronic rejection.[11] Other risk factors include the use of high-viscosity preservation solution (University of Wisconsin solution), PSC as the cause of liver disease necessitating transplantation, hepaticojejunostomy, and postoperative cytomegalovirus infection.[30,34] The use of DCD donors especially increases the risk of NAS by seven-fold, with an "ischemic cholangiopathy" evolving in 9% to 20% of patients following transplantation from a DCD donor.[35] Recipients of grafts from older DCD donors (age >50 years) are at increased risk of developing biliary complications, including biliary strictures and ischemic cholangiopathy (32.3% vs 23.7% for younger donors).[36] Prevention of ischemic cholangiopathy in such patients includes attempts to reduce the cold and warm ischemia times, and the use of fibrinolytic agents (eg, tissue plasminogen activator) to reduce the formation of microthrombi in the graft, which may contribute to ischemia/reperfusion injury.[11,35]

The location of NAS has prognostic and therapeutic implications. In their review of non-HAT-related NAS, Buis and colleagues[30] subdivided the location of NAS into four different zones: (A) extrahepatic bile duct to hilar bifurcation, (B) bile ducts between first- and second-order branches, (C) bile ducts between the second- and third-order branches, and (D) bile ducts in the periphery of the liver. Most NAS occurred in zone A (85%), whereas lesions in zone D were the least common. Intrahepatic lesions (zones B and C) carried the greatest risk of progression to advanced fibrosis/biliary cirrhosis.[29] Peripheral lesions were significantly more common when patients presented more than 1 year from the time of LT.[30]

Management of NAS is not standardized, and there is limited literature available. The approach is often dependent on the given patient's anatomy, and may involve a combination of therapies, including medical therapy with ursodeoxycholic acid, ERCP, percutaneous transhepatic cholangiography (PTC), and occasionally surgical revision.[29] The approach similar to that which is taken with anastomotic strictures may be used, with balloon dilation and serial placement of MPS at 3-month intervals to gradually dilate the site of stricture. The presence of sludge and biliary casts, which occur in 27% of patients, may necessitate more frequent stent exchange, however, because stent occlusion may occur (**Fig. 2**).[37] If NAS are intrahepatic, access via ERCP may be difficult, necessitating an interventional radiographic approach via PTC or via a combination approach (rendezvous technique). Despite endoscopic and radiographic intervention, radiographic progression may occur in up to 48% of patients.[29] Retransplantation has been reported to be necessary in up to 50% of patients, although in one of the largest series examining the outcome of NAS, retransplantation was necessary in only 16% of patients.[29,38]

Bile Leaks

Bile leaks are the second most common biliary complication following DDLT, with an estimated incidence of 8.5% (range, 5%–10%).[5,39] The incidence is higher (up to 25%) among recipients of grafts from live donors.[40] Most bile leaks occur within the first 30 days post-transplant, and are related to technical issues at the site of anastomosis.[41] Most commonly this is related to errors in suturing of the anastomosis or to the development of ischemia at the site of anastomosis, either caused by tension on the anastomosis or by injury of the arterial blood supply to the bile duct. Nonanastomotic leaks also may occur from the cystic duct stump or from minor ducts, including the duct of Luschka.[42] Several nontechnical donor risk factors for bile leak have been identified, including receipt of a graft from a DCD donor, receipt of a graft from a donor with a high donor risk index, and receipt of a steatotic graft.[41] Recipient risk factors for the development of bile leaks include a higher preoperative bilirubin level, model for end-stage liver disease score, and advanced recipient age. Operative risk factors include a prolonged warm ischemia time.[1] The type of biliary reconstruction (duct-to-duct vs RYHJ) does not seem to significantly impact the risk of bile leak after LT.[1,41] Conversely, the use of a T-tube does seem to increase the risk, where leaks develop around the time of T-tube removal, at a median time of 102 days post-LT. This type of bile leak has decreased in incidence over time because T-tube placement is increasingly uncommon.[6] Bile leaks at the cut surface may also occur in the setting of LDLT or with the use of split liver grafts; these complications are discussed later in the living donor transplantation section.

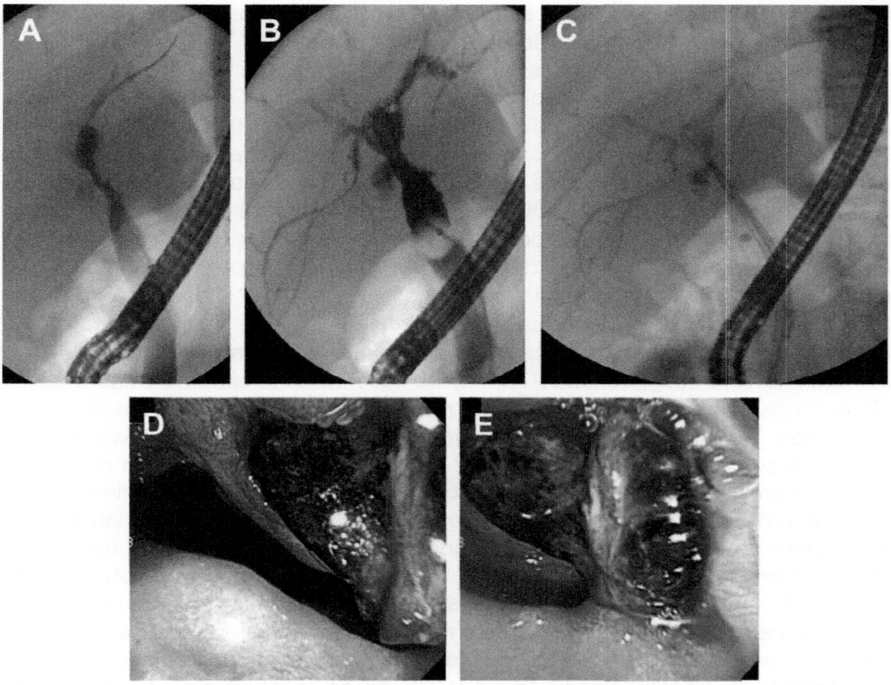

Fig. 2. Ischemic cholangiopathy and a nonanastomotic stricture 2 months after orthotopic liver transplantation. The patient had hepatocellular carcinoma and received a DCD organ. Liver biochemical tests began to rise and the patient developed low-grade fever. No biliary dilation was noted on imaging. (*A*) Wire in the biliary tree with narrowing in the hilar area with irregularity. (*B*) Balloon occlusion and contrast injection demonstrates some filling defects in the donor ducts and some attenuation, particularly on the right. (*C*) A stent has been placed with drainage of contrast. (*D, E*) The endoscopic images show cast and stone material draining through the papilla after a sphincterotomy. (© 2018 Jawad Ahmad, MD, New York.)

Clinically, patients with bile leaks may present with abdominal pain; fever; and if the postoperative drains are still in place, with bilious output. Bile leaks may predispose to peritonitis and sepsis, and if untreated, multiorgan failure and death. Liver enzymes may or may not be elevated. If there is a question about the amount of bile in a patient's drain, the contents may be tested for bilirubin. In the setting of a bile leak, the bilirubin concentration in the drain fluid should be higher than serum bilirubin, with a ratio of greater than 3.25 having a sensitivity and specificity of 73% and 95%, respectively.[43,44] A multimodal approach is used in the diagnosis of post-LT bile leaks. Ultrasound is typically the first test obtained; this may help identify bilomas, although it is often difficult to differentiate these from other postoperative collections. Ultrasound should be performed with Doppler to assess for patency of the hepatic artery, because leaks may occur in the context of ischemic injury.[45,46] Nuclear scintigraphy with hepatobiliary iminodiacetic acid scanning has a diagnostic accuracy for the identification of bile leaks ranging from 83% to 87% after cholecystectomy, although its accuracy seems to be lower following LT.[47,48] Although MRCP has a high sensitivity and specificity for the identification of strictures, its utility in identifying leaks is lower. However, data from small studies with a nontransplant population suggest that MRCP with biliary-specific contrast may be useful.[49]

The gold standard for the diagnosis of bile leaks remains direct cholangiography. If a T-tube is in place, this may be accomplished via a tube study. Otherwise, ERCP is the diagnostic and therapeutic procedure of choice. Although in the general population ERCP is currently reserved only for therapeutic purposes, in the post-LT setting diagnostic ERCP remains valuable. One study revealed a high yield of ERCP done for diagnostic or therapeutic intent (66.3% and 90.1%, respectively).[50] The type of biliary reconstruction (choledochocholedocostomy vs RYHJ) may impact the yield of ERCP. Although more technically difficult, ERCP may be accomplished in most patients (71%) after RYHJ.[51] Among those in whom ERCP fails, PTC may be necessary. This is technically challenging, because bile ducts may not be significantly dilated in the setting of a leak, making percutaneous ultrasound-guided targeting difficult. Available data, however, suggest that PTC may be accomplished effectively and safely.[52]

Endoscopic management involves the diversion of biliary flow from the site of the leak to allow healing and closure of the defect (**Fig. 3**). Most frequently, this is accomplished via placement of a plastic biliary stent across the papilla, with or without sphincterotomy, to decrease the transpapillary gradient and divert the flow of bile. Stent placement alone may result in resolution of the leak in greater than 90% of cases, often obviating sphincterotomy. Indeed, sphincterotomy may be associated with a higher rate of adverse events, including bleeding and perforation.[53] Stents are typically kept in place for 6 to 8 weeks, and removed once closure of the leak is confirmed via repeat ERCP.[54] Plastic stents are recommended, because FCSEMSs have been associated with a high rate of secondary stricture formation.[55] Leaks may occasionally be associated with a downstream biliary stricture; in this case, dilation of the stricture at the time of stent placement may help to ensure closure.[56] Initial endoscopic therapy with plastic stent placement may fail, with up to 40% of patients requiring a repeat intervention. Hepatic artery disease (including thrombosis, stenosis, and pseudoaneurysm) is seen more commonly in such patients; thus, a careful assessment of the hepatic artery in cases of refractory bile leak is essential. Repeat stent placement is successful in resolving the leak in 53% of cases. In the uncommon case where endoscopic or interventional radiologic management fails, surgical revision or even retransplantation may be necessary. Refractory bile leak is associated with significantly decreased survival.[57]

PAPILLARY STENOSIS

Papillary stenosis is uncommon following DDLT, occurring with an incidence of approximately 2% to 5%.[5,58] The pathophysiology is unclear, but may be related to denervation of the recipient duct that occurs in the setting of dissection during transplantation. Infection with cytomegalovirus or other opportunistic infections (eg, cryptosporidium) may also contribute to its development.[59] It presents similarly to papillary stenosis in the nontransplant setting, with dilation of the bile duct and abnormal liver enzymes in the absence of a stricture or other filling defect (**Fig. 4**). The treatment is biliary sphincterotomy, which achieves durable clinical success in up to 80% to 100% of patients.[60]

STONES

As in nontransplant patients, stones may form in patients who have undergone LT (**Fig. 5**). Most commonly, these form in the setting of strictures (anastomotic or nonanastomotic) that lead to biliary stasis. Patients may present with cholestatic liver

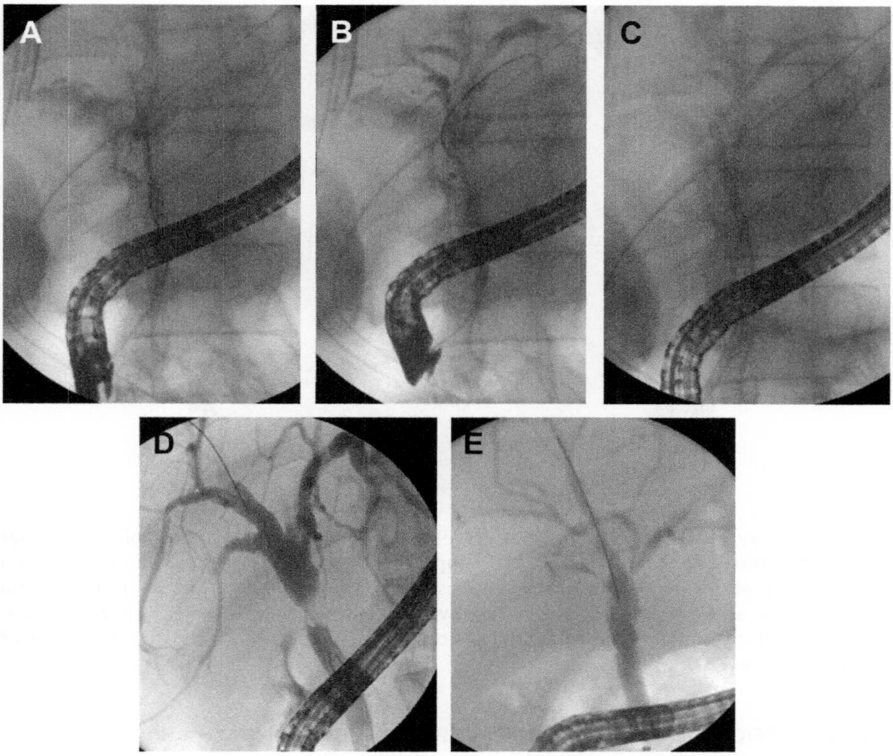

Fig. 3. Bile leak from the duct-to-duct anastomosis 6 weeks after orthotopic liver transplantation. The patient had had a complicated postoperative course and developed fevers with abdominal collections noted on computed tomography scan and bile-stained drainage from his wound. (*A*) Contrast is seen in the recipient and donor ducts with a wire just reaching the hilum. Contrast is extravasating and collecting to the right of the donor system likely from the anastomosis. (*B*) Wire entering the left system and further filling of the intrahepatic ducts. (*C*) Plastic stent has been deployed with the proximal end in the donor system and contrast has drained into the duodenum. The leak healed after several weeks but the patient developed a stricture (*D*) 3 months later that required several ERCPs with balloon dilation and serial stenting to improve (*E*). (© 2018 Jawad Ahmad, MD, New York.)

chemistries alone, or with pain and cholangitis. In one large series, 30.5% of patients developed bile duct stones post-transplant; of these, 73% were associated with a stricture. Patients presented at a mean time of 19.2 months following LT. Stones were cleared from the ducts in 59% of patients after initial ERCP, with the remainder requiring repeat procedures. Recurrence of stone disease was noted in 17% of patients at a median follow-up time of 5.6 months from the last ERCP showing stone clearance.[60] In a more recent single-center study, of 1289 LTs performed, only 49 (3.8%) developed bile duct stones or casts. The median time to development of stones was 613 days post-LT. Risk factors for the development of bile duct stones in this study included concurrent bile duct pathology and hypercholesterolemia and hypertriglyceridemia. Ursodeoxycholic acid use was protective (odds ratio, 0.31; 95% confidence interval, 0.14–0.70). It was again shown that ERCP is generally technically successful using standard stone removal techniques.[61]

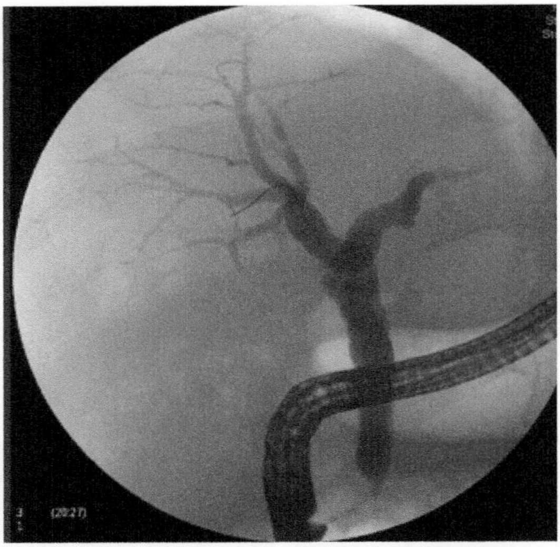

Fig. 4. Papillary stenosis. This patient developed abdominal pain and elevated liver biochemical tests 13 months after orthotopic liver transplantation. Imaging showed mild biliary dilation and a liver biopsy suggested biliary obstruction. At ERCP the papilla looked normal and the cholangiogram is shown. Biliary sphincterotomy led to normalization of liver biochemical tests and alleviation of the abdominal pain. (© 2018 Jawad Ahmad, MD, New York.)

ISSUES SPECIFIC TO LIVING DONOR TRANSPLANTATION

Bile Leaks

Biliary complications are more common following LDLT because of the more complex biliary reconstruction and the risk of cut-surface leaks, with a rate of 40%.[62] Bile leaks comprise two-thirds of all biliary complications following LDLT, whereas strictures make up the remaining one-third.[40] Most bile leaks following LDLT are anastomotic (**Fig. 6**). Somewhat intuitively, the risk of bile leak increases with the complexity of the biliary reconstruction (three or more donor ducts from right lobe vs one or two) and with lower center LDLT volume.[63]

Techniques for diagnosing and treating bile leaks in the setting of LDLT are similar to those in DDLT. The patient may present with abdominal pain, fever, bile noted in surgical drains, and a collection seen on abdominal imaging. If the leak is anastomotic, ERCP may show extravasation of contrast at the site of the leak. In the setting of a cut surface leak, contrast extravasation from the surface of the liver may or may not be appreciated. Therefore, if there is clinical evidence of a bile leak, empiric treatment may be prudent. As in other settings where a bile leak is present, sphincterotomy and plastic stent placement decrease the transpapillary gradient and allow for diversion of bile flow away from the site of leak to allow for healing of the fistula.[64] The ERCP should be repeated in 4 to 6 weeks to assess for resolution of the leak and perform upsizing of the stent if necessary. Resolution of bile leaks with endoscopic methods may be accomplished in 82% to 92% of cases.[62,65]

Biliary Strictures

Like bile leaks, biliary strictures are more common after LDLT when compared with DDLT. In the adult-to-adult LT (A2ALL) study, biliary strictures in LDLT occurred at a

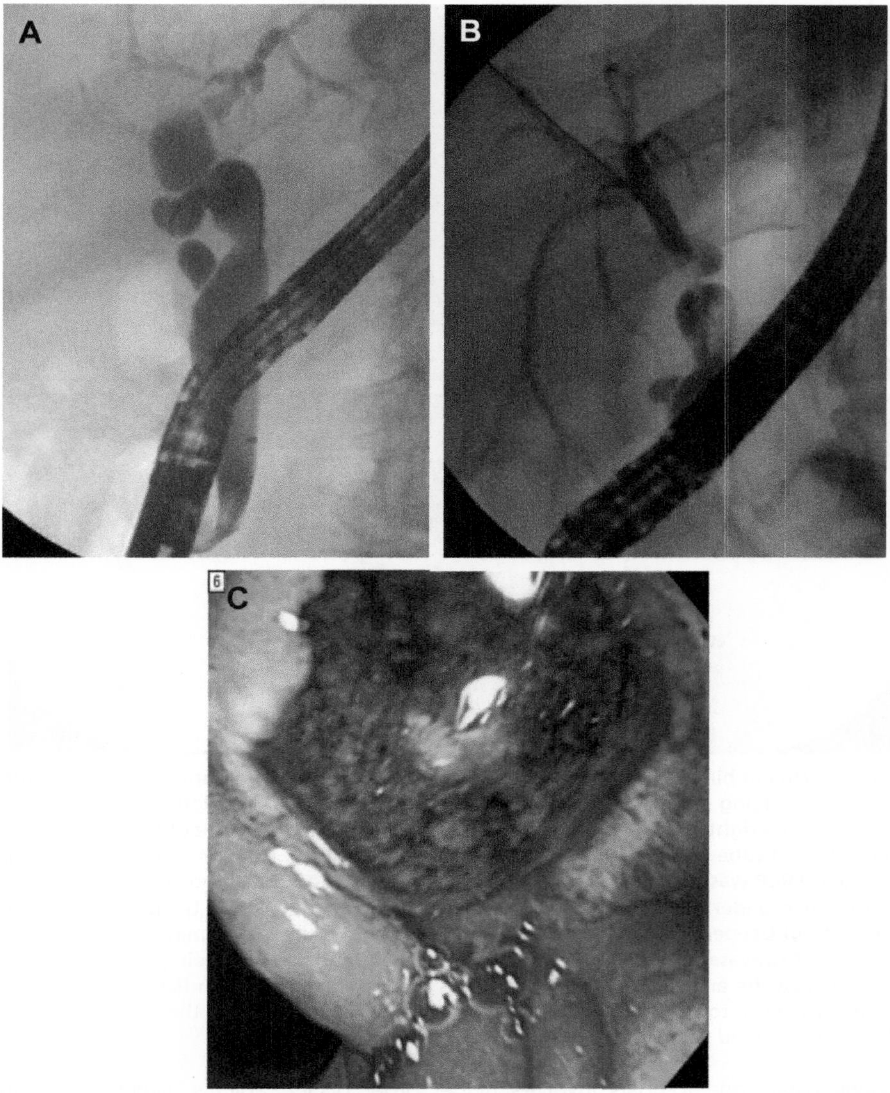

Fig. 5. Bile duct stones after orthotopic liver transplantation. Filling defects are seen in the two cholangiograms in patients many years out from liver transplantation. (*A*) Dilated extrahepatic duct with a filling defect in the very distal recipient duct. (*B*) Filling defect is seen just below the anastomosis. (*C*) The patient was jaundiced and we placed a stent through the anastomosis after removing the mixed cholesterol/black pigment stone and removed the stent several months later. (© 2018 Jawad Ahmad, MD, New York.)

rate of 32%, compared with 21% among patients who underwent DDLT.[62,63] The increased incidence of biliary complications following LDLT may be related to the more complex biliary reconstruction, which involves more than one anastomosis over half of cases, with or without RYHJ.[66] Recent data from the A2ALL group suggest a trend toward a higher incidence of anastomotic biliary strictures among patients

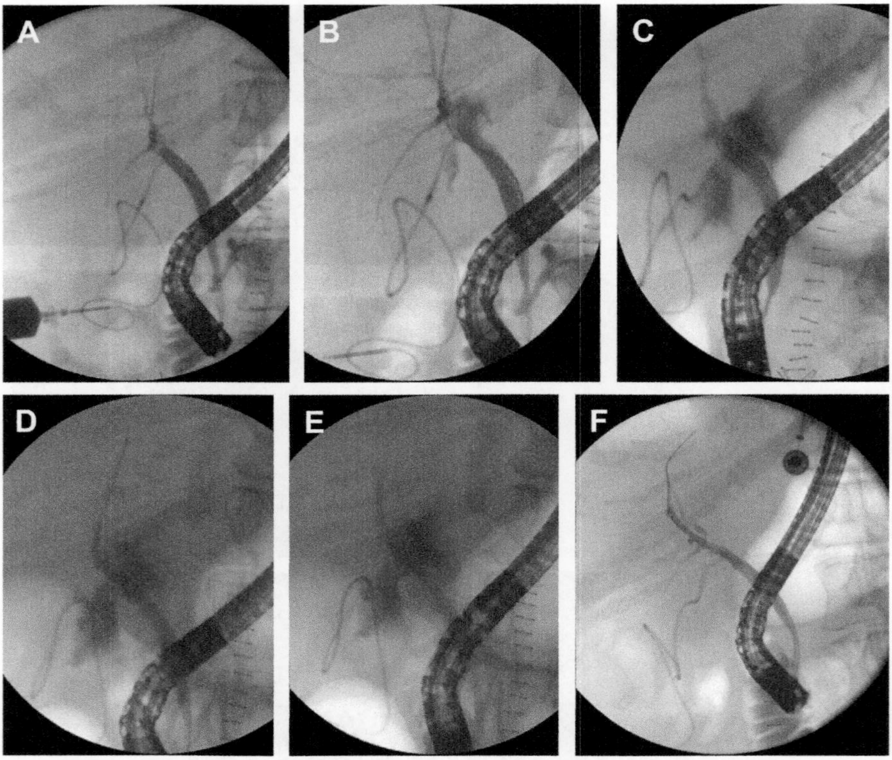

Fig. 6. Recipient bile leak after live donor liver transplantation. This patient presented with fever and imaging showed perihepatic collections 2 weeks after live donor liver transplantation using a right lobe graft. Unusually, a T-tube had been inserted at the time of transplant but a T-tube cholangiogram failed to show a bile leak. However, the suspicion was high and ERCP was performed. (*A*) Cholangiogram shows a normal looking recipient duct and relative underfilling of the donor system even with the T-tube being injected with contrast. (*B*) Deeper cannulation and then injection shows the leak coming off the anastomosis. (*C*) Extravasation of contrast is readily apparent and a wire is being manipulated to try and cross the anastomosis. The wire enters the intrahepatic system (*D*) and a stent has been inserted (into the right anterior system [*E*]). Three weeks later the leak has healed (*F*). (© 2018 Jawad Ahmad, MD, New York.)

whose biliary anastomosis involves higher order biliary radicals, likely related to devascularization of these ducts as they are dissected for reconstruction.[66] Other risk factors for the development of biliary strictures post-LDLT included prolonged operative time, lower center volume for LDLT, and the presence of a concomitant bile leak.[62] As in DDLT, biliary strictures in patients undergoing LDLT may be anastomotic or nonanastomotic. Anastomotic strictures comprise approximately 80% of biliary strictures following LDLT.[67]

As in DDLT, most anastomotic strictures present within 1 year of LT. Clinical presentation is similar, with patients presenting with abnormal liver chemistries, jaundice, anorexia, pruritus, and occasionally abdominal pain. MRCP may be performed to noninvasively assess the bile ducts to look for evidence of a stricture in advance of ERCP.

Endoscopic therapy for biliary strictures post-LDLT includes dilation and stenting (**Fig. 7**). Given the variation in biliary reconstruction among patients who receive

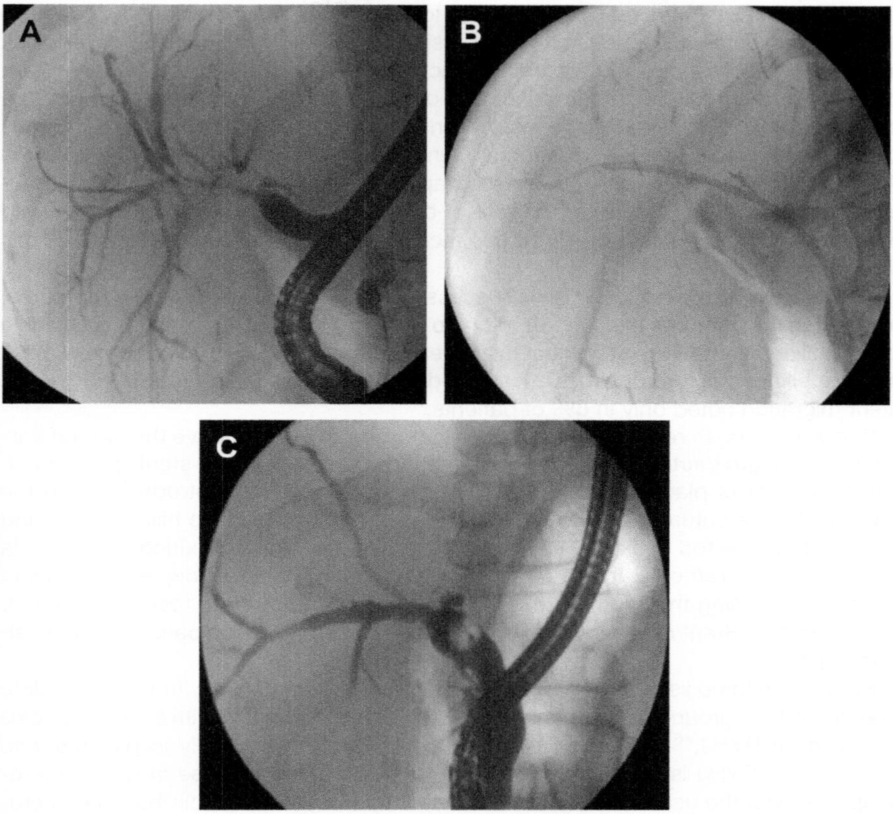

Fig. 7. Recipient stricture after live donor liver transplantation. This patient presented with intense pruritis and elevated cholestatic liver enzymes 4 months after live donor liver transplantation. (*A*) Complex stricture extending from the anastomosis into the donor right lobe. (*B*) After multiple attempts a wire finally made it across the anastomosis into a large duct and a 7F catheter plastic stent was deployed. (*C*) Eventually after multiple procedures and placement of three stents into the three main donor ducts, durable patency was achieved. (© 2018 Jawad Ahmad, MD, New York.)

LDLT, it is essential that the endoscopist review the operative reports before proceeding with ERCP, because the type of biliary reconstruction may impact endoscopic approach (eg, the presence of a Roux limb may necessitate the use of balloon-assisted enteroscopy).[68] After the biliary tree is accessed, passage of a guidewire across the stricture is essential to allow for endoscopic therapy. In LDLT recipients, this may be more difficult because of more complex angulation of the anastomosis. Direct cholangioscopy may be helpful here to guide guidewire passage; in one study, direct cholangioscopy successfully aided guidewire passage in 60% of patients in whom conventional guidewire passage failed.[68,69] Therapy for dilation of most post-LDLT biliary strictures is similar to that which is described previously for DDLT, where balloon dilation is followed by placement of multiple plastic biliary stents across the site of stricture. The procedure is repeated every 2 to 3 months until stricture resolution is achieved. Treatment success using this technique in LDLT patients is variable, with long-term success rates ranging from 51% to 100%.[64,70] The presence of a concomitant bile leak is a strong risk factor for persistence of a biliary stricture.[71] Other risk factors for failure of endoscopic therapy include HAT, multiple biliary anastomoses, prior transarterial chemoembolization, and older donor age.[67,72] The use of prophylactic stenting as a means to reduce the risk of biliary complications in LDLT has been investigated. Here, an intraductal stent (rather than a T-tube) is placed at the time of anastomosis, which exits out the papilla for easy endoscopic retrieval. However, current data suggest that the rate of biliary complications may be higher with the use of prophylactic stenting, so this technique cannot be recommended at this time.[73]

SEMS have also been used with success in treating post-LDLT biliary strictures, most often for strictures that are refractory to standard therapy with the use of multiple plastic biliary stents. One study that evaluated the use of SEMS in 35 patients with refractory biliary strictures post-LDLT showed a stricture resolution rate of 83%, with stent migration noted only in 6% of patients.[74]

Some authors, to reduce the use of sphincterotomy and preserve the natural barrier between gut bacteria and the biliary tree, advocate for "inside stent" placement, where a stent is placed across the stricture, but does not protrude through the papilla. Here, a suture is tied to the distal end of standard plastic biliary stent, and the stent is inserted proximal to the ampulla, with the suture exiting the ampulla for easier stent retrieval. In the largest series studying this technique, 94 patients were treated using this method; 69% of these patients achieved resolution of their strictures.[68,75] Stent migration occurred in 10% of patients, and pancreatitis developed in 19%.

Biliary anastomosis using an RYHJ is common following LDLT. In follow-up data from the A2ALL group, 44% of patients had biliary reconstruction with an anastomosis involving an RYHJ.[66] Accessing the biliary system endoscopically in patients who have had an RYHJ is technically challenging, and requires the use of deep enteroscopy (ie, with the use of a pediatric colonoscopy, single- or double-balloon enteroscope, or a spiral enteroscope). Deep enteroscopy is successful in reaching the biliary anastomosis in 64% to 85% of cases. Typical ERC techniques using these endoscopes, however, are more challenging related to the lack of an elevator mechanism and because of the presence of a smaller working channel than is found on a standard duodenoscope. One small study examining the use of double-balloon ERC for the management of biliary stricture after LDLT with an RYHJ reconstruction showed that the stricture could be successfully treated endoscopically in 78% of patients, with the remaining patients requiring radiologic assistance via a rendezvous technique.[76] Surgical reconstruction is a last resort for the management of post-LDLT biliary strictures.

DONOR BILIARY COMPLICATIONS

Donor surgery for LDLT involves resection of either the left or right lobe of the liver and hence bile leaks from the cut surface or the left or right common hepatic duct can occur but are uncommon. Leaks are recognized early in the postoperative course because abdominal drains are typically left in place for several days. Treatment with transpapillary stents is curative in most cases (**Fig. 8**).

Strictures of the biliary tree after liver resection are uncommon but can occur as the liver regenerates and may not be amenable to endoscopic stenting. Percutaneous drainage can relieve jaundice but surgical correction is usually required (see **Fig. 8**).

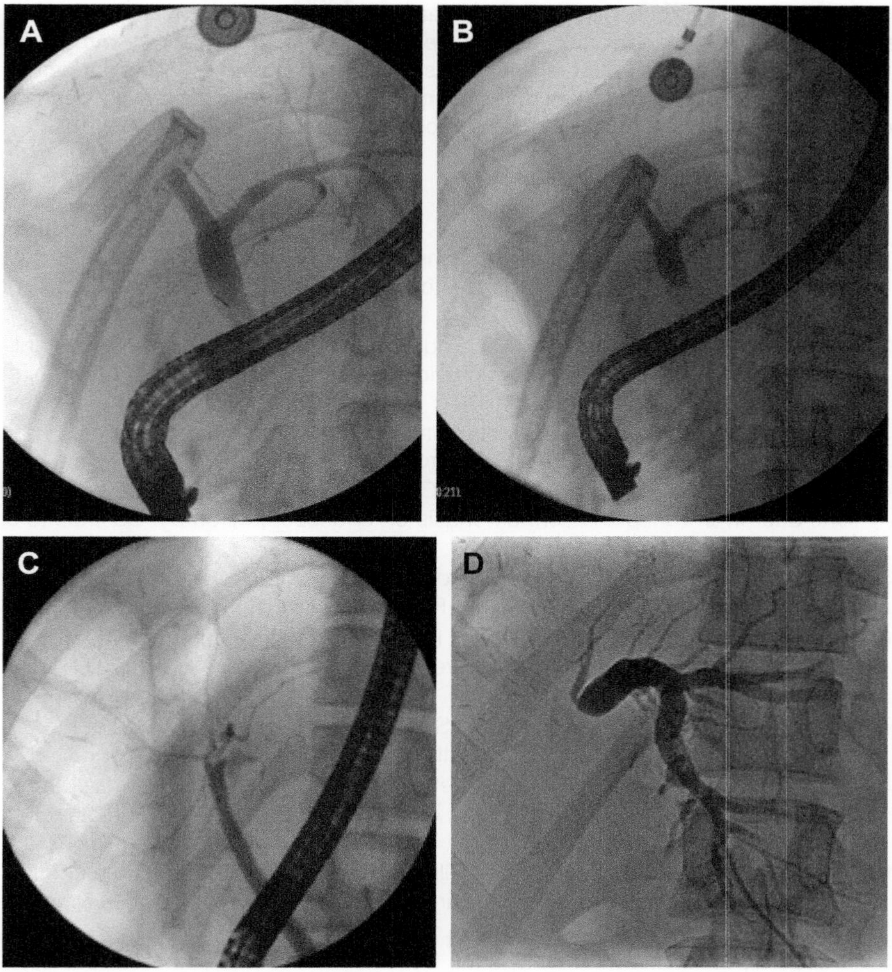

Fig. 8. Biliary complications in live liver donors. (*A, B*) A leak from the right common hepatic duct is shown. A drain is seen adjacent in the space where the right lobe should be and injection of contrast leads to darkening of the drain. This patient had persistent drainage of bile in an abdominal drain for several days after liver donation. A transpapillary stent healed the leak within a week and was removed several weeks later. (*C, D*) This patient developed jaundice 6 weeks after donating his right lobe to his mother. Imaging showed a dilated duct in the remaining left lobe. (*C*) ERCP was performed but despite pressure injection we could not opacify the left system. (*D*) The patient went for percutaneous transhepatic cholangiogram and despite multiple attempts, access to the extrahepatic bile duct could not be obtained and the patient required surgical correction with a Roux hepaticojejunostomy. (© 2018 Jawad Ahmad, MD, New York.)

SUMMARY

The experienced therapeutic endoscopist should be able to successfully manage most biliary complications after LT. Before undertaking the procedure, it is important to understand the anatomy, review appropriate biliary imaging, and discuss the case with the transplant surgeon. Strictures and leaks are the main complications encountered after LT and the techniques involved are similar to regular ERCP with wire placement across the duct-to-duct anastomosis, balloon dilation, and deployment of plastic stents. Several procedures may be required over time to successfully treat patients and percutaneous or surgical correction should seldom be required.

REFERENCES

1. Akamatsu N, Sugawara Y, Hashimoto D. Biliary reconstruction, its complications and management of biliary complications after adult liver transplantation: a systematic review of the incidence, risk factors and outcome. Transpl Int 2011;24(4):379–92.
2. Macías-Gómez C, Dumonceau J-M. Endoscopic management of biliary complications after liver transplantation: an evidence-based review. World J Gastrointest Endosc 2015;7(6):606–16.
3. Chascsa DM, Vargas HE. The gastroenterologist's guide to management of the post-liver transplant patient. Am J Gastroenterol 2018;113(6):819–28.
4. Balderramo D, Navasa M, Cardenas A. Current management of biliary complications after liver transplantation: emphasis on endoscopic therapy. Gastroenterol Hepatol 2011;34(2):107–15.
5. Gastaca M. Biliary complications after orthotopic liver transplantation: a review of incidence and risk factors. Transplant Proc 2012;44(6):1545–9.
6. Sundaram V, Jones DT, Shah NH, et al. Posttransplant biliary complications in the pre- and post-model for end-stage liver disease era. Liver Transpl 2011;17(4):428–35.
7. Baccarani U, Isola M, Adani GL, et al. Steatosis of the hepatic graft as a risk factor for post-transplant biliary complications. Clin Transplant 2010;24(5):631–5.
8. Foley DP, Fernandez LA, Leverson G, et al. Biliary complications after liver transplantation from donation after cardiac death donors: an analysis of risk factors and long-term outcomes from a single center. Ann Surg 2011;253(4):817–25.
9. Maheshwari A, Maley W, Li Z, et al. Biliary complications and outcomes of liver transplantation from donors after cardiac death. Liver Transpl 2007;13(12):1645–53.
10. Koksal AS, Eminler AT, Parlak E, et al. Management of biliary anastomotic strictures after liver transplantation. Transplant Rev (Orlando) 2017;31(3):207–17.
11. Seehofer D, Eurich D, Veltzke-Schlieker W, et al. Biliary complications after liver transplantation: old problems and new challenges. Am J Transplant 2013;13(2):253–65.
12. St Peter S, Rodriquez-Davalos MI, Rodriguez-Luna HM, et al. Significance of proximal biliary dilatation in patients with anastomotic strictures after liver transplantation. Dig Dis Sci 2004;49(7–8):1207–11.
13. Beltrán MM, Marugán RB, Oton E, et al. Accuracy of magnetic resonance cholangiography in the evaluation of late biliary complications after orthotopic liver transplantation. Transplant Proc 2005;37(9):3924–5.
14. Xu YB, Min ZG, Jiang HX, et al. Diagnostic value of magnetic resonance cholangiopancreatography for biliary complications in orthotopic liver transplantation: a meta-analysis. Transplant Proc 2013;45(6):2341–6.
15. Wright H, Sharma S, Gurakar A, et al. Management of biliary stricture guided by the Spyglass Direct Visualization System in a liver transplant recipient: an innovative approach. Gastrointest Endosc 2008;67(7):1201–3.

16. Zoepf T, Maldonado-Lopez EJ, Hilgard P, et al. Balloon dilatation vs. balloon dilatation plus bile duct endoprostheses for treatment of anastomotic biliary strictures after liver transplantation. Liver Transpl 2006;12(1):88–94.
17. Tabibian JH, Asham EH, Han S, et al. Endoscopic treatment of postorthotopic liver transplantation anastomotic biliary strictures with maximal stent therapy (with video). Gastrointest Endosc 2010;71(3):505–12.
18. Lee DW, Jo HH, Abdullah J, et al. Endoscopic management of anastomotic strictures after liver transplantation. Clin Endosc 2016;49(5):457–61.
19. Pasha SF, Harrison ME, Das A, et al. Endoscopic treatment of anastomotic biliary strictures after deceased donor liver transplantation: outcomes after maximal stent therapy. Gastrointest Endosc 2007;66(1):44–51.
20. Costamagna G, Pandolfi M, Mutignani M, et al. Long-term results of endoscopic management of postoperative bile duct strictures with increasing numbers of stents. Gastrointest Endosc 2001;54(2):162–8.
21. Barakat MT, Huang RJ, Thosani NC, et al. Liver transplant-related anastomotic biliary strictures: a novel, rapid, safe, radiation-sparing, and cost-effective management approach. Gastrointest Endosc 2018;87(2):501–8.
22. Morelli G, Fazel A, Judah J, et al. Rapid-sequence endoscopic management of posttransplant anastomotic biliary strictures. Gastrointest Endosc 2008;67(6): 879–85.
23. Kao D, Zepeda-Gomez S, Tandon P, et al. Managing the post-liver transplantation anastomotic biliary stricture: multiple plastic versus metal stents: a systematic review. Gastrointest Endosc 2013;77(5):679–91.
24. Coté GA, Slivka A, Tarnasky P, et al. Effect of covered metallic stents compared with plastic stents on benign biliary stricture resolution: a randomized clinical trial. JAMA 2016;315(12):1250–7.
25. Landi F, de'Angelis N, Sepulveda A, et al. Endoscopic treatment of anastomotic biliary stricture after adult deceased donor liver transplantation with multiple plastic stents versus self-expandable metal stents: a systematic review and meta-analysis. Transpl Int 2018;31(2):131–51.
26. Parlak E, Koksal AS, Kucukay F, et al. A novel technique for the endoscopic treatment of complete biliary anastomosis obstructions after liver transplantation: through-the-scope magnetic compression anastomosis. Gastrointest Endosc 2017;85(4):841–7.
27. Noack K, Bronk SF, Kato A, et al. The greater vulnerability of bile duct cells to reoxygenation injury than to anoxia. Implications for the pathogenesis of biliary strictures after liver transplantation. Transplantation 1993;56(3):495–500.
28. den Dulk AC, Wasser MNJM, Willemssen FEJA, et al. Value of magnetic resonance cholangiopancreatography in assessment of nonanastomotic biliary strictures after liver transplantation. Transplant Direct 2015;1(10):e42.
29. Verdonk RC, Buis CI, van der Jagt EJ, et al. Nonanastomotic biliary strictures after liver transplantation, part 2: management, outcome, and risk factors for disease progression. Liver Transpl 2007;13(5):725–32.
30. Buis CI, Verdonk RC, Van der Jagt EJ, et al. Nonanastomotic biliary strictures after liver transplantation, part 1: radiological features and risk factors for early vs. late presentation. Liver Transpl 2007;13(5):708–18.
31. Campsen J, Zimmerman MA, Trotter JF, et al. Clinically recurrent primary sclerosing cholangitis following liver transplantation: a time course. Liver Transpl 2008;14(2):181–5.

32. Bekker J, Ploem S, de Jong KP. Early hepatic artery thrombosis after liver transplantation: a systematic review of the incidence, outcome and risk factors. Am J Transplant 2009;9(4):746–57.
33. Mourad MM, Liossis C, Gunson BK, et al. Etiology and management of hepatic artery thrombosis after adult liver transplantation. Liver Transpl 2014;20(6): 713–23.
34. Sanni A, Asher J, Wilson C, et al. Predisposing factors for biliary complications following liver transplantation. Transplant Proc 2006;38(8):2677–8.
35. Kubal C, Mangus R, Fridell J, et al. Optimization of perioperative conditions to prevent ischemic cholangiopathy in donation after circulatory death donor liver transplantation. Transplantation 2016;100(8):1699–704.
36. Croome KP, Mathur AK, Lee DD, et al. Outcomes of donation after circulatory death liver grafts from donors 50 years or older: a multicenter analysis. Transplantation 2018;102(7):1108–14.
37. Voigtländer T, Negm AA, Strassburg CP, et al. Biliary cast syndrome post-liver transplantation: risk factors and outcome. Liver Int 2013;33(8):1287–92.
38. Villa NA, Harrison ME. Management of biliary strictures after liver transplantation. Gastroenterol Hepatol (N Y) 2015;11(5):316–28.
39. Nemes B, Gámán G, Doros A. Biliary complications after liver transplantation. Expert Rev Gastroenterol Hepatol 2015;9(4):447–66.
40. Simoes P, Kesar V, Ahmad J. Spectrum of biliary complications following live donor liver transplantation. World J Hepatol 2015;7(14):1856–65.
41. Senter-Zapata M, Khan AS, Subramanian T, et al. Patient and graft survival: biliary complications after liver transplantation. J Am Coll Surg 2018;226(4):484–94.
42. Shin M, Joh J-W. Advances in endoscopic management of biliary complications after living donor liver transplantation: comprehensive review of the literature. World J Gastroenterol 2016;22(27):6173–91.
43. Atwal T, Pastrana M, Sandhu B. Post-liver transplant biliary complications. J Clin Exp Hepatol 2012;2(1):81–5.
44. DeBenedet AT, Scheiman JM, Elta GH, et al. Peritoneal fluid bilirubin to serum bilirubin ratio for the diagnosis of bile leaks in orthotopic liver transplant recipients. Dig Dis Sci 2013;58(10):3044–8.
45. Peñas-Herrero I, Perez-Miranda M. Hepatic artery disease and anastomotic bile leaks after liver transplantation: shining the light on the true Achilles' heel. Gastrointest Endosc 2017;85(5):993–5.
46. Hussaini SH, Sheridan MB, Davies M. The predictive value of transabdominal ultrasonography in the diagnosis of biliary tract complications after orthotopic liver transplantation. Gut 1999;45(6):900–3.
47. Sandoval BA, Goettler CE, Robinson AV, et al. Cholescintigraphy in the diagnosis of bile leak after laparoscopic cholecystectomy. Am Surg 1997;63(7):611–6.
48. Eckenschwiller M, Ackermann H, Bechstein WO, et al. Accuracy of hepatobiliary scintigraphy after liver transplantation and liver resection. Int J Mol Imaging 2016; 2016:7857849.
49. Kul M, Erden A, Düşünceli Atman E. Diagnostic value of Gd-EOB-DTPA-enhanced MR cholangiography in non-invasive detection of postoperative bile leakage. Br J Radiol 2017;90(1072):20160847.
50. Elmunzer BJ, Debenedet AT, Volk ML, et al. Clinical yield of diagnostic endoscopic retrograde cholangiopancreatography in orthotopic liver transplant recipients with suspected biliary complications. Liver Transpl 2012;18(12):1479–84.

51. Chahal P, Baron TH, Poterucha JJ, et al. Endoscopic retrograde cholangiography in post-orthotopic liver transplant population with Roux-en-Y biliary reconstruction. Liver Transpl 2007;13(8):1168–73.
52. Righi D, Franchello A, Ricchiuti A, et al. Safety and efficacy of the percutaneous treatment of bile leaks in hepaticojejunostomy or split-liver transplantation without dilatation of the biliary tree. Liver Transpl 2008;14(5):611–5.
53. Adler DG, Papachristou GI, Taylor LJ, et al. Clinical outcomes in patients with bile leaks treated via ERCP with regard to the timing of ERCP: a large multicenter study. Gastrointest Endosc 2017;85(4):766–72.
54. Morelli J, Mulcahy HE, Willner IR, et al. Endoscopic treatment of post-liver transplantation biliary leaks with stent placement across the leak site. Gastrointest Endosc 2001;54(4):471–5.
55. Phillips MS, Bonatti H, Sauer BG, et al. Elevated stricture rate following the use of fully covered self-expandable metal biliary stents for biliary leaks following liver transplantation. Endoscopy 2011;43(6):512–7.
56. Dolay K, Soylu A, Aygun E. The role of ERCP in the management of bile leakage: endoscopic sphincterotomy versus biliary stenting. J Laparoendosc Adv Surg Tech A 2010;20(5):455–9.
57. DaVee T, Geevarghese SK, Slaughter JC, et al. Refractory anastomotic bile leaks after orthotopic liver transplantation are associated with hepatic artery disease. Gastrointest Endosc 2017;85(5):984–92.
58. Thuluvath PJ, Pfau PR, Kimmey MB, et al. Biliary complications after liver transplantation: the role of endoscopy. Endoscopy 2005;37(9):857–63.
59. Halme L, Hockerstedt K, Lautenschlager I. Cytomegalovirus infection and development of biliary complications after liver transplantation. Transplantation 2003; 75(11):1853–8.
60. Rerknimitr R, Sherman S, Fogel EL, et al. Biliary tract complications after orthotopic liver transplantation with choledochocholedochostomy anastomosis: endoscopic findings and results of therapy. Gastrointest Endosc 2002;55(2):224–31.
61. Spier BJ, Pfau PR, Lorenze KR, et al. Risk factors and outcomes in post-liver transplantation bile duct stones and casts: a case-control study. Liver Transpl 2008;14(10):1461–5.
62. Samstein B, Smith AR, Freise CE, et al. Complications and their resolution in recipients of deceased and living donor liver transplants: findings from the A2ALL cohort study. Am J Transplant 2016;16(2):594–602.
63. Freise CE, Gillespie BW, Koffron AJ, et al. Recipient morbidity after living and deceased donor liver transplantation: findings from the A2ALL retrospective cohort Study. Am J Transplant 2008;8(12):2569–79.
64. Elwir S, Thompson J, Amateau SK, et al. Endoscopic management of biliary leaks and strictures after living donor liver transplantation: optimizing techniques for successful management. Dig Dis Sci 2017;62(1):244–52.
65. Wadhawan M, Kumar A, Gupta S, et al. Post-transplant biliary complications: an analysis from a predominantly living donor liver transplant center. J Gastroenterol Hepatol 2013;28(6):1056–60.
66. Baker TB, Zimmerman MA, Goodrich NP, et al. Biliary reconstructive techniques and associated anatomic variants in adult living donor liver transplantations: the adult-to-adult living donor liver transplantation cohort study experience. Liver Transpl 2017;23(12):1519–30.
67. Rao HB, Prakash A, Sudhindran S, et al. Biliary strictures complicating living donor liver transplantation: problems, novel insights and solutions. World J Gastroenterol 2018;24(19):2061–72.

68. Tsujino T, Isayama H, Kogure H, et al. Endoscopic management of biliary strictures after living donor liver transplantation. Clin J Gastroenterol 2017;10(4):297–311.
69. Woo YS, Lee JK, Noh DH, et al. SpyGlass cholangioscopy-assisted guidewire placement for post-LDLT biliary strictures: a case series. Surg Endosc 2016;30(9):3897–903.
70. Hsieh T-H, Mekeel KL, Crowell MD, et al. Endoscopic treatment of anastomotic biliary strictures after living donor liver transplantation: outcomes after maximal stent therapy. Gastrointest Endosc 2013;77(1):47–54.
71. Kato H, Kawamoto H, Tsutsumi K, et al. Long-term outcomes of endoscopic management for biliary strictures after living donor liver transplantation with duct-to-duct reconstruction. Transpl Int 2009;22(9):914–21.
72. Chang JH, Lee IS, Choi JY, et al. Biliary stricture after adult right-lobe living-donor liver transplantation with duct-to-duct anastomosis: long-term outcome and its related factors after endoscopic treatment. Gut Liver 2010;4(2):226–33.
73. Santosh Kumar KY, Mathew JS, Balakrishnan D, et al. Intraductal transanastomotic stenting in duct-to-duct biliary reconstruction after living-donor liver transplantation: a randomized trial. J Am Coll Surg 2017;225(6):747–54.
74. Jang SI, Sung SY, Park H, et al. Salvage therapy using self-expandable metal stents for recalcitrant anastomotic strictures after living-donor liver transplantation. Therap Adv Gastroenterol 2017;10(3):297–309.
75. Kurita A, Kodama Y, Minami R, et al. Endoscopic stent placement above the intact sphincter of Oddi for biliary strictures after living donor liver transplantation. J Gastroenterol 2013;48(9):1097–104.
76. Tomoda T, Tsutsumi K, Kato H, et al. Outcomes of management for biliary stricture after living donor liver transplantation with hepaticojejunostomy using short-type double-balloon enteroscopy. Surg Endosc 2016;30(12):5338–44.

Endoscopic Management of Complex Biliary Stone Disease

Prashant Kedia, MD*, Paul R. Tarnasky, MD

KEYWORDS

• Choledocholithiasis • ERCP • Cholangioscopy • Lithotripsy • Laser lithotripsy • Bile duct stone

KEY POINTS

- The index success rate of endoscopic retrograde cholangiopancreatography (ERCP) for large or complex stones may range from 77% to 90%.
- Complex stone disease includes large size (>1 cm), irregular shape, multiple number, difficult location (impacted, above a biliary stricture, intrahepatic, or cystic duct), and altered enteral anatomy to reach the ampulla.
- Endoscopic papillary large balloon dilation (EPLBD) is now considered a first-line therapy for large bile duct stones.
- Cholangioscopy-guided lithotripsy is useful for very large stones greater than 2 cm and also stones that are located in challenging positions, such as above biliary strictures, or in intrahepatic/cystic duct segments.
- The clearance rate of complex stones at index ERCP is about 80%, but with subsequent procedures reaches an overall success of 99%.

Video content accompanies this article at http://www.giendo.theclinics.com/.

INTRODUCTION

Bile duct stones are a common problem encountered universally by gastroenterologists. The prevalence of gallstones (ie, cholelithiasis) worldwide ranges from 10% to 20% and causes clinical symptoms in 20% of cases.[1] Approximately 5% to 12% of patients undergoing cholecystectomy (CCX) are found to have concurrent choledocholithiasis.[2–4] Successful stone extraction from the bile duct depends on 2 general

Disclosure Statement: Dr P. Kedia is a consultant for Boston Scientific, Apollo Endosurgery, Endogastric Solutions, and Medtronic. Dr P.R. Tarnasky is a consultant for Boston Scientific.
Division of Gastroenterology, Department of Medicine, Methodist Dallas Medical Center, 221 West Colorado Boulevard, Pavillion II, Suite 630, Dallas, TX 75208, USA
* Corresponding author.
E-mail address: Prashant.kedia@dhat.com

Gastrointest Endoscopy Clin N Am 29 (2019) 257–275
https://doi.org/10.1016/j.giec.2018.11.004
giendo.theclinics.com
1052-5157/19/© 2018 Elsevier Inc. All rights reserved.

principles: one is to decrease the size of the stone and the other is to increase the size of the outflow tract or biliary orifice. Endoscopic retrograde cholangiopancreatography (ERCP) facilitates application of both of these therapeutic goals. The first ERCP was performed in 1968, followed by the first biliary sphincterotomy in 1974, which ushered in an entirely new era of therapeutic endoscopy.[5,6] ERCP has since become the first-line gold-standard intervention for management of bile duct stones. Nationwide registries show that over the past 20 years ERCP accounts for 96.1% of biliary interventions for choledocholithiasis compared with prior more commonly used techniques, such as percutaneous and surgical biliary therapies.[7] In 2009, more than 228,000 ERCPs were performed in the United States, accounting for almost 1 billion dollars in health care costs.[8] ERCP has become ubiquitous for the management of choledocholithiasis because it is highly effective, minimally invasive, and safe.[9–12] Although ERCP is highly effective for managing choledocholithiasis, a variety of reasons (**Box 1**) can make stone extraction challenging, including large size (>1 cm), irregular shape, multiple number, difficult location (impacted, above a biliary stricture, intrahepatic, or cystic duct), and altered enteral anatomy to reach the ampulla. For difficult or complex stones, ERCP with conventional techniques may fail to achieve index biliary clearance in 10% to 15% of cases.[2] Predictors of increasing the technical difficulty of stone extraction include a short distal common bile duct (CBD) arm (<36 mm), acute distal CBD angulation (>135°), very elevated direct bilirubin, and low CBD/stone ratio.[13,14] The goal of this article is to review the endoscopic management of complex bile duct stone disease.

LARGE BILE DUCT STONES

The most common challenge encountered during difficult stone extraction is large size.[13] The definition of a large stone is not standardized. Generally, 10 mm has been considered the lower limit for criteria of a large stone. However, some investigators have argued that large stones should be those that are greater than 15 mm and have a size greater than the diameter of the common bile duct.[15,16] Multiple studies have shown that larger stone size is inversely correlated with successful biliary clearance at ERCP.[13,14,17] Techniques for removing large bile duct stones include biliary sphincterotomy, mechanical lithotripsy (ML), papillary large balloon dilation, and cholangioscopy-guided lithotripsy (CGL).

ENDOSCOPIC BILIARY SPHINCTEROTOMY

The foundation for endoscopic biliary stone extraction is endoscopic biliary sphincterotomy (ES). The sphincter of Oddi is usually positioned in the second portion of the duodenum and is composed of a complex arrangement of muscle fibers. The sphincter choledochus surrounds the bile duct outflow tract, whereas the sphincter pancreaticus

Box 1
Reasons for difficult stone extraction

Large size (>1 cm)

Irregular shape

Multiple number

Difficult location (impacted, above a biliary stricture, intrahepatic, or cystic duct)

Surgically altered enteral anatomy

surrounds the pancreatic duct.[18] There are also sphincter ampullae fibers encompassing the entire structure. The sphincter of Oddi appears as a nodular prominence on the lateral wall of the duodenum and contains muscular fibers in both the intraduodenal and intramural portions of the pancreaticobiliary ducts. ES involves using an electrocautery alternating current to sever the intraduodenal portion of the sphincter choledochus and ampullae, thus leading to a shortening of the sphincter mechanism and reducing the resistance of the outflow tract. After ES, an extraction balloon can be inserted over a wire into the bile duct proximal to a stone, inflated, and then withdrawn to remove a stone from the bile duct. ES with balloon extraction has been shown to be highly effective for stones less than 10 mm (~100% success) but rapidly decline with stone size, approaching 12% success rate for stones greater than 15 mm.[17] Balloon sweep may fail especially when the stone/distal CBD ratio is greater than 1. Therefore, additional techniques have been developed to assist with large stone extraction.

MECHANICAL LITHOTRIPSY

One of the earliest and most commonly used techniques for large stone extraction is ML, which involves using a through-the-scope instrument to fragment large stones inside the bile duct. The first ML was performed in 1982.[19] Mechanical lithotripters are generally 3-layered devices: a metal basket, surrounded by a plastic casing within a metal sheath that can be passed over a wire. After insertion into the bile duct, lithotripters are opened and then used to grasp and crush large stones (Video 1). Modern mechanical lithotripters can withstand high-tensile forces and can fragment large stones in most cases. The benefits of ML are that it is widely available, it is relatively inexpensive, and it is effective. The success rates of complete stone clearance at index ERCP for ML range from 52% to 84%.[20–25] However, with multiple, successive procedures (up to 3 ERCPs), the cumulative success rate reaches 90% to 98%.[20,21,23] Failure rates with ML correlate with stone size and can be as high as 32% in stones greater than 28 mm in diameter.[22] Other predictors of ML failure included impacted stones and higher stone/duct ratio.[24,25] One of the limitations of ML is that it can be a cumbersome technique requiring time and skill to optimize stone capture within the basket wires. Techniques to improve efficacy of ML include opening the basket below the level of the stone and using short-term biliary stenting. A small randomized trial studying basket-opening position showed that opening a basket below the stone rather than above it improved capture rates from 33.3% to 94.1%.[26] Short-term biliary stenting before ML reduced procedure time and improved basket durability.[27] Adverse event (AE) rates associated with ML range from 1.4% to 14.3% and include cholangitis, pancreatitis, and bleeding.[20,23] One unique AE of ML is basket impaction, which can happen after stone capture. Usually with progressive cranking of the ML handle, either the stone will fragment or the basket will rupture at the distal (safety end) or proximal end of the device. In the event that the wires rupture at the proximal end of the instrument while the basket is encased around a stone, it may be impossible to pull the basket out of the bile duct now that the cranking handle is dysfunctional. This situation can be unnerving for the endoscopist, because failure to remove an impacted basket may require surgical intervention. Various techniques to remove impacted baskets have been described, including using a large external mechanical lithotriptor, laser or electrohydraulic lithotripter, second salvage basket, sphincterotomy extension, and grasping forceps.[28–31]

ENDOSCOPIC PAPILLARY BALLOON DILATION

Because of the limitations of ES and ML, endoscopic papillary balloon dilation (EPBD) was proposed as an alternative technique for biliary stone extraction in 1982.[32] EPBD involves inserting and inflating a dilation balloon (up to 10 mm in diameter) across the ampullary orifice to stretch the outflow tract. EPBD differs from ES in that it does not shorten the length of the sphincter mechanism, but instead dilates the entire length, thus reducing the resistance of the outflow tract. The rationale for using EPBD over ES was that it could allow for stone extraction and at the same time preserve the sphincter mechanism, reduce complications such as bleeding and perforation, and prevent long-term intestinal reflux into the bile duct.

Navigating the literature regarding EPBD is challenging because of its considerable inconsistencies, which may be due to variations in study populations, trial designs, and also operator techniques. Early large prospective series and randomized controlled trials were promising and showed equal efficacy of EPBD and ES for stone removal with inconsistent suggestion of higher rates of pancreatitis in the EPBD group traded off with higher bleeding rates in the ES groups.[33–36] However, a multicenter randomized controlled trial conducted in the United States comparing EPBD (without ES) with ES for less than 10 mm stone extraction demonstrated significantly higher rates of AE, 17.9 versus 3.3%, for the EPBD group.[37] These results included clearly higher rates of post-ERCP pancreatitis (15.4 vs 0.8%) with 2 associated mortalities. There was less bleeding intraoperatively in the EPBD group, although neither group had clinically significant delayed bleeding. The limitations of this trial included the variability of operator technique among the 24 included centers, balloon inflation time of 60 seconds, and exclusion of patients with coagulopathy. Subsequent multiple meta-analyses confirmed that EPBD was associated with significantly higher rates of pancreatitis, increased use of ML, and possibly even lower rates of clinical efficacy compared with ES.[38,39] The primary benefit of EPBD per these meta-analyses was a lower risk of bleeding compared with ES. The reason for increased incidence of pancreatitis with EPBD is speculated to be secondary to the dilation balloon applying concentric forces through the ampulla, some of which is felt by the sphincter pancreaticus. These forces may result in tissue edema and outflow obstruction at the pancreatic orifice, which is compounded by additional techniques such as ML for stone extraction, thus triggering pancreatitis. More recent studies postulate that longer dilation times, up to 5 minutes compared with 1 minute, actually reduce this side effect and pancreatitis.[40,41] However, EPBD quickly lost favor due to its risk profile and was relegated as a technique to be used in cases of coagulopathy whereby ES may not be safe.

ENDOSCOPIC PAPILLARY LARGE BALLOON DILATION

The concept of balloon dilation of the biliary orifice evolved over time and was resurrected with endoscopic papillary large balloon dilation (EPLBD), which was first described in 2003.[42] EPLBD entails performing a limited or incomplete ES and combining it with a large balloon dilation (>12 mm) in the same setting. The rationale supporting EPLBD is that clinical outcomes related to EPBD are suboptimal because of insufficient dilation of the bile duct (<10 mm), thus limiting successful stone extraction and also increasing the risk of complications, particularly pancreatitis. EPLBD improves on these shortcomings by further dilating the outflow tract to facilitate stone extraction and redirecting compressive forces of the balloon dilation itself and other stone removal measures (balloon sweep, ML) away from the sphincter pancreaticus because of performance of the prior ES.

Following the report of the initial success with EPLBD, multiple well-designed prospective randomized trials were performed comparing EPLBD with limited ES versus standard ES and conventional stone extraction techniques alone.[43–45] These studies uniformly revealed that EPLBD was equally efficacious as ES alone with possible decreased costs and rates of cholangitis. Some of these studies also showed that EPLBD reduced the need for ML compared with ES alone. Multiple systematic reviews have confirmed these conclusions, including lower risks of bleeding, perforation and overall complications with EPLBD, while maintaining equal therapeutic efficacy.[46–50] Use of ML significantly decreases with EPLBD, especially with stones greater than 15 mm. Some centers have also restudied the utility of performing EPLBD without a prior limited ES, because it may reduce procedure complexity, time, and possibly complications related to a combined inadvertent large ES with large balloon dilation.[51,52] Recent comparisons of large balloon dilation alone with EPLBD have shown similar stone clearance rates without significantly increased rates of complications.[53,54] Multivariate analysis in a cohort of almost 1000 EPLBD patients showed that cirrhosis, full-length ES, and stone size greater than 16 mm were risk factors for bleeding, whereas common bile duct stricture was an independent predictor for perforation.[55] Overwhelming results of these studies led to international consensus guidelines, including expert endoscopists from 8 different countries regarding the role and utility of EPLBD being published in 2016.[56] Some of the primary conclusions of this consensus report based on level 1 evidence were that (1) EPLBD can be used at a primary method of extraction of large or difficult bile duct stones identified on ERCP or cross-sectional imaging; (2) the initial and overall success rates of EPLBD with limited ES are comparable to ES alone; and (3) the AE rate of EPLBD with limited ES is lower than that of ES alone when removing large or difficult bile duct stones. Therefore, EPLBD is now considered a first-line therapy for large bile duct stones, but should be avoided in cases of CBD stricture. Nuances of the technique, including positioning of the balloon, duration and size of balloon dilation, and need for preceding ES, are still not certain. Although it seems reasonable to perform an ES to one-third or one-half of the intraduodenal segment and use the maximal bile duct diameter as a gauge for safe balloon size, EPLBD may be particularly useful in cases of altered anatomy and periampullary diverticulum where conventional ES may be difficult and/or dangerous.

CHOLANGIOSCOPY-GUIDED LITHOTRIPSY

In cases where fragmentation of the stone is needed for removal, CGL is an alternative option to ML. Cholangioscopy is the technique of inserting an endoscopic device into the bile duct to allow for direct visualization and treatment of intraductal lesions. Currently, there are 2 primary methods to perform cholangioscopy: one is direct peroral cholangioscopy (DPOC) with a forward viewing high-definition ultraslim endoscope and the other is a single-operator catheter-based digital cholangioscope (Spyglass DS; Boston Scientific, Natick, MA, USA) (SCBC) that inserts through the duodenoscope.

Effective DPOC requires endoscopic expertise to manipulate a forward viewing scope into the bile duct to maintain position and apply therapy without the help of an elevator mechanism. DPOC advantages include that it is a single endoscope system, it is cost-effective, it allows for improved imaging (ie, resolution, narrow-band imaging), and it uses large instrument channels (2 mm).[57] The primary limitations of DPOC are that it is technically difficult to perform in terms of obtaining and maintaining biliary access (due to the size and limitations of the endoscope), only allows for evaluation of the subhilar biliary system, and carries unique risks of AEs, such as air embolism. DPOC cannulation success is suboptimal because of the excessive looping of ultraslim scopes in the stomach and duodenum, and published experience is limited.[58,59] Various supportive maneuvers using anchoring balloons, overtubes, and snares have been studied to improve successful DPOC biliary access and intervention.[60–63] One unique and dreaded AE of DPOC is gaseous embolism due to either air or carbon dioxide insufflation within the biliary tree itself.[64,65]

The other more widely used method of intraductal visualization is SCBC. This concept was originally developed as a multioperator "mother-baby" system in which a baby endoscope was inserted through a standard duodenoscope and operated by 2 separate endoscopists.[66] This procedure was a technically challenging procedure that was not widely performed. SCBC was slow to gain recognition until development of single operator systems that allowed for a 10-French catheter that contained a channel for passage of a fiber-optic probe and utilization of a 1.2-mm working channel with associated irrigation port and to be inserted into the duodenoscope directly and controlled with 4-way steering by a single endoscopist (Spyglass DVS; Boston Scientific). Although this system was a step forward, it was fragile, difficult to use, and did not provide optimal resolution, thus tempering its popularity. The second generation of this device has incorporated these features in a 10-French digital cholangioscope with high-resolution imaging, easy setup, and continued 4-way steering with a 1.2-mm working channel. This newest iteration has gained widespread popularity because of its ease of use and high-resolution images and is being used more frequently for assessment and treatment of intraductal lesions. The benefits of SCBC are that it allows for high cannulation and biliary intervention success through catheter stability possibly even in the hands of less experienced users, whereas its limitations may include availability and cost.

CGL involves applying direct energy inside the bile duct to fragment stone burden. There are 2 energy modalities, electrohydraulic lithotripsy (EHL) and pulsed laser lithotripsy (LL), which can be delivered through either the DPOC or the SCBC systems. EHL is a coaxial bipolar device that generates underwater sparks and subsequent hydraulic pressure waves, which induce stone fragmentation. Thus, EHL requires a fluid-based medium and for the catheter tip to be about 2 mm from the target to be effective. During LL, a flexible quartz fiber is advanced to deliver pulsed laser energy at a specific wavelength that generates a mechanical shockwave adjacent to the stone (see Video 1).[67] As with EHL, physical contact of the laser tip with the stone is not required.

Multiple series regarding SCBC outcomes have reported index procedure biliary stone clearance rates of 71% to 90% with overall clearance rates after multiple procedures reaching up to 100%.[68–70] However, much of the published literature on CGL with SCBC is based on the first-generation system, which is technologically outdated. A large multicenter international series involving 407 patients using the digital cholangioscope system was recently reported.[71] This study showed that EHL was used 3 times more often than LL as the energy modality, but resulted in longer procedure times (74 vs 50 minutes). Index and overall biliary clearance was achieved in 77.4% (74.5% EHL and 86.1% LL) and 97.3% (96.7% EHL and 99% LL) of patients. The severe and overall AE rate was 0.5% and 3.7%. Outcomes regarding DPOC with large stone extraction are limited to small case series with limited experience. One meta-analysis reviewing DPOC CGL studies, none of which contained more than 40 subjects, showed success rates anywhere from 78% to 100%, although not all studies included or reported large stone size.[72] The overall stone clearance rate and AE rate across all forms of cholangioscopy were 88% and 7%, respectively.

CGL seems to be particularly useful in very large stones greater than 2 cm, where ML is likely to fail, and also in stones that are located in challenging positions for extraction, such as Mirizzi syndrome (MS), above biliary strictures, or in intrahepatic/cystic duct segments (see later discussion). CGL has rapidly gained popularity because it allows the endoscopist to directly visualize the target and precisely deliver therapy with the improved high-resolution imaging capabilities of the new-generation SCBC system. In experienced hands, CGL can fragment stones to the necessary size required for extraction and avoid bile duct wall damage, unlike the cruder "trial-and-error" technique of ML. The possible limitation of CGL, particularly SCBC compared with other extraction techniques, is the cost of the device, although this may be offset if CGL can prove itself to be a more efficient procedure compared with conventional ERCP stone removal techniques. One cost-analysis report showed that SCBC CGL was significantly less costly than conventional ERCP extraction techniques.[73]

When performing CGL, it is important to consider practices to optimize outcomes. One is to minimize the amount of contrast injected during cholangiography because this obscures visualization. Aspiration through the cholangioscope can be useful to clear contrast during the procedure. Flushing water through the instrument port may also be helpful if debris occludes the camera. Passage of an EHL or LL catheter through the device can be challenging occasionally because of the distal angulation of the duodenoscope during ERCP. This problem can be overcome by reducing the angle of the duodenoscope using the large dial. Other troubleshooting options for catheter passage are to insert the cholangioscope deeper into the bile duct, which relieves pressure at the elevator mechanism, or pass the catheter through the cholangioscope before inserting the cholangioscope into the bile duct. For anticipated longer or challenging procedures where significant intraductal irrigation may be needed during lithotripsy of large stone burden, it is prudent to intubate the patient for airway protection. Antibiotic prophylaxis is recommended for all cases of CGL because there is an increased reported rate of cholangitis with this technique compared with standard ERCP.[74]

BILIARY STENTING

Currently, the role for nonendoscopic (ie, surgical or percutaneous) interventions for complex bile duct stones is minimal given the overall success of endoscopic therapy. The clearance rate of complex stones at index ERCP is about 80%, but with subsequent procedures reaches an overall success of 99%.[75] Endoscopists should be prudent to acknowledge the limitations of index procedures and not overextend their efforts to a point that may cause harm to the patient without significant clinical benefit. If it is deemed that complete stone extraction cannot be achieved in one setting, especially in elderly or medically precarious patients, then establishing drainage with placement of a biliary stent with intended repeat ERCP is a very reasonable option. This strategy assures flow of bile along with mechanical friction of the stents with stones, which facilitates drainage, prevents cholangitis, and increases chances of successful clearance on subsequent procedures. The addition of choleretic agents between procedures may be useful for additional stone dissolution. Combination treatment of biliary stenting with ursodeoxycholic acid (UDCA) and terpene resulted in 92% biliary clearance at 6 months with a mean of 1.7 ERCPs.[76] One study showed a higher rate of stone clearance for plastic stenting combined with UDCA and terpene compared with stenting alone.[77] Other adjuncts to assist with stone dissolution with biliary stenting include extracorporeal shockwave lithotripsy (ESWL), which directs high-intensity shockwaves from outside the body at various specific targets. ESWL studies showed stone clearance rates up to 90%, and an increased clearance of stone burden with subsequent procedures with the addition of ESWL to ERCP.[78–80] The limitations of ESWL are that it may not be widely available, may have difficulty targeting bile duct stones that are radiolucent, and is less effective in obese patients. The concept of longer-term stent indwell time up to 6 months using fully covered self-expanding metal stents has also been proposed and shown to have reasonable success in small trials.[81,82] The cost-effectiveness of this strategy requires further evaluation, although logically there may be a role for metal stenting with longer indwell times in cases of difficult stone extraction due to benign distal biliary strictures. Thus, it is not necessary for the endoscopist to "be a hero" in every stone case. Considering a treat and repeat strategy for very difficult stones especially in medically suboptimal candidates has been shown to be effective and practical.

CHOLEDOCHOLITHIASIS IN DIFFICULT LOCATIONS

Treatment of CDL can be challenging when it is difficult to achieve close proximity to stones with therapeutic devices or when it is not possible to gain sufficient ductal access proximal to impacted stones. Occasionally, access to "capture" stones is difficult when small stones are floating within a very dilated bile duct. More common reasons for difficult direct stone access are when stones are proximally located, for example, within intrahepatic ducts, proximal to bile duct strictures, or above narrowed acute duct angulations.

Compared with all other CDL scenarios, hepatolithiasis (HL) presents the greatest challenges. HL is about 20-fold more common in East Asia when compared with the low prevalence (1%) observed in Western countries.[83–85] Recurrent pyogenic cholangitis represents a distinct clinical subset of HL characterized by repeated bacterial and parasitic infections of the biliary tract.[86] In addition to being difficult to offer primary therapy, HL is associated with refractory and recurrent stones, liver abscess, cirrhosis, and risk for cholangiocarcinoma.[83]

Most of the data regarding therapy of HL are derived from surgical experience from Southeast Asia. Residual HL is strongly related to the risk for biliary complications after surgical or percutaneous transhepatic cholangioscopy-directed lithotripsy.[87] The frequency of therapeutic ERCP increased from almost never to 23% of cases in a 40-year Japanese survey, but residual and recurrent stones were more common (**Fig. 1**).[88] Nevertheless, partial hepatectomy is generally recommended when the stone burden is localized to one lobe, there are associated strictures, and/or lobar atrophy is present.[87] In the absence of lobar atrophy, known intrahepatic cholangiocarcinoma, and intrahepatic strictures, either percutaneous or endoscopic cholangioscopy-

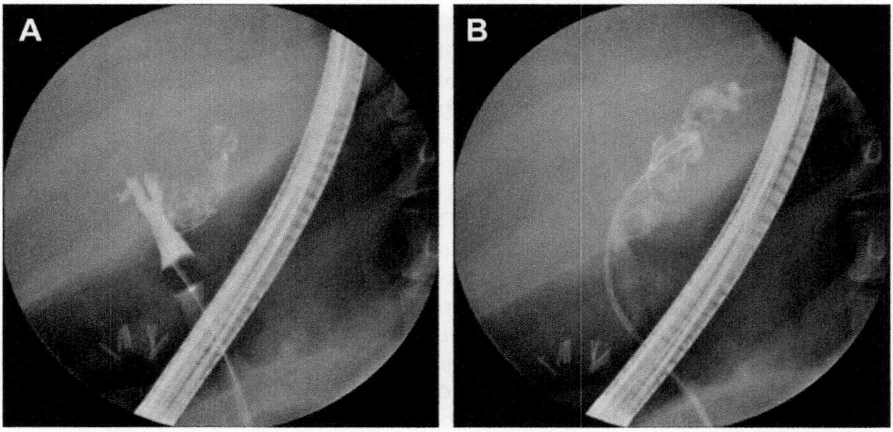

Fig. 1. (*A*) Occlusion cholangiogram revealing HL of the left intrahepatic system. (*B*) Wire access of the left intrahepatic system to attempt endoscopic therapy.

directed therapy has been suggested as reasonable.[89] However, others recommend segmental resection to prevent intrahepatic cholangiocarcinoma even if stone clearance can be achieved.[90] Laparoscopic bile duct exploration with choledochoscopy and LL is proposed for patients with bilateral stones or cirrhosis.[91] Although surgical therapy is most often definitive, additional treatment is occasionally still required to treat residual HL.[92,93] Adding to the complexity, HL is often characterized by intrahepatic bile duct strictures that create access challenges and are a major cause for treatment failure.[87]

HL in the West is more commonly seen in immigrants from Asia, but also in conditions whereby strictures are unrelated to infections. Stones can migrate from the gallbladder into intrahepatic ducts, form primarily in the liver, for example, hemolytic disorders, or be associated with stasis due to strictures.[84] Operative bile duct injuries, foreign bodies (eg, surgical clips or sutures), primary sclerosing cholangitis, or any cause for hepatic artery ischemia may result in HL.

Impacted cystic duct stones causing compression or obstruction of the extrahepatic bile duct are known as MS. Classifications of MS depend on whether or not there is an associated cholecystobiliary fistula. Type I MS involves external compression of the bile duct; all other types (II–V) are associated with fistulization.[94] Although considered a rare event (<6% of CCX), MS may now be more commonly encountered due to more frequent laparoscopic partial cholecystectomies.[94]

A scoring system based on clinical, laboratory, and imaging criteria may be helpful to predict MS, but it is generally not difficult to diagnose when considered in the appropriate setting.[95] The classic presentation includes history of biliary colic, jaundice, and a "meniscus sign" on imaging. For example, Magnetic resonance cholangiopancreatography (MRCP) will typically reveal a dilated bile duct proximal to a curvilinear filling defect at the cystic duct takeoff. It is not uncommon at tertiary centers that a patient referred for a "difficult bile duct stone" is found to have MS. The typical scenario is whereby a patient with jaundice undergoes an ERCP, and a filling defect is seen on cholangiography, but the stone "cannot be captured" and/or the stone "cannot be extracted" due to "a stricture" (**Fig. 2**). In such cases, the typical imaging findings are not recognized so the diagnosis of MS is not considered. Still,

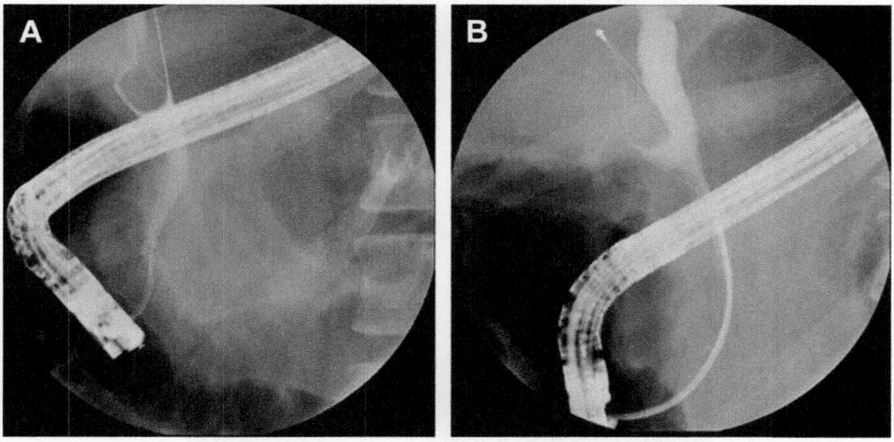

Fig. 2. (*A*) Large cystic duct stone overlaying the bile duct with wire in the common bile duct. (*B*) Capture of the cystic duct stone with a mechanical basket after cystic duct access achieved.

about half of MS cases are diagnosed at the time of CCX.[96,97] It is important to recognize and define the type of MS preoperatively whenever possible for several reasons. First, there is an increased risk of operative bile duct injuries and need for conversion from laparoscopic to open CCX in the setting of MS.[94] Second, CCX should be initially an open procedure for MS with fistulization, whereas a laparoscopic approach is generally deemed safe in the setting of type I MS.[89] Last, preoperative ERCP should be considered when MS is suspected.

Normally, ERCP is recommended before CCX only when there is cholangitis, biliary pancreatitis with an impacted gallstone, and/or if otherwise a high likelihood for CDL and ERCP expertise is low.[98] When MS is suspected, however, preoperative ERCP can be endorsed to both confirm the diagnosis and to provide biliary drainage.[89] Laparoscopic CCX has even been shown to be safe in the setting of type II MS when combined with preoperative ERCP and endotherapy that involves drainage.[99] It is also easier to treat CDL when ductal access proximal to stones is not limited. If there is a short cystic duct remnant after CCX, there may not be enough room proximal to the stone or stones to allow a retrieval balloon and/or basket (**Fig. 3**).

CGL is commonly required to fracture stones when stones are proximal to strictures or when there is minimal ductal length proximal to stones as can occur with HL or MS. From a large multicenter retrospective study of the management of patients with difficult CDL (N = 407), the indications for cholangioscopy included impacted extrahepatic stones (38%), nonimpacted cystic duct stones (12%), HL (18%), and MS (9%).[71] Binmoeller and colleagues[100] described the first series of CGL in 1993. It has been stated that CGL may be too difficult for type I MS.[101] However, CGL of cystic duct stones ± MS by experts is universally successful, most often in a single setting.[102]

As noted above, bile duct stenting may be required urgently for treatment of cholangitis, to ensure drainage after endotherapy for CDL, or even as primary therapy.[89] It also is important to consider the potential need for bile duct stenting to treat strictures and/or leaks.

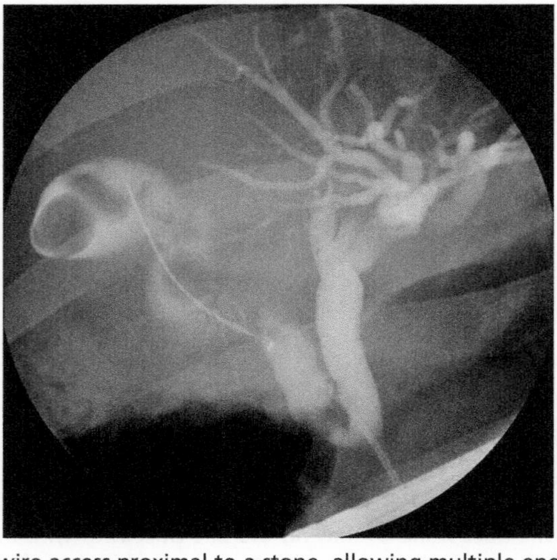

Fig. 3. Cystic duct wire access proximal to a stone, allowing multiple endoscopic modalities of therapy.

CHOLEDOCHOLITHIASIS IN SURGICALLY ALTERED ANATOMY

Encountering benign biliary stone disease in surgically altered enteral anatomy is not infrequent and poses unique challenges for endoscopists. Because of the difficulty in obtaining ampullary access in anatomies such as Roux-en-Y gastric bypass (RYGB), Billroth 2, Whipple procedure, and Roux-en-Y hepaticojejunostomy (HJ), conventional ERCP with standard duodenoscopes may be less effective or not possible at all. Challenges of endoscopic biliary intervention in altered anatomy can include the need for specialized deep enteroscope access, lower ampullary cannulation success, and the restricted use of standard ERCP devices through deep enteroscopes. A prerequisite to maximize success in any of these procedures is to first understand the anatomy that is to be negotiated, using patient history, operative reports, and imaging. Generally, with post-Whipple anatomy the bilioenteric anastomosis can be cannulated with a pediatric colonoscope in 84% of cases.[103] In Billroth 2 anatomy, however, cannulation rates with a duodenoscope range anywhere from 49% to 92% with the added challenge of approaching the ampulla with inverted orientation.[104] Often, straight cannulating catheters or rotating sphincterotomes are required to access the bile duct. Performing a sphincterotomy may also be challenging in this orientation; thus, EPLBD can be a useful technique for Billroth 2 with efficacious and safe outcomes.[104] The other dreaded AE of ERCP in Billroth 2 is bowel perforation at the gastrojejunal anastomosis, which has been found to range from 3.0% to 3.6% in a large systemic review.[105] In anatomies such as HJ and RYGB, deep enteroscopy-assisted ERCP is necessary to reach the ampulla, and that with only a 63% success rate and as high as a 12.4% AE rate.[106] Thus in Roux-en-Y reconstructions, alternative methods for biliary therapy, such as percutaneous biliary access or laparoscopy-assisted ERCP (LA-ERCP), through a surgically fashioned gastrostomy tract have become standards of care due to higher success rates.[107,108] However, both options have significant drawbacks. Percutaneous therapy has been shown to have procedure-related AE rates of 10% with long-term catheter-related complications up to 25%.[108,109] LA-ERCP is fraught with limitations of being an invasive and expensive procedure, associated with significant risk, and logistically challenging due to the need to coordinate multiple teams. Case series have reported AE rates up to 36% with conversion to open gastrostomy in 13% of patients.[107,110,111] Therefore, efforts to develop and perform minimally invasive, completely endoscopic procedures using endoscopic ultrasound (EUS) guidance for biliary access have been put forth. One novel technique that has been conceived is EUS-directed transgastric ERCP (EDGE) procedure, which temporarily reverses an RYGB by creating a gastrogastric or jejunogastric fistula with a lumen-apposing metal stent, through which a conventional ERCP with a standard duodenoscope can be performed.[112] EDGE has been shown to be noninferior to LA-ERCP in terms of efficacy and safety and provide added benefits of significantly shorter procedure time and hospital stays.[113] One theoretic concern regarding EDGE is the possibility of weight regain with temporary reversal of the RYGB. However, current series have shown the opposite that patients usually lose weight following EDGE.[113,114] In HJ anatomy, an alternate technique known as EUS-guided hepaticoenterostomy (EUS-HE) has also been described. EUS-HE involves using EUS to locate and access left-sided intrahepatic ducts from the stomach or jejunum and create a hepaticoenterostomy usually with a 10-mm fully covered metal stent. Through this fistula, endoscopically directed treatment of benign stone disease can be performed in an antegrade fashion with ultraslim endoscopes or cholangioscopes. Early experiences with EUS-HE have been reported with reasonable success and AE rates.[115,116] Although EUS-guided biliary access techniques are still somewhat early

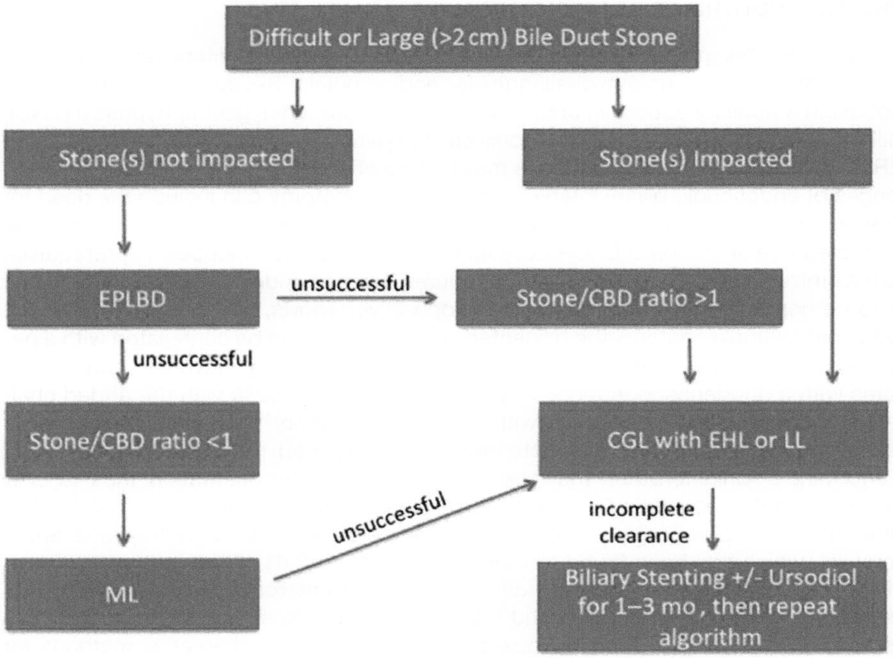

Fig. 4. Proposed algorithm for endoscopic management of difficult bile duct stones.

in their maturity and are only performed at expert centers, a comparative meta-analysis showed better clinical outcomes than percutaneous biliary drainage and with fewer AEs and repeat interventions.[117] The ability to avoid a transcutaneous catheter and its associated complications is also likely to improve the quality of life of patients. EUS-guided therapies are promising area of endoscopic innovation that requires further study to determine its role in the choledocholithiasis treatment algorithm for altered anatomy patients.

SUMMARY

Endoscopic intervention is now the gold standard for management of CDL and has largely replaced percutaneous and surgical interventions. Although effective, the index success rate of ERCP for large or complex stones may range from 77% to 90%. Thus, advanced techniques for stone removal, including ML, ESLBD, CGL, and EUS-guided techniques, and serial biliary stenting have been developed and implemented with excellent success rates. Because of a wide variety of endoscopic technical options available, practices vary greatly around the world. A proposed clinical algorithm based on the authors' own clinical experience is shown in **Fig. 4**. Further studies are needed to optimize an algorithm by which these techniques maximize technical and clinical success while minimizing AE and costs.

SUPPLEMENTARY DATA

Supplementary data related to this article can be found online at https://doi.org/10.1016/j.giec.2018.11.004.

REFERENCES

1. Lammert F, Gurusamy K, Ko CW, et al. Gallstones. Nat Rev Dis Primers 2016;2: 16024.
2. Trikudanathan G, Arain MA, Attam R, et al. Advances in the endoscopic management of common bile duct stones. Nat Rev Gastroenterol Hepatol 2014; 11(9):535–44.
3. Collins C, Maguire D, Ireland A, et al. A prospective study of common bile duct calculi in patients undergoing laparoscopic cholecystectomy: natural history of choledocholithiasis revisited. Ann Surg 2004;239(1):28–33.
4. Koo KP, Traverso LW. Do preoperative indicators predict the presence of common bile duct stones during laparoscopic cholecystectomy? Am J Surg 1996; 171(5):495–9.
5. McCune WS, Shorb PE, Moscovitz H. Endoscopic cannulation of the ampulla of vater: a preliminary report. Gastrointest Endosc 1988;34(3):278–80.
6. Kawai K, Akasaka Y, Murakami K, et al. Endoscopic sphincterotomy of the ampulla of Vater. Gastrointest Endosc 1974;20(4):148–51.
7. Huang RJ, Thosani NC, Barakat MT, et al. Evolution in the utilization of biliary interventions in the United States: results of a nationwide longitudinal study from 1998 to 2013. Gastrointest Endosc 2017;86(2):319–26.e5.
8. Peery A, Dellon E, Lund J. Burden of gastrointestinal disease in the United States: 2012 update. Gastroenterology 2012;143(5):1179–87.
9. Carr-Locke DL. Therapeutic role of ERCP in the management of suspected common bile duct stones. Gastrointest Endosc 2002;56(6):S170–4.
10. Chathadi KV, Chandrasekhara V, Acosta RD, et al. The role of ERCP in benign diseases of the biliary tract. Gastrointest Endosc 2015;81(4):795–803.
11. Chandrasekhara V, Khashab MA, Muthusamy VR, et al. Adverse events associated with ERCP. Gastrointest Endosc 2017;85(1):32–47.
12. Seitz U, Bapaye A, Bohnacker S, et al. Advances in therapeutic endoscopic treatment of common bile duct stones. World J Surg 1998;22:1133–44.
13. Kim HJ, Choi HS, Park JH, et al. Factors influencing the technical difficulty of endoscopic clearance of bile duct stones. Gastrointest Endosc 2007;66(6): 1154–60.
14. Üsküdar O, Parlak E, Dişibeyaz S, et al. Major predictors for difficult common bile duct stone. Turk J Gastroenterol 2013;24(5):423–9.
15. Doshi B, Yasuda I, Ryozawa S, et al. Current endoscopic strategies for managing large bile duct stones. Dig Endosc 2018;30(30):59–66.
16. Sharma SS, Jain P. Should we redefine large common bile duct stone? World J Gastroenterol 2008;14(4):651–2.
17. Lauri A, Horton RC, Davidson BR, et al. Endoscopic extraction of bile duct stones: management related to stone size. Gut 1993;34(12):1718–21.
18. Ding J, Li F, Zhu H-Y, et al. Endoscopic treatment of difficult extrahepatic bile duct stones, EPBD or EST: an anatomic view. World J Gastrointest Endosc 2015;7(3):274–7.
19. Demling L, Seuberth KRJ. A mechical lithotriptor. Endoscopy 1982;14(3):100–1.
20. Hintze RE, Adler AVW. Outcome of mechanical lithotripsy of bile duct stones in an unselected series of 704 patients. Hepatogastroenterology 1996;43(9): 473–6.
21. Siegel JH, Ben-Zvi JS, Pullano WE. Mechanical lithotripsy of common duct stones. Gastrointest Endosc 1990;36(4):351–6.

22. Cipolletta L, Costamagna G, Bianco MA, et al. Endoscopic mechanical lithotripsy of difficult common bile duct stones. Br J Surg 1997;84(10):1407–9.
23. Chang WH, Chu CH, Wang TE, et al. Outcome of simple use of mechanical lithotripsy of difficult common bile duct stones. World J Gastroenterol 2005;11(4):593–6.
24. Garg PK, Tandon RK, Ahuja V, et al. Predictors of unsuccessful mechanical lithotripsy and endoscopic clearance of large bile duct stones. Gastrointest Endosc 2004;59(6):601–5.
25. Lee SH, Park JK, Yoon WJ, et al. How to predict the outcome of endoscopic mechanical lithotripsy in patients with difficult bile duct stones? Scand J Gastroenterol 2007;42(8):1006–10.
26. Shi D, Yu C-G. Comparison of two capture methods for endoscopic removal of large common bile duct stones. J Laparoendosc Adv Surg Tech A 2014;24(7):457–61.
27. Sharma SS, Jhajharia AMS. Short-term biliary stenting before mechanical lithotripsy for difficult bile duct stones. Indian J Gastroenterol 2014;33(3):237–40.
28. Liu W, Zhang LP, Xu M, et al. "Post-cut": an endoscopic technique for managing impacted biliary stone within an entrapped extraction basket. Arab J Gastroenterol 2018;19(1):37–41.
29. Fenner J, Croglio MP, Tzimas D, et al. Successful treatment of an impacted lithotripter basket in the common bile duct with intracorporeal electrohydraulic lithotripsy. Endoscopy 2018;50(4):447–8.
30. Benatta MA, Desjeux A, Barthet M, et al. Case Report impacted and fractured biliary basket : a second basket rescue technique. Case Rep Med 2016;1–2. https://doi.org/10.1155/2016/6210646.
31. Wong JC, Wong MY, Lam KL, et al. Second-generation peroral cholangioscopy and holmium:YAG laser lithotripsy for rescue of impacted biliary stone extraction basket. Gastrointest Endosc 2016;83(4):837–8.
32. Staritz M, Ewe KM, zum BK. Endoscopic papillary dilation, a possible alternative to endoscopic papillotomy. Lancet 1982;1(8284):1306–7.
33. Fujita N, Maguchi H, Komatsu Y, et al. Endoscopic sphincterotomy and endoscopic papillary balloon dilatation for bile duct stones: a prospective randomized controlled multicenter trial. Gastrointest Endosc 2003;57(2):151–5.
34. Bergman JJ, Rauws EAJ, Fockens P, et al. Randomised trial of endoscopic balloon dilation versus endoscopic sphincterotomy for removal of bileduct stones. Lancet 1997;349(9059):1124–9.
35. Komatsu Y, Kawabe T, Toda N, et al. Endoscopic papillary balloon dilation for the management of common bile duct stones: experience of 226 cases. Endoscopy 1998;30(1):12–7.
36. Mathuna PM, White P, Clarke E, et al. Endoscopic balloon sphincteroplasty (papillary dilation) for bile duct stones: efficacy, safety, and follow-up in 100 patients. Gastrointest Endosc 1995;42(5):468–74.
37. Disario JA, Freeman ML, Bjorkman DJ, et al. Endoscopic balloon dilation compared with sphincterotomy for extraction of bile duct stones. Gastroenterology 2004;127(5):1291–9.
38. Baron TH, Harewood GC. Endoscopic balloon dilation of the biliary sphincter compared to endoscopic biliary sphincterotomy for removal of common bile duct stones during ERCP: a metaanalysis of randomized, controlled trials. Am J Gastroenterol 2004;99(8):1455–60.

39. Weinberg BM, Shindy W, Lo S. Endoscopic balloon sphincter dilation (sphincteroplasty) versus sphincterotomy for common bile duct stones. Cochrane Database Syst Rev 2006;(4). https://doi.org/10.1002/14651858.CD004890.pub2.
40. Liao WC, Lee CT, Chang CY, et al. Randomized trial of 1-minute versus 5-minute endoscopic balloon dilation for extraction of bile duct stones. Gastrointest Endosc 2010;72(6):1154–62.
41. Liao WC, Tu YK, Wu MS, et al. Balloon dilation with adequate duration is safer than sphincterotomy for extracting bile duct stones: a systematic review and meta-analyses. Clin Gastroenterol Hepatol 2012;10(10):1101–9.
42. Ersoz G, Tekesin O, Ozutemiz AO. Biliary sphincterotomy plus dilation with a large balloon for bile duct stones that are difficult to extract. Gastrointest Endosc 2003;57(2):156–9.
43. Heo JH, Kang DH, Jung HJ, et al. Endoscopic sphincterotomy plus large-balloon dilation versus endoscopic sphincterotomy for removal of bile-duct stones. Gastrointest Endosc 2007;66(4):720–6.
44. Stefanidis G, Viazis N, Pleskow D, et al. Large balloon dilation vs. mechanical lithotripsy for the management of large bile duct stones: a prospective randomized study. Am J Gastroenterol 2011;106(2):278–85.
45. Teoh AYB, Cheung FKY, Hu B, et al. Randomized trial of endoscopic sphincterotomy with balloon dilation versus endoscopic sphincterotomy alone for removal of bile duct stones. Gastroenterology 2013;144(2):341–5.
46. Feng Y, Zhu H, Chen X, et al. Comparison of endoscopic papillary large balloon dilation and endoscopic sphincterotomy for retrieval of choledocholithiasis: a meta-analysis of randomized controlled trials. J Gastroenterol 2012;47(6):655–63.
47. Yang XM, Hu B. Endoscopic sphincterotomy plus large-balloon dilation vs endoscopic sphincterotomy for choledocholithiasis: a meta-analysis. World J Gastroenterol 2013;19(48):9453–60.
48. Liu Y, Su P, Lin Y, et al. Endoscopic sphincterotomy plus balloon dilation versus endoscopic sphincterotomy for choledocholithiasis: a meta-analysis. J Gastroenterol Hepatol 2013;28(6):937–45.
49. Sakai Y, Tsuyuguchi T, Kawaguchi Y, et al. Endoscopic papillary large balloon dilation for removal of bile duct stones. World J Gastroenterol 2014;20(45):17148–54.
50. Xu L, Kyaw MH, Tse YK, et al. Endoscopic sphincterotomy with large balloon dilation versus endoscopic sphincterotomy for bile duct stones: a systematic review and meta-analysis. Biomed Res Int 2015;2015:673103.
51. Jeong S, Ki SH, Lee DH, et al. Endoscopic large-balloon sphincteroplasty without preceding sphincterotomy for the removal of large bile duct stones: a preliminary study. Gastrointest Endosc 2009;70(5):915–22.
52. Omuta S, Maetani I, Saito M, et al. Is endoscopic papillary large balloon dilatation without endoscopic sphincterotomy effective? World J Gastroenterol 2015;21(23):7289–96.
53. Hwang JC, Kim JH, Lim SG, et al. Endoscopic large-balloon dilation alone versus endoscopic sphincterotomy plus large-balloon dilation for the treatment of large bile duct stones. BMC Gastroenterol 2013;13(1). https://doi.org/10.1186/1471-230X-13-15.
54. Cheon YK, Lee TY, Kim SN, et al. Impact of endoscopic papillary large-balloon dilation on sphincter of Oddi function: a prospective randomized study. Gastrointest Endosc 2017;85(4):782–90.

55. Park SJ, Kim JH, Hwang JC, et al. Factors predictive of adverse events following endoscopic papillary large balloon dilation: results from a multicenter series. Dig Dis Sci 2013;58(4):1100–9.
56. Kim TH, Kim JH, Seo DW, et al. International consensus guidelines for endoscopic papillary large-balloon dilation. Gastrointest Endosc 2016;83(1):37–47.
57. Parsi MA. Biliary papillomatosis: diagnosis with direct peroral cholangioscopy. Gastrointest Endosc 2015;81(1):231–2.
58. Terheggen G, Neuhaus H. New options of cholangioscopy. Gastroenterol Clin North Am 2010;39(4):827–44.
59. Moon JH, Ko BM, Choi HJ, et al. Direct peroral cholangioscopy using an ultraslim upper endoscope for the treatment of retained bile duct stones. Am J Gastroenterol 2009;104(11):2729–33.
60. Article O, Li J, Guo S, et al. A new hybrid anchoring balloon for direct peroral cholangioscopy using an ultraslim upper endoscope. Dig Endosc 2018;30(3): 364–71.
61. Huang YH, Chang H, Yao W, et al. A snare-assisted peroral direct choledochoscopy and pancreatoscopy using an ultra-slim upper endoscope: a case series study. Dig Liver Dis 2017;49(6):657–63.
62. Choi HJ, Moon JH, Ko BM, et al. Overtube-balloon-assisted direct per- oral cholangioscopy by using an ultra-slim upper endoscope (with videos). Gastrointest Endosc 2009;69(4):935–40.
63. Moon JH, Ko BM, Choi HJ, et al. Intraductal balloon-guided direct peroral cholangioscopy with an ultraslim upper endoscope (with videos). Gastrointest Endosc 2009;70(2):297–302.
64. Efthymiou M, Raftopoulos S, Chirinos JA, et al. Air embolism complicated by left hemiparesis after direct cholangioscopy with an intraductal balloon anchoring system. Gastrointest Endosc 2012;75(1):221–3.
65. Kondo H, Naitoh I, Nakazawa T, et al. Development of fatal systemic gas embolism during direct peroral cholangioscopy under carbon dioxide insufflation. Endoscopy 2016;48:E215–6.
66. Bogardus ST, Hanan I, Ruchim M, et al. "Mother-baby" biliary endoscopy: the University of Chicago experience. Am J Gastroenterol 1996;91(1):105–10.
67. Shah RJ. Innovations in intraductal endoscopy. cholangioscopy and pancreatoscopy. Gastrointest Endosc Clin N Am 2015;25(4):779–92.
68. Maydeo A, Kwek BEA, Bhandari S, et al. Single-operator cholangioscopy-guided laser lithotripsy in patients with difficult biliary and pancreatic ductal stones (with videos). Gastrointest Endosc 2011;74(6):1308–14.
69. Fishman DS, Tarnasky PR, Patel SN, et al. Management of pancreaticobiliary disease using a new intra-ductal endoscope: the Texas experience. World J Gastroenterol 2009;15(11):1353–8.
70. Chen YK, Parsi MA, Binmoeller KF, et al. Single-operator cholangioscopy in patients requiring evaluation of bile duct disease or therapy of biliary stones (with videos). Gastrointest Endosc 2011;74(4):805–14.
71. Brewer Gutierrez OI, Bekkali NLH, Raijman I, et al. Efficacy and safety of digital single-operator cholangioscopy for difficult biliary stones. Clin Gastroenterol Hepatol 2018;16(6):918–26.e1.
72. Korrapati P, Ciolino J, Wani S, et al. The efficacy of peroral cholangioscopy for difficult bile duct stones and indeterminate strictures: a systematic review and meta-analysis. Endosc Int Open 2016;04(03):E263–75.
73. Deprez PH, Garces Duran R, Moreels T, et al. The economic impact of using single-operator cholangioscopy for the treatment of difficult bile duct stones

and diagnosis of indeterminate bile duct strictures. Endoscopy 2018;50(2):109–18.
74. Sethi A, Chen YK, Austin GL, et al. ERCP with cholangiopancreatoscopy may be associated with higher rates of complications than ERCP alone: a single-center experience. Gastrointest Endosc 2011;73(2):251–6.
75. Brown NG, Camilo J, Nordstrom E, et al. Advanced ERCP techniques for the extraction of complex biliary stones: a single referral center's 12-year experience. Scand J Gastroenterol 2018;53(5):626–31.
76. Han J, Moon JH, Koo HC, et al. Effect of biliary stenting combined with ursodeoxycholic acid and terpene treatment on retained common bile duct stones in elderly patients: a multicenter study. Am J Gastroenterol 2009;104(10):2418–21.
77. Lee TH, Han JH, Kim HJ, et al. Is the addition of choleretic agents in multiple double-pigtail biliary stents effective for difficult common bile duct stones in elderly patients? A prospective, multicenter study. Gastrointest Endosc 2011;74(1):96–102.
78. Tao T, Zhang M, Zhang Q-J, et al. Outcome of a session of extracorporeal shock wave lithotripsy before endoscopic retrograde cholangiopancreatography for problematic and large common bile duct stones. World J Gastroenterol 2017;23(27):4950.
79. Lenze F, Heinzow HS, Herrmann E, et al. Clearance of refractory bile duct stones with extracorporeal shockwave lithotripsy: higher failure rate in obese patients. Scand J Gastroenterol 2014;49(2):209–14.
80. Cecinato P, Fuccio L, Azzaroli F, et al. Extracorporeal shock wave lithotripsy for difficult common bile duct stones: a comparison between 2 different lithotripters in a large cohort of patients. Gastrointest Endosc 2015;81(2):402–9.
81. García-Cano J, Reyes-Guevara AK, Martínez-Pérez T, et al. Fully covered self-expanding metal stents in the management of difficult common bile duct stones. Rev Esp Enferm Dig 2013;105(1):7–12.
82. Hartery K, Lee CS, Doherty GA, et al. Covered self-expanding metal stents for the management of common bile duct stones. Gastrointest Endosc 2017;85(1):181–6.
83. Kim HJ, Kim JS, Joo MK, et al. Hepatolithiasis and intrahepatic cholangiocarcinoma: a review. World J Gastroenterol 2015;21(48):13418–31.
84. Pausawasdi A, Watanapa P. Hepatolithiasis: epidemiology and classification. Hepatogastroenterology 1997;44(14):314–6.
85. Li C, Wen T. Surgical management of hepatolithiasis: a minireview. Intractable Rare Dis Res 2017;6(2):102–5.
86. Tsui WMS, Chan YK, Wong CT, et al. Hepatolithiasis and the syndrome of recurrent pyogenic cholangitis: clinical, radiologic, and pathologic features. Semin Liver Dis 2011;31(1):33–48.
87. Park J-S, Jeong S, Lee DH, et al. Risk factors for long-term outcomes after initial treatment in hepatolithiasis. J Korean Med Sci 2013;28(11):1627–31.
88. Suzuki Y, Mori T, Yokoyama M, et al. Hepatolithiasis: analysis of Japanese nationwide surveys over a period of 40 years. J Hepatobiliary Pancreat Sci 2014;21(9):617–22.
89. Tazuma S, Unno M, Igarashi Y, et al. Evidence-based clinical practice guidelines for cholelithiasis 2016. J Gastroenterol 2017;52(3):276–300.
90. Suzuki Y, Toshiyuki M, Masaaki Y, et al. A proposed severity classification system for hepatolithiasis based on an analysis of prognostic factors in a Japanese patient cohort. J Gastroenterol 2018;53(7):854–60.

91. Pu Q, Zhang C, Ren R, et al. Choledochoscopic lithotripsy is a useful adjunct to laparoscopic common bile duct exploration for hepatolithiasis: a cohort study. Am J Surg 2016;211(6):1058–63.
92. Wen XD, Xiao L, Wang T, et al. Routine guidewire application facilitates cholangioscopy in the management of postoperative residual hepatolithiasis. Dig Endosc 2018;30(3):372–9.
93. Wen XD, Wang T, Huang Z, et al. Step-by-step strategy in the management of residual hepatolithiasis using post-operative cholangioscopy. Therap Adv Gastroenterol 2017;10(11):853–64.
94. Chen H, Siwo EA, Khu M, et al. Current trends in the management of Mirizzi Syndrome A review of literature. Medicine (Baltimore) 2018;97(4):e9691.
95. Tataria RD, Salgaonkar HP, Maheshwari GHP. Mirizzi's syndrome: a scoring system for preoperative diagnosis. Saudi J Gastroenterol 2018;24(5):274–81.
96. Shirah BH, Shirah HA, Albeladi KB. Mirizzi syndrome: necessity for safe approach in dealing with diagnostic and treatment challenges. Ann Hepatobiliary Pancreat Surg 2017;21(3):122.
97. Kumar A, Senthil G, Prakash A, et al. Mirizzi's syndrome: lessons learnt from 169 patients at a single center. Korean J Hepatobiliary Pancreat Surg 2016;20(1):17.
98. Tarnasky PR. ERCP peri-cholecystectomy. In: Cotton PB, Leung J, editors. ERCP: the fundamentals. 2nd edition. Hoboken (NJ): John Wiley & Sons, Ltd; 2015. p. 228–49.
99. Yuan H, Yuan T, Sun X. A minimally invasive strategy for mirizzi syndrome type II : combined endoscopic with laparoscopic approach. Surg Laparosc Endosc Percutan Tech 2016;26(3):248–52.
100. Binmoeller KF, Thonke F, Soehendra N. Endoscopic treatment of Mirizzi's syndrome. Gastrointest Endosc 1993;39(4):532–6.
101. Tsuyuguchi T, Sakai Y, Sugiyama H, et al. Long-term follow-up after peroral cholangioscopy-directed lithotripsy in patients with difficult bile duct stones, including Mirizzi syndrome: an analysis of risk factors predicting stone recurrence. Surg Endosc 2011;25(7):2179–85.
102. Bhandari S, Bathini R, Sharma A, et al. Usefulness of single-operator cholangioscopy-guided laser lithotripsy in patients with Mirizzi syndrome and cystic duct stones: experience at a tertiary care center. Gastrointest Endosc 2016;84(1):56–61.
103. Chahal P, Baron T, Topazian M. Endoscopic retrograde cholangiopancreatography in post–Whipple patients background. Endoscopy 2006;38:1241–5.
104. Nakai Y, Kogure H, Yamada A, et al. Endoscopic management of bile duct stones in patients with surgically altered anatomy. Dig Endosc 2018;30:67–74.
105. Park TY, Bang CS, Choi SH, et al. Forward-viewing endoscope for ERCP in patients with Billroth II gastrectomy: a systematic review and meta-analysis. Surg Endosc 2018;32(11):4598–613.
106. Shah RJ, Smolkin M, Yen R, et al. A multicenter, U.S. experience of single-balloon, double-balloon, and rotational overtube-assisted enteroscopy ERCP in patients with surgically altered pancreaticobiliary anatomy (with video). Gastrointest Endosc 2013;77(4):593–600.
107. Schreiner MA, Chang L, Gluck M, et al. Laparoscopy-assisted versus balloon enteroscopy-assisted ERCP in bariatric post-Roux-en-Y gastric bypass patients. Gastrointest Endosc 2012;75(4):748–56.
108. Kint JF, van den Bergh JE, van Gelder RE, et al. Percutaneous treatment of common bile duct stones: results and complications in 110 consecutive patients. Dig Surg 2015;32(1):9–15.

109. Kedia P, Sharaiha RZ, Kumta N a, et al. Endoscopic gallbladder drainage compared with percutaneous drainage. Gastrointest Endosc 2015;82(6): 1031–6.
110. Frederiksen NA, Tveskov L, Helgstrand F, et al. Treatment of common bile duct stones in gastric bypass patients with laparoscopic transgastric endoscopic retrograde cholangiopancreatography. Obes Surg 2017. https://doi.org/10.1007/s11695-016-2524-2.
111. Gutierrez JM, Lederer H, Krook JC, et al. Surgical gastrostomy for pancreatobiliary and duodenal access following Roux en Y gastric bypass. J Gastrointest Surg 2009;13(12):2170–5.
112. Kedia P, Sharaiha RZ, Kumta N a, et al. Internal EUS-directed transgastric ERCP (EDGE): game over. Gastroenterology 2014;147(3):566–8.
113. Kedia P, Tarnasky PR, Nieto J, et al. EUS-directed transgastric ERCP (EDGE) versus laparoscopy-assisted ERCP (LA-ERCP) for Roux-en-Y Gastric bypass (RYGB) anatomy: a multicenter early comparative experience of clinical outcomes. J Clin Gastroenterol 2018. https://doi.org/10.1097/MCG.0000000000001037.
114. Tyberg A, Nieto J, Salgado S, et al. Endoscopic ultrasound (EUS)-directed transgastric endoscopic retrograde cholangiopancreatography or eus: mid-term analysis of an emerging procedure. Clin Endosc 2017;50(2):185–90.
115. James TW, Fan YC, Baron TH, et al. EUS-guided hepaticoenterostomy as a portal to allow de fi nitive antegrade treatment of benign biliary diseases in patients with surgically altered anatomy. Gastrointest Endosc 2018. https://doi.org/10.1016/j.gie.2018.04.2353.
116. Iwashita T, Nakai Y, Hara K, et al. Endoscopic ultrasound-guided antegrade treatment of bile duct stone in patients with surgically altered anatomy: a multicenter retrospective cohort study. J Hepatobiliary Pancreat Sci 2016;23(4): 227–33.
117. Sharaiha RZ, Khan MA, Kamal F, et al. Efficacy and safety of EUS-guided biliary drainage in comparison with percutaneous biliary drainage when ERCP fails: a systematic review and meta-analysis. Gastrointest Endosc 2017;85(5):904–14.

Endoscopic Ultrasound-Guided Biliary Drainage

Jeremy S. Nussbaum, BS, Nikhil A. Kumta, MD, MS*

KEYWORDS

- Therapeutic endoscopic ultrasound • Endoscopic ultrasound • Biliary drainage
- Choledochoduodenostomy • Hepaticogastrostomy • Rendezvous procedure

KEY POINTS

- Endoscopic ultrasound-guided biliary drainage seems is a safe and effective means of biliary decompression after failed conventional endoscopic retrograde cholangiopancreatography, with cost and quality of life benefits comparable with surgery and percutaneous transhepatic drainage.
- There are multiple approaches, stent directions, and drainage routes with which endoscopic ultrasound-guided biliary drainage seems can be performed. We propose an algorithm to determine the appropriate options based on patient anatomy and imaging results.
- Further studies are required on the optimal method of performing endoscopic ultrasound-guided biliary drainage seems, as well as whether it is a viable alternative to endoscopic retrograde cholangiopancreatography as a primary means of biliary decompression in malignant biliary obstruction.

INTRODUCTION

Endoscopic retrograde cholangiopancreatography (ERCP) is the preferred method for gaining biliary access, and managing both benign and malignant biliary obstructions. However, biliary cannulation can fail in 4% to 16% of ERCPs.[1] Failure can occur owing to altered anatomy, periampullary diverticulum, ampullary pathology, tumor infiltration of the papilla, or gastric outlet obstruction. When ERCP fails, other options include surgical drainage, percutaneous transhepatic drainage (PTBD), and endoscopic ultrasound-guided biliary drainage (EUS-BD).

Surgical options to restore bile flow include choledochoenteric drainage or the more complex Roux-en-Y hepaticojejunostomy.[2] A 2014 metaanalysis found the technical success of surgically drained biliary obstruction patients to be 89.5%. However, the 30-day mortality rate was 15% and up to 39% of patients experienced major

Disclosures: Dr Kumta is a consultant for Apollo Endosurgery, Boston Scientific, Olympus.

Dr. Henry D. Janowitz Division of Gastroenterology, Icahn School of Medicine at Mount Sinai, Mount Sinai Hospital, One Gustave L. Levy Place, Box 1069, New York, NY 10029, USA
* Corresponding author.
E-mail address: Nikhil.Kumta@gmail.com

Gastrointest Endoscopy Clin N Am 29 (2019) 277–291
https://doi.org/10.1016/j.giec.2018.11.005
1052-5157/19/© 2018 Elsevier Inc. All rights reserved.

complications.[3] A 2016 matched cohort study of patients with pancreatic cancer showed that undergoing endoscopic stent placement had a significantly shorter length of stay and cost of care compared with those undergoing surgical bypass.[4] Endoscopic biliary stent placement also increased the likelihood of being discharged home and was associated with an increase in quality of life.

PTBD is a minimally invasive procedure performed by interventional radiologists. The bile duct is accessed through the skin and liver under fluoroscopic (sometimes combined with ultrasound) guidance, and can be drained internally or externally.[5] Biliary stenting can be accomplished with PTBD. A 2015 retrospective cohort analysis comparing PTBD and EUS-BD after failed ERCP found EUS-BD to be associated with decreased adverse events, lower cost, and fewer reinterventions.[6] Including repeat interventions, the complication rates for PTBD were 80.4% compared with 15.7% for the EUS-BD group. Other advantages to EUS-BD over PTBD include multiple routes of access to the biliary tree, the lack of an external catheter (improving patient comfort and quality of life), and the ability to be performed in the same session after a failed ERCP.[7]

The development of EUS imaging allowed for the visualization of the biliary tree, and the use of EUS-guided cholangiography was first described by Wiersema and colleagues[8] in 1996. In 2001, Giovannini and colleagues[9] described the first EUS-BD via a transduodenal stent. Then in 2004, Mallery and colleagues[10] described the first biliary rendezvous (RV) with transpapillary EUS-guided ERCP. Since then, various approaches and drainage routes have been explored to access the biliary tree depending on stricture location, patient anatomy, and endoscopist experience.

INDICATIONS AND CONTRAINDICATIONS

The accepted indications for EUS-BD are failed ERCP, altered anatomy, tumor preventing access into the biliary tree, and contraindication to percutaneous access such as large ascites.[11] Relative contraindications to EUS-BD are ascites, recent surgery, and anticoagulation therapy. Specifically, right intrahepatic bile duct drainage is contraindicated with a complicated hilar stricture, and PTBD should be used.[12]

MATERIALS AND INSTRUMENTS

1. Fluoroscopy. Fluoroscopy can be used to facilitate the angle of the bile duct puncture, which should be in a cephalad to caudad direction to facilitate transpapillary passage of the guidewire.
2. Contrast dye for cholangiography.
3. Water to flush the catheters and hydrophilic wires.
4. Therapeutic linear echoendoscope with a 3.8-mm working channel to avoid being limited in catheter and stent diameter. In addition, a duodenoscope should be available for a possible RV technique and conversion to a retrograde procedure.
5. Fine needle aspiration (FNA) needles: 19-G needles are preferred to allow for manipulation of 0.035-inch guidewires.
6. Hydrophilic 0.035-in guidewire is preferred owing to ease of manipulation and ability to support a variety of catheters and stents.
7. Bougie catheters and dilating balloons: Either a 4- to 6-mm wire-guided hydrostatic dilating balloon catheter or a 6F to 8F dilating bougie catheter.
8. Rotatable sphincterotome or bending catheter to help redirect wire to facilitate transpapillary passage.
9. Stents. Both plastic (straight, double-pigtail) or metal (covered, uncovered, lumen apposing) can be used.[13]

TECHNIQUE

EUS-BD can be performed in several ways. In terms of approach, an extrahepatic or intrahepatic technique can be used. For both approaches, stents can then be placed in an antegrade fashion across the stricture or directly at the access site. Alternatively, both approaches allow for the use of a RV technique for conversion to ERCP. For both approaches, biliary drainage can be achieved via transmural or transpapillary drainage route.

The intrahepatic approach requires gaining access to the biliary tree via the stomach, esophagus, or jejunum (in altered anatomy). From one of these sites, access is gained via needle puncture into the left hepatic duct system under direct vision with echoendoscopy. Most endoscopists prefer performing initial entry with a 19-G EUS-FNA needle for easier wire manipulation.[14] Biliary access is confirmed with aspiration of bile, and contrast is injected to perform a cholangiogram.[13] Water should then be flushed through the needle channel to decrease the risk of friction and wire shearing.[15] The guidewire is then inserted through the FNA needle. Dilation of the fistula tract is performed to allow for the passing of a stent. This step can be done with balloon catheter, needle knife, or graded diameter stiff catheter.[16] Hepaticogastrostomy (EUS-HGS) can be performed by inserting a stent over the guidewire with the distal end in the left hepatic duct and the proximal end in the stomach, creating a transhepatic–transgastric fistula and allowing for transmural drainage.[15] An alternative option is antegrade stent placement (EUS-AS). This maneuver requires the wire to be passed beyond the point of obstruction to allow stent placement within the biliary system. Drainage occurs in a transpapillary fashion. A third option, possible for both the intrahepatic and extrahepatic approach, is the RV technique (EUS-RV). In this technique, the guidewire is directed past the stricture and into the duodenum. The guidewire is left in place and the echoendoscope is removed over the guidewire. A duodenoscope is inserted, advanced to the papilla, and used to retrieve the EUS-guided transpapillary guidewire. An ERCP catheter can then be advanced over the guidewire into the bile duct, and conventional ERCP can be performed.[17]

The extrahepatic approach involves transduodenal or transenteric needle puncture into the common bile duct. The same steps as in the intrahepatic approach can then be used to confirm location and direct the wire. Again, access is gained via 19-G FNA needle puncture into the common bile duct, confirmed with bile aspiration, and followed by injection of contrast. Water is flushed through the needle channel, followed by the guidewire. Dilation of the fistula tract, to allow for stent placement, is accomplished by a balloon catheter, needle knife, or graded diameter stiff catheter. The antegrade stent placement and RV techniques are the same as in intrahepatic approach. For antegrade stent placement (EUS-AS), the guidewire is passed beyond the stricture for stent placement within the bile duct and transpapillary drainage. For the RV technique (EUS-RV), the guidewire is passed beyond the stricture, and advanced into the duodenum. The echoendoscope is swapped for a duodenoscope, which is used to retrieve the guidewire and perform conventional ERCP. Drainage is again transpapillary. Transmural drainage differs between the intrahepatic and extrahepatic approaches. For transmural stent placement via choledochoduodenostomy (EUS-CDS), a fistula is created between the duodenal bulb and the extrahepatic bile duct, allowing for drainage into the duodenum rather than the stomach (as in the hepaticogastrostomy intrahepatic approach).

There is currently no consensus on which approach and drainage route is best. A systematic review of 42 studies found no significant differences between the intrahepatic and extrahepatic approaches.[18] However, the 2 approaches have different limitations. In the extrahepatic approach, antegrade stent placement can be difficult owing to the angle of needle puncture.[13] The intrahepatic approach can be limited by displacement between the gastric wall and intrahepatic bile duct, liver cirrhosis, risk of puncture of the intrahepatic portal vein, risk of mediastinitis with the transesophageal approach, and an inability to drain the right side of the liver.[19] Several algorithms have been proposed to choose a strategy based on imaging results and expected difficulties.[1,20–24] We prefer the algorithm provided in **Fig. 1**. After failed ERCP, cross-sectional imaging or endoscopic ultrasound examination is used to determine whether the intrahepatic biliary tree is dilated. If it is dilated, an intrahepatic approach is preferred. If the intrahepatic biliary tree is not dilated, or if the intrahepatic approach fails, an extrahepatic approach is used. In either approach, transpapillary drainage (RV technique or antegrade stenting) is preferred to preserve patient anatomy and avoid creation of a new anastomosis.[21] If the papilla is accessible to duodenoscope, then conversion to ERCP via an RV technique (EUS-RV) is preferred. If not, antegrade stenting (EUS-AS) should be used. If these techniques fail, then transmural drainage can be accomplished via hepaticogastrostomy (EUS-HGS) for the intrahepatic approach or choledochoduodenostomy (EUS-CDS) for the extrahepatic approach. It should be noted that this algorithm is for nonsurgical candidates after failed ERCP. If the patient is a possible candidate for surgery, multidisciplinary discussions should take place to decide whether preoperative biliary drainage should be performed and whether PTBD or an endoscopic approach should be used. There is currently no consensus about the benefits of preoperative biliary drainage versus direct surgery, with some studies showing that preoperative biliary drainage increases morbidity with no effect on mortality,[25] and others showing that preoperative biliary drainage significantly decreased adverse effects.[26]

DISCUSSION

EUS-BD has emerged as a safe and effective means of biliary decompression following failed ERCP. Although it is a complicated procedure requiring skilled

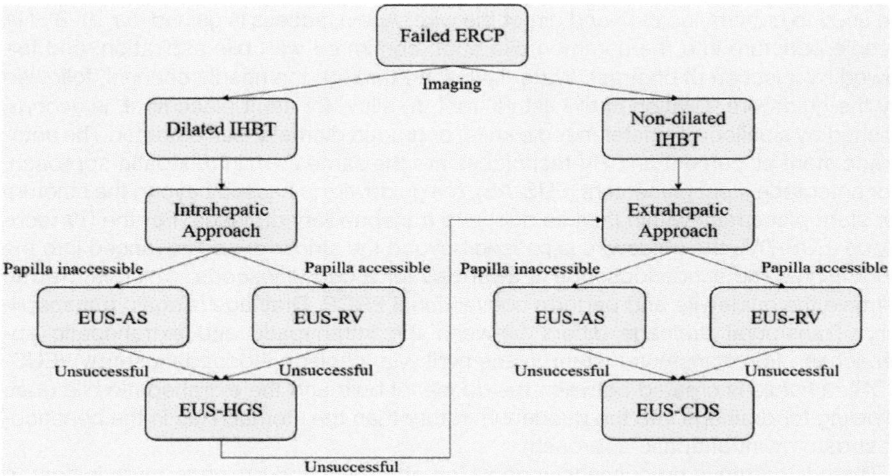

Fig. 1. Algorithm approach to endoscopic ultrasound-guided biliary drainage (EUS-BD). AS, anterograde stent; CDS, choledochoduodenostomy; ERCP, endoscopic retrograde cholangiopancreatography; HGS, hepaticogastronomy; IHBT, intrahepatic biliary tree; RV, rendezvous.

Table 1
Published data on EUS-BD using extrahepatic approach

Author, Year	Number/ Total Sample	Method	Disease	Approach	Initial Stent	Percent Success Rate	Complications
Yamao et al,[32] 2008	3/3	Direct (n = 3)	Malignant (n = 3)	Duodenum (n = 3)	PS (n = 3)	100	Pneumoperitoneum (n = 1)
Tarantino et al,[33] 2008	8/8	Direct (n = 4), rendezvous (n = 4)	Malignant (n = 7), benign (n = 1)	Duodenum (n = 8)	PS (n = 8)	100	None
Itoi et al,[34] 2008	4/4	Direct (n = 4)	Malignant (n = 4)	Duodenum (n = 4)	PS (n = 3), NBD (n = 1)	100	Focal peritonitis (n = 1), bleeding (n = 1)
Brauer et al,[35] 2009	12/12	Direct (n = 4), rendezvous (n = 7)	Malignant (n = 8), benign (n = 4)	N/A	PS (n = 5), SEMS (n = 5)	92	Pneumoperitoneum (n = 1), respiratory failure (n = 1)
Horaguchi et a,[36] 2009	9/16	N/A	Malignant (n = 9)	Duodenum (n = 8), stomach (n = 1)	PS (n = 14), plastic PT (n = 1), NBT (n = 1)	100	Peritonitis (n = 1)
Hanada et al,[37] 2009	4/4	Direct (n = 4)	Malignant (n = 4)	Duodenum (n = 4)	PS (n = 4)	100	None
Maranki et al,[38] 2009	14/49	Direct (n = 6), rendezvous (n = 8)	Malignant (n = 9), benign (n = 5)	N/A	N/A	86	Biliary peritonitis (n = 1), abdominal pain (n = 1), pneumoperitoneum (n = 1)
Kim et al,[39] 2010	15/15	Rendezvous (n = 15)	Malignant (n = 10), benign (n = 5)	Duodenum (n = 15)	PS (n = 4), MS (n = 8)	80	Pancreatitis (n = 1)

(*continued on next page*)

Table 1
(continued)

Author, Year	Number/Total Sample	Method	Disease	Approach	Initial Stent	Percent Success Rate	Complications
Nguyen-Tang et al,[40] 2010	1/5	Rendezvous (n = 1)	Malignant (n = 1)	N/A	MS (n = 1)	100	None
Iwamuro et al,[41] 2010	7/7	Direct (n = 7)	Malignant (n = 7)	Duodenum (n = 5), stomach (n = 2)	PS (n = 7)	100	Bile peritonitis (n = 2)
Artifon et al,[42] 2010	3/3	Direct (n = 3)	Malignant (n = 3)	Duodenum (n = 3)	MS (n = 3)	100	None
Belletrutti et al,[43] 2010	1/1	Direct (n = 1)	Malignant (n = 1)	Duodenum (n = 1)	MS (n = 1)	100	None
Park et al,[44] 2011	31/57	Direct (n = 31)	Malignant (n = 51), benign (n = 6)	Duodenum (n = 31)	PS (n = 6), MS (n = 25)	87	Pneumoperitoneum (n = 6), mild bleeding (n = 2)
Fabbri et al,[45] 2011	16/16	Direct (n = 13), rendezvous (n = 3)	Malignant (n = 16)	Duodenum (n = 15), stomach (n = 1)	PS (n = 4), MS (n = 8)	80	Pancreatitis (n = 1)
Hara et al,[46] 2011	18/18	Direct (n = 18)	Malignant (n = 18)	N/A	PS (n = 17)	94	Peritonitis (n = 2), bleeding (n = 1)
Ramirez-Luna et al,[47] 2011	9/11	Direct (n = 9)	Malignant (n = 9)	Duodenum (n = 9)	Plastic DPT (n = 9)	89	Biloma (n = 1)
Siddiqui et al,[48] 2011	8/8	Direct (n = 8)	Malignant (n = 8)	Duodenum (n = 8)	MS (n = 8)	100	Stent migration (n = 1), duodenal perforation (n = 1)
Komaki et al,[49] 2011	15/15	Direct (n = 14), rendezvous (n = 1)	Malignant (n = 15)	Duodenum (n = 15)	PS (n = 15)	100	None

Prachayakul et al,[50] 2011	1/1	Direct (n = 1)	Malignant (n = 1)	Duodenum (n = 1)	PS (n = 1)	100	None
Artifon et al,[51] 2012	13/13	Direct (n = 13)	Malignant (n = 13)	Duodenum (n = 13)	MS (n = 13)	100	Bile leak (n = 1), bleeding (n = 1)
Attasaranya et al,[52] 2012	10/31	Direct (n = 9), antegrade (n = 1)	Malignant (n = 23), benign (n = 8)	Duodenum	N/A	60	4/10 (40%)
Katanuma et al,[53] 2012	1/1	Direct (n = 1)	Benign (n = 1)	Duodenum (n = 1)	PS (n = 1)	100	None
Kawakubo et al,[54] 2012	2/2	Direct (n = 2)	Malignant (n = 2)	Duodenum (n = 2)	PS (n = 2)	100	None
Khashab et al,[55] 2012	7/9	Direct (n = 2), antegrade (n = 2), rendezvous (n = 3)	Malignant (n = 7)	Duodenum (n = 6), gastric (n = 1)	MS (n = 7)	100	Pancreatitis (n = 1), cholecystitis (n = 1), abdominal pain (n = 1)
Kim et al,[56] 2012	9/13	Direct (n = 9)	Malignant (n = 9)	Duodenum (n = 9)	MS (n = 9)	100	Pneumoperitoneum (n = 2), migration (n = 2), peritonitis (n = 1)
Song et al,[57] 2012	15/15	Direct (n = 15)	Malignant (n = 15)	Duodenum (n = 15)	MS (n = 15)	100	Pneumoperitoneum (n = 2), cholangitis (n = 1)
Dhir et al,[58] 2012	58/58	Rendezvous (n = 58)	Malignant (n = 43), benign (n = 15)	Duodenum (n = 58)	N/A	98	Bile leak (n = 2)
Hara et al,[23] 2013	18/18	Direct (n = 18)	Malignant (n = 18)	Duodenum (n = 18)	MS (n = 18)	94	Bile peritonitis (n = 2)
Park et al,[59] 2013	16/45	Direct (n = 2), rendezvous (n = 14)	Malignant (n = 39), benign (n = 6)	Duodenum (n = 16)	MS (n = 16)	88	Pancreatitis (n = 1), bile peritonitis (n = 1)

(*continued on next page*)

Table 1
(continued)

Author, Year	Number/ Total Sample	Method	Disease	Approach	Initial Stent	Percent Success Rate	Complications
Itoi et al,[60] 2013	1/1	Direct (n = 1)	Malignant (n = 1)	Stomach (n = 1)	MS (n = 1)	100	None
Will et al,[61] 2015	9/95	Antegrade (n = 9)	Malignant (n = 77), benign (n = 15)	Stomach (n = 9)	MS (n = 9)	85	15/95 (16%)
Brückner et al,[62] 2015	5/5	Direct (n = 5)	Malignant (n = 5)	Duodenum (n = 5)	MS (n = 5)	100	None
Tyberg et al,[21] 2016	17/52	Direct (n = 6), rendezvous (n = 11)	Malignant (n = 42), benign (n = 5)	Duodenum (n = 17)	MS (n = 41), PS (n = 11)	96	Liver abscess (n = 1), bleeding (n = 2)
Guo et al,[63] 2016	14/21	Direct (n = 14)	Malignant (n = 14)	Duodenum (n = 14)	MS (n = 14)	100	Sepsis (n = 1)
Makmun et al,[64] 2017	23/24	Direct (n = 23)	Malignant (n = 23)	Duodenum (n = 23)	PS (n = 20), MS (n = 3)	78	Pneumoperitoneum (n = 1), cholangitis (n = 3)
Rai et al,[65] 2018	30/30	Direct (n = 30)	Malignant (n = 30)	Duodenum (n = 30)	MS (n = 28)	93	Bile leak (n = 1), bleeding (n = 1), stent block (n = 1)
Total	427					394/427 (92.3%)	63/427 (15%)

Abbreviations: DPT, double pigtail stent; EUS-BD, endoscopic ultrasound-guided biliary drainage; MS, metal stent; N/A, not applicable; NBD, naso-biliary drain; NBT, naso-biliary tube; PT, pigtail stent; SEMS, self-expandable metal stent.

Table 2
Published data on EUS-BD using intrahepatic approach

Author, Year	Number/ Total Sample	Method	Disease	Approach	Initial Stent	Percent Success Rate	Complications
Horaguchi et al,[36] 2009	7/16	N/A	Malignant	Stomach (n = 5), esophagus (n = 2)	PS (n = 2), MS (n = 5)	100	None
Maranki et al,[38] 2009	35/49	Direct (n = 9), antegrade (n = 24)	Malignant (n = 26), benign (n = 9)	N/A	N/A	83	Bleeding (n = 1), pneumoperitoneum (n = 3), aspiration pneumonia (n = 1)
Nguyen-Tang et al,[40] 2010	4/5	Rendezvous (n = 4)	Malignant (n = 3), benign (n = 1)	Duodenum (n = 1), stomach (n = 3)	MS (n = 5)	100	None
Park et al,[44] 2011	31/57	Direct (n = 31)	Malignant (n = 51), benign (n = 6)	Duodenum (n = 31)	PS (n = 6), MS (n = 25)	87	Pneumoperitoneum (n = 1), bile peritonitis (n = 2)
Ramirez-Luna et al,[47] 2011	2/11	Direct (n = 2)	Malignant (n = 2)	Stomach (n = 2)	PS (n = 2)	100	Stent migration (n = 1)
Attasaranya et al,[52] 2012	16/31	Direct (n = 16)	Malignant (n = 23), benign (n = 8)	N/A	N/A	81	6/16 (38%)
Khashab et al,[55] 2012	2/9	Antegrade (n = 1), rendezvous (n = 1)	Malignant (n = 2)	Stomach	MS (n = 2)	100	Nausea (n = 1)
Kim et al,[56] 2012	4/13	Direct (n = 4)	Malignant (n = 4)	Stomach (n = 4)	MS (n = 3)	75	Peritonitis (n = 1), stent migration (n = 1)
Park et al,[59] 2013	29/45	Direct (n = 9), antegrade (n = 14), rendezvous (n = 5)	Malignant (n = 39), benign (n = 6)	Stomach (n = 29)	N/A	66	Biloma (n = 1)

(*continued on next page*)

Table 2
(continued)

Author, Year	Number/ Total Sample	Method	Disease	Approach	Initial Stent	Percent Success Rate	Complications
Iwashita et al,[66] 2013	6/6	Direct (n = 1)	Malignant (n = 1), benign (n = 5)	N/A	MS (n = 1)	100	Pancreatitis (n = 1), abdominal pain (n = 1)
Will et al,[61] 2015	61/95	Direct (n = 43), antegrade (n = 7), rendezvous (n = 11)	Malignant (n = 77), benign (n = 15)	Stomach (n = 46), jejunum (n = 8), esophagus (n = 7)	MS (n = 46), PS (n = 15)	85	15/95 (16%)
Tyberg et al,[21] 2016	35/52	Antegrade (n = 27), direct (n = 8)	Malignant (n = 42), benign (n = 5)	Stomach (n = 35)	MS (n = 41), PS (n = 11)	96	Bleeding (n = 2), cardiac arrest (n = 1)
Guo et al,[63] 2016	7/21	Direct (n = 7)	Malignant (n = 7)	Stomach (n = 7)	MS (n = 7)	100	Sepsis (n = 1), bile leak (n = 1)
Makmun et al,[64] 2017	1/24	Rendezvous (n = 1)	Malignant (n = 1)	Stomach (n = 1)	PS (n = 1)	100	None
Imai et al,[67] 2017	79/145	Direct (n = 42), antegrade (n = 37)	Malignant (n = 79)	Stomach (n = 79)	MS (n = 79)	91	Bile leak (n = 8), stent migration (n = 2), cholangitis (n = 3), pancreatitis (n = 2)
Oh et al,[29] 2017	129/129	Direct (n = 129)	Malignant (n = 113), benign (n = 16)	Stomach (n = 129)	MS (n = 118), PS (n = 2)	93	32/129 (25%)
Ogura et al,[68] 2018	49/49	Antegrade (n = 40), direct (n = 7)	Malignant (n = 49)	Stomach (n = 49)	MS (n = 47)	96	Pancreatitis (n = 4), bleeding (n = 1)
Total	497					444/497 (89.3%)	93/497 (19%)

Abbreviations: EUS-BD, endoscopic ultrasound-guided biliary drainage; MS, metal stent; N/A, not applicable; PS, plastic stent.

endoscopists, it has several demonstrated advantages over surgical biliary drainage and PTBD.

A review of published EUS-BD data (**Tables 1** and **2**) including 40 studies and 924 patients demonstrates an overall technical success rate of 90.7% and adverse event rate of 17.0%. A recent metaanalysis of 16 studies reports the overall cumulative success rate of EUS-BD as 88% to 93%.[7] Although the procedure is efficacious, the metaanalysis found complications occurring in 13% to 20% of cases. Another recent systematic review, including 42 studies and 1192 patients, reported technical and clinical success rates of 94.71% and 91.66%, respectively.[18] This analysis also found the adverse event rate to be 23.32%. Complications associated with EUS-BD include infection (peritonitis, cholangitis, cholecystitis, and pancreatitis), pneumoperitoneum, bile leak, bleeding, abdominal pain, and stent migration. In our review of the published literature, infection was the most common at 2.1%, followed by pneumoperitoneum at 1.9%, bleeding at 1.2%, and stent migration at 0.6%. Another review examined the occurrence of complications, with the most common being infection (3.5%) and bile leak (3.0%).[27]

A recent review of 9 studies including 483 patients found that EUS-BD was associated with better clinical success, fewer adverse events, and a lower rate of reintervention than PTBD.[27] Although the review found no difference in technical success between the 2 procedures, EUS-BD was more cost effective. One advantage of EUS-BD over PTBD is the ability to personalize the procedure owing to the many combinations of approach, stent placement, and drainage routes that allow the technique to adapt to the individual patient.

Another study compared the outcomes of surgery versus endoscopy for biliary obstruction owing to metastatic pancreatic cancer.[28] The study included 273 patients and found that endoscopy was associated with a lower cost of care (both for the procedure and after care until death), as well as a better quality of life.

One limitation of EUS-BD is that it is a complex procedure that requires experienced, skilled endoscopists to perform effectively. One study analyzed the number of procedures required for a single provider to stabilize their procedure time and adverse event rate in performing EUS-HGS. The study found that more than 33 cases were required to reach a plateau in success rates.[29] This finding demonstrates that EUS-BD can be a complex procedure that requires a learning curve for endoscopists to optimize their results. To this effect, a consortium of advanced endoscopists met in 2011 to review EUS-BD.[14] The consortium recommended that endoscopists perform at least 200 to 300 EUS and ERCP each year for 4 to 5 years, have a 95% success rate for ERCP cannulation with normal anatomy, and be located in a center with interventional radiology and surgery as backups to perform EUS-BD.

EUS-BD has been shown to be safe and effective in multiple studies. In the majority of these studies, EUS-BD was used as rescue procedure when ERCP has failed. Recently, EUS-BD and ERCP have been compared in randomized, controlled studies for primary biliary drainage for malignant obstruction. Both studies showed no significant difference in rates of technical or therapeutic success, or rate of adverse effects.[30,31] EUS-BD may be a safe and effective alternative to ERCP as a primary means of malignant biliary decompression, but further studies are warranted.

SUMMARY

In conclusion, EUS-BD is an effective, safe, and innovative technique for biliary drainage when conventional ERCP fails. It has been demonstrated that EUS-BD offers advantages over surgery and PTBD in terms of clinical success, reintervention, and cost effectiveness. However, it is a complicated procedure that requires careful patient selection, highly skilled endoscopists, and has a learning curve. Although success has been found with an individualized approach to EUS-BD, further studies are needed to ascertain the optimal approach, stent direction, and drainage route.

REFERENCES

1. Holt BA, Hawes R, Hasan M, et al. Biliary drainage: role of EUS guidance. Gastrointest Endosc 2016;83(1):160–5.
2. Maire F, Sauvanet A. Palliation of biliary and duodenal obstruction in patients with unresectable pancreatic cancer: endoscopy or surgery? J Visc Surg 2013; 150(3):S27–31.
3. Glazer ES, Hornbrook MC, Krouse RS. A meta-analysis of randomized trials: immediate stent placement vs. surgical bypass in the palliative management of malignant biliary obstruction. J Pain Symptom Manage 2014;6(8):307–14.
4. Bliss LA, Eskander MF, Kent TS, et al. Early surgical bypass versus endoscopic stent placement in pancreatic cancer. HPB (Oxford) 2016;18(8):671–7.
5. Chandrashekhara SH, Gamanagatti S, Singh A, et al. Current status of percutaneous transhepatic biliary drainage in palliation of malignant obstructive jaundice: a review. Indian J Palliat Care 2016;22(4):378–87.
6. Khashab MA, Valeshabad AK, Afghani E, et al. A comparative evaluation of EUS-guided biliary drainage and percutaneous drainage in patients with distal malignant biliary obstruction and failed ERCP. Dig Dis Sci 2015;60(2):557–65.
7. Moole H, Bechtold ML, Forcione DG, et al. Comparing endoscopic ultrasound guided versus percutaneous biliary stenting in patients with inoperable malignant biliary strictures and a failed ERCP: a systematic review and meta-analysis. Gastroenterology 2016;150(4):S656.
8. Wiersema M, Sandusky D, Carr R, et al. Endosonography-guided cholangiopancreatography. Gastrointest Endosc 1996;43(2):102–6.
9. Giovannini M, Moutardier V, Pesenti C, et al. Endoscopic ultrasound-guided bilioduodenal anastomosis: a new technique for biliary drainage. Endoscopy 2001; 33(10):898–900.
10. Mallery S, Matlock J, Freeman ML. EUS-guided rendezvous drainage of obstructed biliary and pancreatic ducts: report of 6 cases. Gastrointest Endosc 2004;59(1):100–7.
11. Kedia P, Gaidhane M, Kahaleh M. Endoscopic guided biliary drainage: how can we achieve efficient biliary drainage? Clin Endosc 2013;46(5):543–51.
12. Itoi T, Dhir V, Moon JH. EUS-guided biliary drainage: moving into a new era of biliary drainage. Gastrointest Endosc 2017;85(5):915–7.
13. Kumta NA, Kedia P, Kahaleh M. Endoscopic ultrasound-guided biliary drainage: an update. Curr Opin Gastroenterol 2014;12(2):154–68.
14. Kahaleh M, Artifon EL, Perez-Miranda M, et al. Endoscopic ultrasonography guided biliary drainage: summary of consortium meeting, May 7th, 2011, Chicago. World J Gastroenterol 2013;19(9):1372–9.
15. Sarkaria S, Lee H-S, Gaidhane M, et al. Advances in endoscopic ultrasound-guided biliary drainage: a comprehensive review. Gut Liver 2013;7(2):129–36.
16. Boulay BR, Lo SK. Endoscopic ultrasound–guided biliary drainage. Gastrointest Endosc Clin N Am 2018;28(2):171–85.
17. Tsuchiya T, Itoi T, Sofuni A, et al. Endoscopic ultrasonography-guided rendezvous technique. Dig Endosc 2016;28:96–101.

18. Wang K, Zhu J, Xing L, et al. Assessment of efficacy and safety of EUS-guided biliary drainage: a systematic review. Gastrointest Endosc 2016;83(6):1218–27.
19. Itoi T, Sofuni A, Itokawa F, et al. Endoscopic ultrasonography-guided biliary drainage. J Hepatobiliary Pancreat Sci 2010;17(5):611–6.
20. Paik WH, Park DH. Endoscopic ultrasound-guided biliary access, with focus on technique and practical tips. Clin Endosc 2017;50(2):104–11.
21. Tyberg A, Desai AP, Kumta NA, et al. EUS-guided biliary drainage after failed ERCP: a novel algorithm individualized based on patient anatomy. Gastrointest Endosc 2016;84(6):941–6.
22. Baars JE, Kaffes AJ, Saxena P. Review article EUS - guided biliary drainage: a comprehensive review of the literature. Endosc Ultrasound 2018;7(1):4–9.
23. Hara K, Yamao K, Hijioka S, et al. Prospective clinical study of endoscopic ultrasound- guided choledochoduodenostomy with direct metallic stent placement using a forward-viewing echoendo- scope. Endoscopy 2013;45:392–6.
24. Iwashita T, Doi S, Yasuda I. Endoscopic ultrasound-guided biliary drainage: a review. Clin J Gastroenterol 2014;7(2):94–102.
25. Fang Y, Gurusamy KS, Wang Q, et al. Meta-analysis of randomized clinical trials on safety and efficacy of biliary drainage before surgery for obstructive jaundice. Br J Surg 2013;100(12):1589–96.
26. Moole H, Bechtold M, Puli SR. Efficacy of preoperative biliary drainage in malignant obstructive jaundice: a meta-analysis and systematic review. World J Surg Oncol 2016;14(1):1–11.
27. Sharaiha RZ, Khan MA, Kamal F, et al. Efficacy and safety of EUS-guided biliary drainage in comparison with percutaneous biliary drainage when ERCP fails: a systematic review and meta-analysis. Gastrointest Endosc 2017;85(5):904–14.
28. Artifon ELA, Sakai P, Cunha JEM, et al. Surgery or endoscopy for palliation of biliary obstruction due to metastatic pancreatic cancer. Am J Gastroenterol 2006;101(9):2031–7.
29. Oh D, Park DH, Song TJ, et al. Optimal biliary access point and learning curve for endoscopic ultrasound-guided hepaticogastrostomy with transmural stenting. Therap Adv Gastroenterol 2017;10(1):42–53.
30. Bang JY, Navaneethan U, Hasan M, et al. Stent placement by EUS or ERCP for primary biliary decompression in pancreatic cancer: a randomized trial (with videos). Gastrointest Endosc 2018;88(1):9–17.
31. Park JK, Woo YS, Noh DH, et al. Efficacy of EUS-guided and ERCP-guided biliary drainage for malignant biliary obstruction: prospective randomized controlled study. Gastrointest Endosc 2018;88(2):277–82.
32. Yamao K, Bhatia V, Mizuno N, et al. EUS-guided choledochoduodenostomy for palliative biliary drainage in patients with malignant biliary obstruction: results of long-term follow-up. Endoscopy 2008;40(4):340–2.
33. Tarantino I, Barresi L, Repici A, et al. EUS-guided biliary drainage: a case series. Endoscopy 2008;40(4):336–9.
34. Itoi T, Itokawa F, Sofuni A, et al. Endoscopic ultrasound-guided choledochoduodenostomy in patients with failed endoscopic retrograde cholangiopancreatography. World J Gastroenterol 2008;14(39):6078.
35. Brauer BC, Chen YK, Fukami N, et al. Single-operator EUS-guided cholangiopancreatography for difficult pancreaticobiliary access (with video). Gastrointest Endosc 2009;70(3):471–9.
36. Horaguchi J, Fujita N, Noda Y, et al. Endosonography-guided biliary drainage in cases with difficult transpapillary endoscopic biliary drainage. Dig Endosc 2009; 21(4):239–44.

37. Hanada K, Iiboshi T, Ishii Y. Endoscopic ultrasound-guided choledochoduodenostomy for palliative biliary drainage in cases with inoperable pancreas head carcinoma. Dig Endosc 2009;21(SUPPL. 1):75–8.
38. Maranki J, Hernandez a J, Arslan B, et al. Interventional endoscopic ultrasound-guided cholangiography: long-term experience of an emerging alternative to percutaneous transhepatic cholangiography. Endoscopy 2009;41(6):532–8.
39. Kim YS, Gupta K, Mallery S, et al. Endoscopic ultrasound rendezvous for bile duct access using a transduodenal approach: cumulative experience at a single center. A case series. Endoscopy 2010;42:496–502.
40. Nguyen-Tang T, Binmoeller KF, Sanchez-Yague A, et al. Endoscopic ultrasound (EUS)-guided transhepatic anterograde self-expandable metal stent (SEMS) placement across malignant biliary obstruction. Endoscopy 2010;42(3):232–6.
41. Iwamuro M, Kawamoto H, Harada R, et al. Combined duodenal stent placement and endoscopic ultrasonography-guided biliary drainage for malignant duodenal obstruction with biliary stricture. Dig Endosc 2010;22(3):236–40.
42. Artifon EL, Takada J, Okawa L, et al. EUS-guided choledochoduodenostomy for biliary drainage in unresectable pancreatic cancer: a case series. JOP 2010; 11(6):597–600.
43. Belletrutti PJ, Gerdes H, Schattner MA. Successful endoscopic ultrasound-guided transduodenal biliary drainage through a pre-existing duodenal stent. JOP 2010;11(3):234–6.
44. Park DH, Jang JW, Lee SS, et al. EUS-guided biliary drainage with transluminal stenting after failed ERCP: predictors of adverse events and long-term results. Gastrointest Endosc 2011;74(6):1276–84.
45. Fabbri C, Luigiano C, Fuccio L, et al. EUS-guided biliary drainage with placement of a new partially covered biliary stent for palliation of malignant biliary obstruction: a case series. Endoscopy 2011;43(5):438–41.
46. Hara K, Yamao K, Niwa Y, et al. Prospective clinical study of EUS-guided choledochoduodenostomy for malignant lower biliary tract obstruction. Am J Gastroenterol 2011;106(7):1239–45.
47. Ramirez-Luna M, Tellez-Avila F, Giovannini M, et al. Endoscopic ultrasound-guided biliodigestive drainage is a good alternative in patients with unresectable cancer. Endoscopy 2011;43:826–30.
48. Siddiqui AA, Sreenarasimhaiah J, Lara LF, et al. Endoscopic ultrasound-guided transduodenal placement of a fully covered metal stent for palliative biliary drainage in patients with malignant biliary obstruction. Surg Endosc 2011; 25(2):549–55.
49. Komaki T, Kitano M, Sakamoto H, et al. Endoscopic ultrasonography-guided biliary drainage: evaluation of a choledochoduodenostomy technique. Pancreatology 2011;11(Suppl 2):47–51.
50. Prachayakul V, Aswakul P, Kachintorn U. EUS-guided choledochoduodenostomy for biliary drainage using tapered-tip plastic stent with multiple fangs. Endoscopy 2011;43(Suppl 2):E109–10.
51. Artifon EL, Ferreira FC, Sakai P. Endoscopic ultrasound-guided biliary drainage. Korean J Radiol 2012;13(Suppl 1):S74–82.
52. Attasaranya S, Netinasunton N, Jongboonyanuparp T, et al. The spectrum of endoscopic ultrasound intervention in biliary diseases: a single center's experience in 31 cases. Gastroenterol Res Pract 2012;2012:680753.
53. Katanuma A, Maguchi H, Osanai M, et al. Endoscopic ultrasound-guided biliary drainage performed for refractory bile duct stenosis due to chronic pancreatitis: a case report. Dig Endosc 2012;24(Suppl 1):34–7.

54. Kawakubo K, Isayama H, Nakai Y, et al. Simultaneous duodenal metal stent placement and EUS-guided choledochoduodenostomy for unresectable pancreatic cancer. Gut Liver 2012;6(3):399–402.
55. Khashab MA, Fujii LL, Baron TH, et al. EUS-guided biliary drainage for patients with malignant biliary obstruction with an indwelling duodenal stent (with videos). Gastrointest Endosc 2012;76(1):209–13.
56. Kim TH, Kim SH, Oh HJ, et al. Endoscopic ultrasound-guided biliary drainage with placement of a fully covered metal stent for malignant biliary obstruction. World J Gastroenterol 2012;18(20):2526–32.
57. Song TJ, Hyun YS, Lee SS, et al. Endoscopic ultrasound-guided choledochoduodenostomies with fully covered self-expandable metallic stents. World J Gastroenterol 2012;18(32):4435–40.
58. Dhir V, Bhandari S, Bapat M, et al. Comparison of EUS-guided rendezvous and precut papillotomy techniques for biliary access (with videos). Gastrointest Endosc 2012;75(2):354–9.
59. Park DH, Jeong SU, Lee BU, et al. Prospective evaluation of a treatment algorithm with enhanced guidewire manipulation protocol for EUS-guided biliary drainage after failed ERCP (with video). Gastrointest Endosc 2013;78(1):91–101.
60. Itoi T, Binmoeller K, Itokawa F, et al. Endoscopic ultrasonography-guided cholecystogastrostomy using a lumen-apposing metal stent as an alternative to extrahepatic bile duct drainage in pancreatic cancer with duodenal invasion. Dig Endosc 2013;25 Suppl 2:137–41.
61. Will U, Fueldner F, Kern C, et al. EUS-guided bile duct drainage (EUBD) in 95 patients. Ultraschall Med 2015;36(3):276–83.
62. Brückner S, Arlt A, Hampe J. Endoscopic ultrasound-guided biliary drainage using a lumen-apposing self-expanding metal stent: a case series. Endoscopy 2015;47(9):858–61.
63. Guo J, Sun S, Liu X, et al. Endoscopic ultrasound-guided biliary drainage using a fully covered metallic stent after failed endoscopic retrograde cholangiopancreatography. Gastroenterol Res Pract 2016;2016:9469472.
64. Makmun D, Fauzi A, Abdullah M, et al. The role of EUS-BD in the management of malignant biliary obstruction: the Indonesian perspective. Diagn Ther Endosc 2017;2017:4856276.
65. Rai P, Goel A. Endoscopic ultrasound-guided choledochoduodenostomy using partially-covered self-expandable metal stent in patients with malignant distal biliary obstruction and unsuccessful ERCP. Endosc Int Open 2018;6(1):E67–72.
66. Iwashita T, Yasuda I, Doi S, et al. Endoscopic ultrasound-guided antegrade treatments for biliary disorders in patients with surgically altered anatomy. Dig Dis Sci 2013;58(8):2417–22.
67. Imai H, Takenaka M, Omoto S, et al. Utility of endoscopic ultrasound-guided hepaticogastrostomy with antegrade stenting for malignant biliary obstruction after failed endoscopic retrograde cholangiopancreatography. Oncology 2017;93(1):69–75.
68. Ogura T, Kitano M, Takenaka M, et al. Multicenter prospective evaluation study of endoscopic ultrasound-guided hepaticogastrostomy combined with antegrade stenting (with video). Dig Endosc 2018;30(2):252–9.

Endoscopic Retrograde Cholangiopancreatography and Endoscopic Ultrasound-Guided Gallbladder Drainage

Habeeb Salameh, MD, MS, Christopher J. DiMaio, MD*

KEYWORDS

- Endoscopic ultrasound (EUS)
- Endoscopic retrograde cholangiopancreatography (ERCP) • Gallbladder drainage
- Cholecystitis

KEY POINTS

- Surgical cholecystectomy remains the gold-standard definitive therapy for management of acute cholecystitis.
- Percutaneous gallbladder drainage remains a widely available and effective alternative to surgery, particularly in critically ill patients.
- For patients who are not ideal candidates for either surgical or percutaneous gallbladder drainage, several endoscopic therapeutic options exist.
- Endoscopic retrograde cholangiopancreatography–guided transpapillary gallbladder drainage can allow for simultaneous therapy of choledocholithiasis and can provide safe, effective, and long-term drainage of the gallbladder.
- Endoscopic ultrasound–guided gallbladder drainage is an alternative minimally invasive endoscopic option for acute cholecystitis. This modality can allow for direct endoscopic cholecystoscopy and subsequent diagnostic and therapeutic maneuvers.

Gallbladder disease is one of the most common gastrointestinal diseases encountered in clinical practice. Traditionally, the gold standard for definitive treatment has been surgical intervention, namely cholecystectomy. When surgery is contraindicated or not feasible, percutaneous gallbladder drainage is a widely accepted, effective, and widely available treatment modality. Several endoscopic approaches exist as an alternative to either surgical or percutaneous intervention. These include transpapillary

Disclosure Statement: H. Salameh: No disclosures. C.J. DiMaio: Consultant/Teaching for Boston Scientific.
Icahn School of Medicine at Mount Sinai, Dr. Henry D. Janowitz Division of Gastroenterology, One Gustave L. Levy Place, Box 1069, New York, NY 10029, USA
* Corresponding author.
E-mail address: Christopher.DiMaio@MountSinai.org

Gastrointest Endoscopy Clin N Am 29 (2019) 293–310
https://doi.org/10.1016/j.giec.2018.12.002 **giendo.theclinics.com**
1052-5157/19/© 2018 Elsevier Inc. All rights reserved.

approaches via ERCP, transmural drainage and access approaches via endoscopic ultrasound (EUS), and endoscopic surgical approaches using natural orifice transluminal endoscopic surgery (NOTES) techniques. This article reviews the epidemiology and pathophysiology of gallbladder diseases and discusses the various percutaneous, surgical, and endoscopic approaches to managing gallbladder disease.

EPIDEMIOLOGY AND PATHOPHYSIOLOGY OF GALLBLADDER DISEASE

It is estimated that 12% of all US adults have gallstones with 1 million new cases annually.[1–3] Obesity, insulin resistance, and metabolic syndrome have contributed to the increase of gallstone disease in western countries. Seventy-five percent of all gallstones are of cholesterol type, 24.5% are pigment stones (20% black and 4.5% brown), and 0.5% rare stones.[4] These contribute to most of all cholecystectomies in the United States with acalculous/necrotizing cholecystitis accounting for 5% to 10%.[5]

Regardless of their type, all gallstones can result in cholecystitis when a stone embeds in the cystic duct and causes chronic obstruction.[6] There are differences in the underlying conditions or factors predisposing to the development of different types of stones. For example, cholesterol stones result from a complex interaction between hepatic cholesterol hypersecretion, gallbladder hypomotility, genetic factors, cholesterol rapid phase transitions, and intestinal factors. Increasing age, female sex, western diet, obesity, insulin resistance, diabetes mellitus, ileal diseases, rapid weight loss, total parenteral nutrition, biliary sludge, and variety of medications are all factors that have been implicated in the development of cholesterol gallstones.[4,7–16] Black pigment stones result from either hepatic bilirubin hypersecretion as seen in hemolysis or increased enterohepatic bilirubin circulation seen with chronic ileal diseases. Brown pigment stones result from biliary stasis and infections with pathogens such as *Escherichia coli*, Clonorchis sinensis, and roundworms.

Calculous cholecystitis is uncomplicated in most of the cases. However, severe complications can develop, including gangrenous cholecystitis (7%), empyema (6%), perforation (3%), and emphysematous disease (<1%).[17] Acalculous cholecystitis is seen in hospitalized and severely ill patients with prolonged fasting, immobility, and hemodynamic instability.[18–20] As calculous cholecystitis, a series of inflammatory conditions precedes gallbladder wall bacterial infection.[21] Although calculous cholecystitis is typically a disease of younger women, acalculous disease affects elderly patients more frequently. In contrast to calculous disease, almost half of acalculous cholecystitis patients have gangrenous or confined perforation by the time of diagnosis.[22,23] The mortality rate of acute acalculous cholecystitis is high (10%–50%) as compared with a 1% with calculous cholecystitis.[24]

Complications of cholecystitis and gallstones themselves vary in severity and outcomes. These include gangrenous cholecystitis in which vascular insufficiency and ischemia result in necrosis and perforation of the gallbladder wall with 15% to 50% mortality rate and Mirizzi syndrome in which a stone embeds in the neck of the gallbladder or cystic duct, causing extrinsic compression of the common hepatic duct resulting in bile duct obstruction (type I) and in some cases a fistula (type II) with 7% mortality rate.[25–30]

Large gallstones (>25 mm) may erode through the gallbladder wall into an adjacent enteric structure causing a cholecystoenteric fistula, with the duodenum being the most common site of fistulization. In some cases, the stone can migrate through the fistula and subsequently obstruct either the ileocecal valve resulting in small intestinal obstruction, known as gallstone ileus, or the duodenum, resulting in gastric outlet obstruction, known as Bouveret syndrome.[31,32] Unfortunately, diagnosis of gallstone ileus is often delayed and carries a 12% to 27% mortality.[33] Finally, gallstones are present in about 85% of patients with gallbladder cancer, with larger stones (>2–3 cm) having a higher association with gallbladder carcinoma.[34–38] The natural history of the disease supports prophylactic cholecystectomy in patients with very large stones ($\geq$3 cm) and perhaps elderly American Indian women with cholelithiasis.[38,39]

MANAGEMENT OF CHOLECYSTITIS

Traditional Approaches to Treating Cholecystitis

Antibiotic therapy

Physicians routinely place acute cholecystitis patients on antimicrobial therapy until the gallbladder is removed or the cholecystitis clinically resolves. This is likely due to fear of secondary gallbladder infection, which can progress into empyema, pericholecystic abscess, and life-threatening gram-negative sepsis. In a randomized clinical trial, intravenous antibiotics did not improve the hospital length of stay, rates of percutaneous cholecystostomy tube placement, or readmission rates in a cohort of mild acute calculus cholecystitis.[40] However, this remains controversial.[40–44] Current guidelines of the Infectious Disease Society of America suggest that patients with suspected infection (high white cell count >12.5–16$\times$10^3 per mm^3 or temperature >38.5°C), those with complicated gallbladder disease (eg, emphysematous, abscess, ischemia, or necrosis), older patients, and those with diabetes or immunodeficiency should receive antibiotics at the outset of diagnosis.[42,45]

The 2018 Tokyo guidelines for the management of acute cholangitis and cholecystitis recommend that selected antimicrobial therapy should cover gram-negative rods and anaerobes until the infection source is controlled (usually by surgical removal of the gallbladder) for mildly and moderately severe cholecystitis. Antibiotic therapy is extended for 4 to 7 days after source control in severe cholecystitis (those with end organ dysfunction) and for 2 weeks in health care associated biliary infections.[46]

Surgical approaches

When feasible, surgical cholecystectomy is the definitive gold-standard treatment option for cholecystitis and its complications. This is achieved through laparoscopic approach in nearly 90% of the cases in the United States. An open approach is usually reserved for patients with complicated disease.[47,48]

Open cholecystectomy The first known open cholecystectomy was performed by a Berlin surgeon, Karl Langenbuch, in 1882. Since then, symptomatic relief following surgery can be achieved in up to 95% of the cases.[49] It is associated with 4% to 5% perioperative morbidity.[50,51] Bile duct injury is the most dreaded adverse event with a rate of 1 in 200 to 600 cases.[52,53] The mortality rate associated with open cholecystectomy has decreased steadily over the last few decades. It is lower for patients operated for biliary pain (0.02%–0.5%) as compared with acute cholecystitis (0.26%–2.9%).[54–57] This rate increasess to 2.3% to 3.5% when there is need for concomitant bile duct exploration.[55,56] Overall, mortality rate is directly proportional to the patient's age, with cardiac diseases leading the cause of death.[56,57]

Laparoscopic cholecystectomy Over the last 4 decades, the laparoscopic approach has become the technique of choice for managing patients with biliary pain, cholecystitis and gallstone disease due to lower overall costs, morbidity and mortality, and quicker return to normal activities.[56,58–62] In a large series in the United States, rates of operative mortality was 0.06%, major morbidity was 5.4%, bile duct injury was 0.5%, and conversion to an open procedure was 2.2%.[63] Most elective cases were discharged home on the same day of the procedure and returned to full activities within 1 week.

On the introduction of laparoscopic cholecystectomy, there was an unacceptably high rate of bile duct injuries as compared with the historical rates with the open approach. However, as a surgeons gained more experience, the rate declined over time and is somewhat similar to the open approach.[64,65] The use of routine intraoperative cholangiography has resulted in lower bile duct injury rate.[66] Of note, the adoption of laparoscopic techniques resulted in 30% to 60% increase in the number of cholecystectomies performed over a short period of time without a clear and true increase in gallbladder diseases, suggesting that there has been an overutilization of this procedure, perhaps in the management of patients with unexplained abdominal pain or other weak indications.[62,67]

Percutaneous approaches

The primary goal of any surgical intervention is source control. However, in many critically ill and high surgical risk cholecystitis patients, surgery carries an unacceptably high risk of morbidity and mortality. In such patients, 2 interventional percutaneous transhepatic gallbladder drainage (PTGBD) approaches provide such source control with low morbidity and mortality. These include percutaneous transhepatic gallbladder aspiration (PTGBA) and percutaneous transhepatic cholecystostomy tube placement (PTCT). They provide bridge therapy to an elective and delayed cholecystectomy when patient's surgical risks improve.[68,69] Contraindications to interventional approaches include massive ascites and severe coagulopathy.

Percutaneous transhepatic cholecystostomy tube placement Percutaneous cholecystostomy tube placement, typically performed with a local anesthetic or under moderate sedation, allows gallbladder decompression, collection of bile for Gram stain and culture, and cholangiography to assess for concomitant bile duct obstruction. A systematic review reported technical success, clinical success, and the adverse events rates of 98%, 90%, and 3.7%, respectively.[70] Such an approach can be used in calculous cholecystitis for percutaneous stone extraction after maturation and dilation of the tract. Unfortunately, 10-year stone recurrence rate can be up to 40%.[71]

Percutaneous transhepatic gallbladder aspiration An even less invasive approach as compared with PTCT is simple aspiration of the gallbladder. A systematic review reported technical success, clinical success, and adverse events rates of 93%, 83%, and 0.8%, respectively.[70] A more recent analysis of 7 studies on PTGBA found that source control success rate was higher with repetitive aspiration, as compared with single aspiration (76%–96% vs 50%–93%), with low procedure-related morbidity 2%.[72] Only 10% of patients required salvage percutaneous cholecystostomy, and 1% needed urgent surgery. When antibiotics were instilled during aspiration procedure, clinical success rate was 95% to 96%.[72]

Endoscopic Approaches

For patients in whom surgical risk is high and when percutaneous drainage is contraindicated due to coagulopathy, or ascites, endoscopic approaches to gallbladder drainage can provide a good alternative management strategy.[73] Endoscopic gallbladder treatment can be performed with transpapillary approaches via ERCP, transmural drainage and access approaches via EUS, and endoscopic surgical approaches using NOTES techniques (**Table 1**).

ERCP (transpapillary)-guided gallbladder drainage

This technique was first reported in 1990 and uses standard ERCP techniques.[74] The bile duct is cannulated in the usual fashion and an obliquely angled guidewire

Table 1
Endoscopic approaches for managing gallbladder disease

ERCP (transpapillary)-guided gallbladder drainage	Nasogallbladder drain (NGBD)	
	Transpapillary cystic duct stent (TPCDS)	
EUS-guided gallbladder drainage	Nasogallbladder drain (NGBD)	
	Transmural stents	Plastic stents (PS)
		Self-expanding metal stents (SEMS)
		Lumen-apposing metal stents (LAMS)
	Direct cholecystoscopy	Gastrocholecystostomy
		Duodenocholecystostomy
NOTES		

is advanced to the cystic duct and into the gall bladder where it is coiled. Two drainage methods have been described. In nasogallbladder drainage (NGBD), a nasobiliary catheter is advanced over the guidewire to drain the gallbladder. This catheter can also be used to flush and irrigate the gallbladder. The other method is transpapillary cystic duct stent (TPCDS) placement. In the latter approach, a dilatation catheter can be used to fragment any residual cystic duct stones and then a transcystic double pigtail catheter is placed over the guidewire with one end in the gallbladder and the other end in the duodenum (**Fig. 1**). A systematic review reported technical success, clinical success, and adverse events rates in endoscopic NGBD (n = 194) and TPCDS (n = 127): 81%, 75%, and 3.6% versus 96%, 88%, and 6.3%, respectively.[70]

More recently, a retrospective analysis of consecutive TPCDS in a referral center reported a technical success rate of 76% and a sustained clinical response rate on a mean follow-up of 1 year of 90% without any reported periprocedural complications.[75] Another retrospective study evaluated similar outcomes of TPCDS in 46 elderly patients (>65 years) with acute cholecystitis in a Japanese referral center.[76] Technical success rate was 77.5% without any immediate postprocedural complications.[76] Cholecystitis recurrence rate was low at 3.3% and most patients (93.5%) remained asymptomatic until death or the end of the study period (1 month–5 years).[76] A report

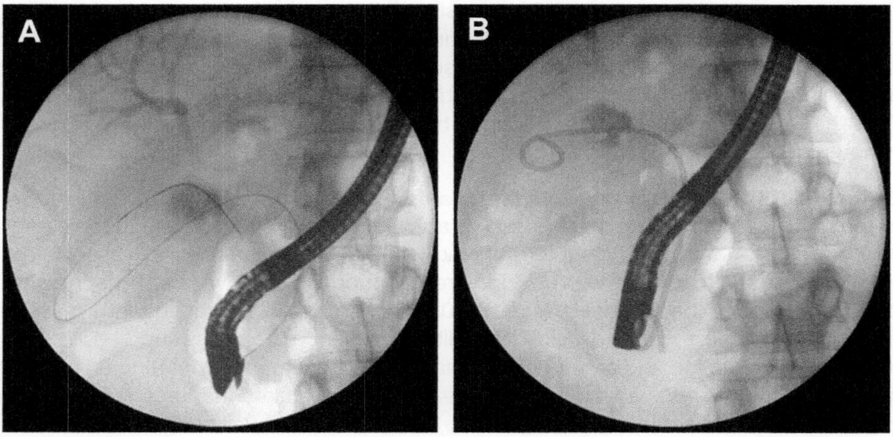

Fig. 1. ERCP-guided transpapillary wire placement (*A*) and transcystic stent placement (*B*) for gallbladder drainage.

of prospectively collected data from 2 tertiary referral centers using TPCDS in 29 patients with symptomatic gallbladder disease who were poor surgical candidates showed technical success rate of 79.3% and a mean procedure time of 22.4 minutes. Mild pancreatitis (8.7%) and cholestasis (8.7%) were the main adverse events. Late adverse events include distal stent migration (10%), cholangitis (5%), and recurrent biliary pain (5%). Median stent patency was 760 days.[77]

Overall, the technical success rate is relatively low and is likely due to difficulty in accessing the cystic duct using standard fluoroscopic guidance. Peroral cholangioscopy can improve direct visualization of the cystic duct take-off and subsequent advancement of a wire into the gallbladder under direct visualization, thus facilitating NGBD and cystic duct stent placement.[76,78–82]

Nasogallbladder drain versus transpapillary cystic duct stent In one randomized control trial (RCT) comparing NGBD and TPCDS for patients with acute cholecystitis, the overall rates of technical success (91.9% vs 86.1%), clinical success (86.5% vs 77.8%), adverse events (5.4% vs 2.7%), and mean procedure time (20.3 minutes vs 22.2 minutes) were statistically similar in both arms.[83] In another RCT no significant differences were found between the NGBD and TPCDS groups in the rates of technical success, clinical success, and adverse events (82.4%, 70.6%, and 17.6% vs 88.9%, 83.3%, and 12.5%, respectively), with similar procedure times between both arms.[84]

Each method has its own advantages. TPCDS allows for internalized drainage, without need for nasodrainage tubes. On the other hand, NGBD allows for irrigation of the gallbladder, whether with normal saline or 1% N-acetylcysteine, and removal of debris is possible.[83,85,86] However, NGBD is associated with higher postprocedure pain.[83]

Transpapillary cystic duct stent versus percutaneous transhepatic gallbladder drainage When TPCDS was compared with percutaneous gallbladder drainage, technical success rate was similar but cholecystitis recurrence rate was higher in the percutaneous approach (17.2%) as compared with the endoscopic one (0%) with overall biliary event rate of 24.1% versus 9.1%, respectively.[87] Another study showed that the endoscopic approach was associated with shorter hospitalization as compared with percutaneous drainage.[88]

Endoscopic ultrasound–guided transmural drainage

Transpapillary techniques may not be feasible if the cystic duct cannot be opacified during a cholangiogram and/or the guidewire cannot be advanced through the cystic duct due to tortuosity or obstruction. In such cases, EUS-guided approaches can achieve source control and gallbladder drainage. Since it was first described in 2007,[89] EUS-guided gallbladder drainage has gained increasing popularity and with various technical approaches available.

Endoscopic ultrasound–nasogallbladder drains Given the proximity of the gallbladder to the gastrointestinal tract on endosonography, endoscopists can introduce needles into the gallbladder under Doppler imaging while avoiding interposing vessels. The initial puncture is made at the prepyloric area or duodenal bulb with a 19-gauge needle. Cultures can be obtained and a 0.035-inch guidewire subsequently passed through the needle and coiled inside the gallbladder. Once the wire is secured in place, the needle is removed and a 6-Fr or 7-Fr biliary bougie dilator or a triple-lumen needle-knife with a 7-Fr shaft is advanced over the guidewire to dilate the tract. A 5-Fr nasobiliary drainage tube can be advanced into the gallbladder over the guidewire.[90,91]

Two recent pooled analyses of different modalities of EUS-guided transmural drainage showed cumulative EUS-NGBD technical and clinical success rates of

98% to 100% and 95% to 100% with adverse event rates of 10% to 12.5%.[92,93] Data on treatment duration, long-term follow-up, or cholecystitis recurrence are lacking.[92] Patency of these drains can be maintained by flushing and irrigation.[90]

There is risk of bile leakage associated with this approach due to the presence of free space between the gallbladder and the stomach or duodenum and the need to dilate the tract to a size larger than the nasobiliary tube.[94–96] However, none of the 2 large series reported such complication or biliary peritonitis.[90,91] This is likely due to the adherence of the inflamed gallbladder wall to the adjacent structures and the use of small diameter catheters minimizing this risk.[90,91] Another self-limiting complication reported was pneumoperitoneum.[90,91]

Endoscopic ultrasound–plastic stents The technique here follows similar principles to the EUS-NGBD technique mentioned earlier. After securing the guide wire in the gallbladder, the tract can be dilated using a dilation balloon or biliary bougie dilation catheters or by using a microtome, cystoenterostome, or cystotome with cutting current. Subsequently, a 7-Fr or 8.5-Fr straight or double pigtail PS can be deployed over the guidewire.[89,97–100]

Two recent pooled analyses of different modalities of EUS-guided transmural drainage showed cumulative EUS-PS technical and clinical success rates of 100% and adverse events rate of 16% to 18.2%.[92,93] Mean follow-up period was less than 6 months without cholecystitis recurrence.[92] Reported complications include bile leak and peritonitis, stent migration, and pneumoperitoneum.[97–99] Double pigtail plastic stents are preferred, and these are less likely to migrate compared with straight stents.[92]

Endoscopic ultrasound–self-expanding metal stents The technique here follows similar principles to EUS-NGBD and EUS-PS techniques except for the last step in which a self-expanding metal stents (SEMS) is advanced over the guidewire and deployed. The length of the SEMS is determined based on the thickness of the interposed tissue with an extra 1 to 1.5 cm to secure the stent in the gallbladder.[96,101–103]

Two recent pooled analyses of different modalities of EUS-guided transmural drainage reported cumulative EUS-SEMS technical and clinical success rates of 99% to 100% with adverse events rate of 6% to 12.3%.[92,93] Recurrence of gallbladder disease was reported in 2% of the cases with an overall follow-up period, while the stent was still in place, of less than 9 months.[92] Reported complications include pneumoperitoneum and duodenal perforation.[96,101] However, SEMS allow the use of coaxial double pigtail PS to maintain its position and patency or nasogallbladder drainage catheters to irrigate and flush out thick bile content.[101–103] Another advantage is the lower theoretic risk for bile leak or peritonitis because these stents expand and seal the tract between the gallbladder and the stomach/duodenum and they have a larger diameter, which allows longer patency time due to lower chance of being occluded by the thick and/or purulent bile.[96,101,102]

Long-term data of EUS-SEMS approach, although scarce, are promising. In one retrospective study in which 56 surgically unsuitable patients with acute calculous cholecystitis underwent EUS-SEMS, 4% had acute cholecystitis recurrence.[101] These were due to food impaction in one patient and stent fracture in another patient. Stent patency of 190 days was reported over a median follow-up of 275 days.[101] More recently, Kamata and colleagues[104] reported 100% technical and clinical success rate and 0% adverse events when SEMS were removed at 4 weeks or replaced with double pigtail plastic stents. Early removal and replacement may have helped in avoiding stent migration and cholecystitis recurrence due to food impaction.[104]

Lumen-apposing metal stents The most recent development in the technique of EUS-guided gallbladder drainage is the use of lumen-apposing metal stents (LAMS). These stents were originally designed for EUS-guided drainage of pancreatic fluid collections. However, given the similarity in endoscopic technique, there has been rapid adoption of using them for EUS-guided gallbladder drainage. These short, "dumbbell-shaped" fully covered metal stents are designed such that on deployment, the 2flanges of the stent bring the gallbladder wall in close contact with the stomach/ duodenum wall (**Fig. 2**). This has the advantage of minimizing leakage into the peritoneum and facilitating rapid fistula formation. In addition, the radial force applied by the expanding stent may theoretically provide a tamponade effect and minimize tract site bleeding. Lastly, the LAMS deployment system is designed to allow for quick and simple stent placement, thus avoiding the need for numerous needle and device exchanges over a wire. LAMS come in a variety of diameters, all of which are larger than plastic stents. This has the potential advantage of rapid drainage of the gallbladder. In addition, the LAMS luminal diameter is wide enough to allow passage of the scope across it directly into the gallbladder lumen, thus allowing further diagnostic or therapeutic maneuvers.

There are multiple types of LAMS available, all with the same basic design as previously described. In the United States, there is only one available LAMS system (Axios, Boston Scientific, Natick, MA, USA), and it is only Food and Drug Administration–approved for EUS-guided drainage of pancreatic fluid collections. Two versions of these are available; the earliest version is commonly referred to as the "Cold LAMS," whereas the newer version is electrocautery-enhanced and

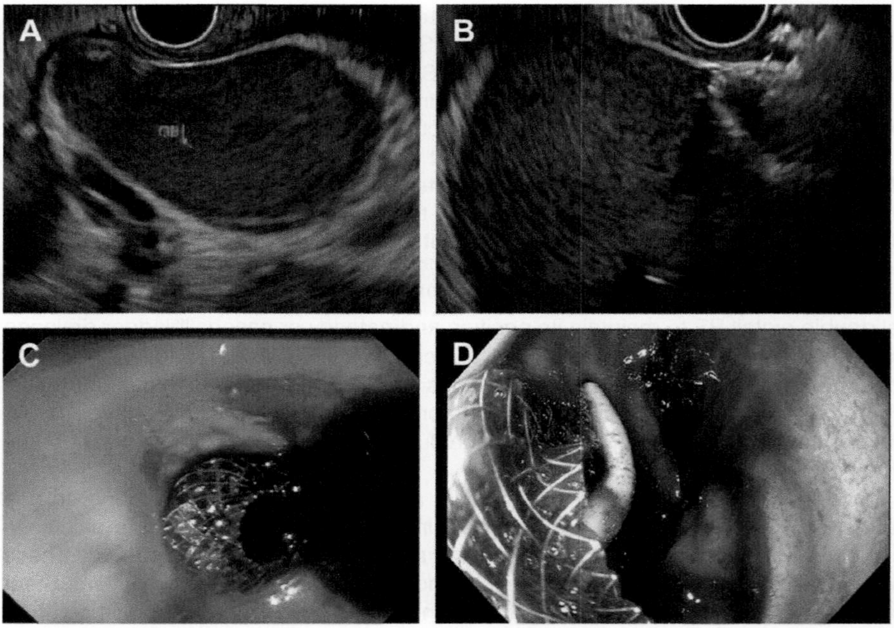

Fig. 2. EUS-guided transduodenal cholecystoduodenostomy for gallbladder drainage. A distended, debris-filled gallbladder in close proximity to the duodenal bulb (*A*). EUS-guided placement of an LAMS (*B*) with subsequent drainage into the gastrointestinal lumen (*C*). A coaxial double pigtail plastic stent is placed to maintain patency of the LAMS and decrease risk of bleeding (*D*).

commonly referred to as “Hot LAMS.” Placement of LAMS follows the same technique as have been previously described for other EUS-guided gallbladder drainage procedures. EUS-guided needle puncture of the gallbladder is performed. A long guidewire is inserted through the needle, and the needle is exchanged over the wire. Tract dilation can be performed using bougies, balloons, or cystotomes. The LAMS deployment system is then advanced over the guidewire and deployed. The Hot LAMS can be placed without need for tract dilation, because the electrocautery-enhanced tip delivers a cutting current to provide easy puncture across the stomach/duodenal wall. Hot LAMS can be placed using a freehand technique, without prior needle puncture or guidewire placement.[105,106] At the discretion of the endoscopist, a continuous radial expansion balloon dilator can be inflated within the LAMS lumen to achieve rapid expansion and prevent potential dislodgement while immediate therapeutic maneuvers through the stent are attempted.[106]

Two recent pooled analyses examining various modalities of EUS-guided transmural drainage showed cumulative EUS-LAMS technical and clinical success rates of 93% to 96% and 90% to 93%, respectively with adverse events rate of 7% to 10%.[92,93] Recurrence rate of gallbladder disease was 0% amongst 16 cases that were followed-up to 5 months.[92] Postprocedure complications included fever, abdominal pain, aspiration pneumonia, pancreatitis, hemobilia, stent migration, and bleeding.[105,107–110] The latter is the most serious complication and can be fatal at times.

Long-term data have been reported with EUS-LAMS in 1 prospective and 2 retrospective studies.[108,109,111] In their prospective study of patients with acute cholecystitis deemed too high risk for surgery, Walter and colleagues[109] reported recurrent cholecystitis in 2 out of 30 patients after 1-year follow-up. A retrospective study by Irani and colleagues[108] reported no disease recurrence or stent occlusion in 15 patients with various gall bladder diseases after a median follow-up of 5 months. However, a retrospective study from Dollhopf and colleagues[111] demonstrated that complications occurred in 6 out of 50 patients, including recurrent cholecystitis in 3 patients, stent migration in 2 patients, and Bouveret syndrome in 1 patient. Garcia-Alonso and colleagues[105] studied bleeding and stent migration risks in 250 patients who underwent LAMS placement for pancreatic fluid collections, gallbladder disease, biliary obstruction, and enteral anastomotic strictures. Median follow-up period was 78.5 days. They estimated that LAMSs placed for longer durations for enteral anastomoses and biliary and gallbladder drainage indications had 8.4% stent migration risk at 12 months as compared with 48.9% for patients with pancreatic fluid collections. There were a total of 13 LAMS-related gastrointestinal hemorrhages (5.2%): 2 of them were fatal, presenting a median of 3 days with cumulative 12 months risk of 6.9%.[105]

One unique issue with LAMS is that the tissue overgrowth can occur at the proximal flange, resulting in the stent becoming embedded or “buried” in the lumen wall.[107,112,113] Endoscopic retrieval of a buried LAMS is possible with the assistance of forced argon plasma coagulation, needle-knife incision, dilation of the stent, and traction removal using a Rat-tooth forceps to remove the stent either from the enteral side or in an inside-out fashion after dilating the tract to allow cholecystoscopy.[107,113] It has been suggested that LAMS placement at the gastric antral location may induce rapid development of tissue overgrowth due to the presence of vigorous gastric contractions and thus might be to blame as the reason for buried LAMS and outward migration. Placement of a double-pigtail plastic stent across the LAMS may help in prevention of such complications if an antral location cannot be avoided.[107]

One unique aspect of LAMS is that they can be used as a conduit for direct cholecystoscopy through either a gastrocholecystostomy or a duodenocholecystostomy. As previously mentioned, the luminal diameter of LAMS is such that an ultraslim, standard, or even a therapeutic gastroscope (with larger LAMS diameters) can be inserted directly into the gallbladder allowing for diagnostic examination, irrigation and lavage, electrohyrdaulic or laser lithotripsy of stones, as well as stone extraction.[106,110,114–116] Cholecystoscopy can be done immediately after LAMS deployment,[110,116,117] weeks after deployment,[118] or after fistula tract maturation and LAMS retrieval.[119] Finally, SEMS, PS, or PS-in-SEMS can be inserted coaxially through the LAMS lumen to prevent dislodgement or migration especially in patients with very thick gallbladder walls or when position stability is in question.[96,98,101–103,106,107,120] However, others argue against usefulness of such approaches in decreasing risk of either bleeding or migration.[121]

Cholecystectomy following Endoscopic ultrasound-GBD

Given the lack of extensive short-term and long-term data, it remains unclear what the impact of EUS-gallbladder drainage, particularly with LAMS, has on subsequent surgical intervention. Some suggested that the fistula created by transduodenal EUS-GBD approaches may interfere with subsequent cholecystectomy as compared with those created by transgastric ones.[92,122] However, limited data suggest that transgastric small drainage catheters, namely EUS-NGBD drains, may carry less effects on subsequent cholecystectomy as compared with percutaneous drainage approach.[90] Baron and colleagues[123,124] reported a case of a complicated posttransplant course in a cirrhotic patient who underwent LAMS for purulent cholecystitis almost 6 months before her transplant. She had a challenging transplant procedure due to difficult dissection, and duodenal defect closure, and developed posttransplant leak and abscess. Subsequently, she had hepatic artery pseudoaneurysm and required bypass graft that was complicate with graft thrombosis. Eventually, she was stabilized and leak healed after total parenteral nutrition.[123] With these reports, data on feasibility and outcomes of surgical procedures including cholecystectomy and transplant are still limited. Larger observational studies are needed to identify whether a transgastric or transduodenal GBD are similar in outcomes and whether drain size and duration after GBD have any effects on surgical outcomes.

Natural Orifice Transluminal Endoscopic Surgery

The final frontier of endoscopic management of gallbladder disease involves endoscopic removal of the organ using an entry tract through the gastrointestinal lumen. In NOTES, the endoscopist uses a transgastric, transrectal, or transvaginal approach to obtain access to the peritoneal cavity, allowing for minimally invasive cholecystectomy. This technique avoids cutaneous scarring and may result in less pain because the surgical sample is not extracted through the skin.[125]

The first NOTES cholecystectomy was reported by Tsin and colleagues[126] in 2003 when a transvaginal approach was used. Since then multiple groups have reported on better aesthetic outcomes, shorter procedure duration, shorter hospital stay, and less pain with NOTES as compared with standard laparoscopic approach.[127–131] However, 2 randomized controlled trials showed no differences in postoperative pain, hospital stay, or adverse events.[132,133] In addition, NOTES was associated with longer procedure duration when using a transvaginal approach[133] or a flexible endoscope.[132] Of note, there are no reports of sexual dysfunction following the transvaginal approach.[132,134]

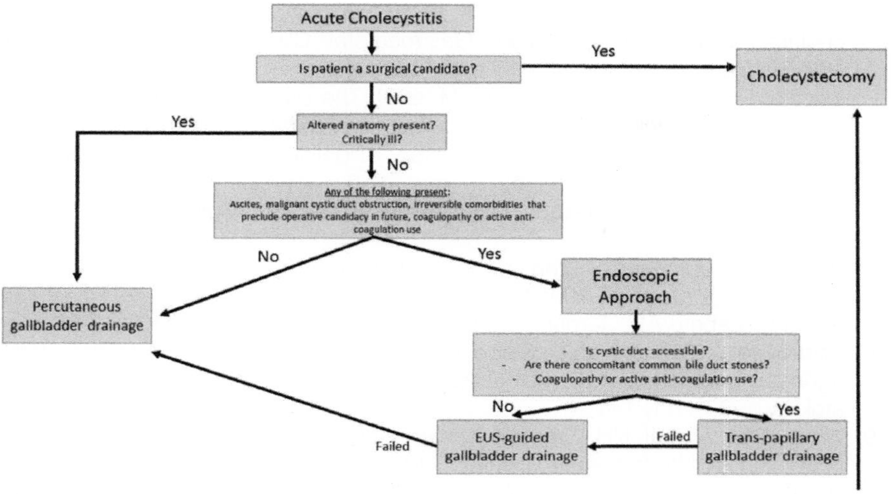

Fig. 3. Suggested algorithm for cholecystitis management. For abbreviations refer to **Table 1**. CCY, cholecystectomy.

NOTES remains in its infancy, because its widespread adoption and dissemination is severely limited by the expected technical difficulties due to the absence of dedicated NOTES scopes and accessories.[125]

SUMMARY

Gallbladder disease is one of the most common gastrointestinal conditions facing health care providers and can be associated with significant morbidity and mortality. In patients who are appropriate surgical candidates, surgical cholecystectomy remains the gold-standard, first-line, definitive therapy for cholecystitis. For patients who are not deemed appropriate for surgery, multiple other management options exist. Percutaneous gallbladder drainage has the advantage of being relatively safe, very effective, and widely available. However, the need for chronic indwelling catheters in a subset of patients can limit the overall attractiveness of this approach. Endoscopic management options include ERCP-guided transpapillary gallbladder drainage and EUS-guided transmural gallbladder drainage and have the advantage of providing internal, physiologic drainage. At this time, it remains unclear which method is more effective or safer and which has the best overall long-term clinical outcomes. The authors suggest the following algorithm for managing acute cholecystitis patients (**Fig. 3**). NOTES cholecystectomy is an emerging endoscopic management option but remains in its infancy due to lack of dedicated scopes and accessories. It remains to be seen whether any of these endoscopic approaches can be deemed definitive management strategies, because robust, prospective, long-term data are sorely lacking. Until further studies are performed, endoscopic gallbladder drainage will likely remain limited to experienced endoscopists at tertiary referral centers.

REFERENCES

1. Krawczyk M, Wang DW, Portincasa P, et al. Semin Liv Dis 2011;31:157–72.

2. Wang HH, Portincasa P, Afdhal NH, et al. Lith genes and genetic analysis of cholesterol gallstone formation. Gastroenterol Clin North Am 2010;39(2):185–207.
3. Sandler RS, Everhart JE, Donowitz M, et al. The burden of selected digestive diseases in the United States. Gastroenterology 2002;122(5):1500–11.
4. Diehl A. Epidemiology and natural history of gallstone disease. Gastroenterol Clin North Am 1991;20(1):1–19.
5. Barie PS, Fischer E. Acute acalculous cholecystitis. J Am Coll Surg 1995;180(2):232–44.
6. Turner MA, Fulcher AS. The cystic duct: normal anatomy and disease processes. Radiographics 2001;21(1):3–22.
7. Sama C, Labate AM, Taroni F, Barabara L. Semin Liv Dis 1990;10:149–58.
8. Valdivieso V, Covarrubias C, Siegel F, et al. Pregnancy and cholelithiasis: pathogenesis and natural course of gallstones diagnosed in early puerperium. Hepatology 1993;17(1):1–4.
9. Wang DQ, Afdhal NH. Genetic analysis of cholesterol gallstone formation: searching for Lith (gallstone) genes. Curr Gastroenterol Rep 2004;6(2):140–50.
10. Tsai C-J, Leitzmann M, Willett W, et al. Central adiposity, regional fat distribution, and the risk of cholecystectomy in women. Gut 2006;55(5):708–14.
11. Nervi F, Miquel JF, Alvarez M, et al. Gallbladder disease is associated with insulin resistance in a high risk Hispanic population. J Hepatol 2006;45(2):299–305.
12. Ruhl CE, Everhart JE. Association of diabetes, serum insulin, and c-peptide with gallbladder disease. Hepatology 2000;31(2):299–303.
13. Lapidus A, Bångstad M, Åström M, et al. The prevalence of gallstone disease in a defined cohort of patients with Crohn's disease. Am J Gastroenterol 1999;94(5):1261–6.
14. Shiffman ML, Sugerman HJ, Kellum JM, et al. Gallstone formation after rapid weight loss: a prospective study in patients undergoing gastric bypass surgery for treatment of morbid obesity. Am J Gastroenterol 1991;86(8):1000–5.
15. Pitt HA, King W III, Mann LL, et al. Increased risk of cholelithiasis with prolonged total parenteral nutrition. Am J Surg 1983;145(1):106–12.
16. Lee SP, Maher K, Nicholls JF. Origin and fate of biliary sludge. Gastroenterology 1988;94(1):170–6.
17. Bedirli A, Sakrak O, Sözüer EM, et al. Factors effecting the complications in the natural history of acute cholecystitis. Hepatogastroenterology 2001;48(41):1275–8.
18. Warren B. Small vessel occlusion in acute acalculous cholecystitis. Surgery 1992;111(2):163–8.
19. Hakala T, Nuutinen P, Ruokonen E, et al. Microangiopathy in acute acalculous cholecystitis. Br J Surg 1997;84(9):1249–52.
20. Lee SP. Pathogenesis of biliary sludge. Hepatology 1990;12(3 Pt 2):200S–3S [discussion: 203S–5S].
21. Claesson B, Holmlund D, Mätzsch TW. Microflora of the gallbladder related to duration of acute cholecystitis. Surg Gynecol Obstet 1986;162(6):531–5.
22. Barie PS, Eachempati SR. Acute acalculous cholecystitis. Gastroenterol Clin North Am 2010;39(2):343–57.
23. Huffman JL, Schenker S. Acute acalculous cholecystitis: a review. Clin Gastroenterol Hepatol 2010;8(1):15–22.
24. Boland GW, Lee MJ, Leung J, et al. Percutaneous cholecystostomy in critically ill patients: early response and final outcome in 82 patients. AJR Am J Roentgenol 1994;163(2):339–42.

25. Stefanidis D, Bingener J, Richards M, et al. Gangrenous cholecystitis in the decade before and after the introduction of laparoscopic cholecystectomy. JSLS 2005;9(2):169.
26. Önder A, Kapan M, Ülger BV, et al. Gangrenous cholecystitis: mortality and risk factors. Int Surg 2015;100(2):254–60.
27. Abou-Saif A, Al-Kawas FH. Complications of gallstone disease: Mirizzi syndrome, cholecystocholedochal fistula, and gallstone ileus. Am J Gastroenterol 2002;97(2):249.
28. Yeh C-N, Jan Y-Y, Chen M-F. Laparoscopic treatment for Mirizzi syndrome. Surg Endosc 2003;17(10):1573–8.
29. McSherry C. The Mirizzi syndrome: suggested classification and surgical therapy. Surg Gastroenterol 1982;1:219–25.
30. Gomez D, Rahman SH, Toogood GJ, et al. Mirizzi's syndrome–results from a large western experience. HPB (Oxford) 2006;8(6):474–9.
31. Lassandro F, Gagliardi N, Scuderi M, et al. Gallstone ileus analysis of radiological findings in 27 patients. Eur J Radiol 2004;50(1):23–9.
32. Gencosmanoglu R, Inceoglu R, Baysal C, et al. Bouveret's syndrome complicated by a distal gallstone ileus. World J Gastroenterol 2003;9(12):2873.
33. Ravikumar R, Williams JG. The operative management of gallstone ileus. Ann R Coll Surg Engl 2010;92(4):279–81.
34. Shaffer EA. Gallbladder cancer: the basics. Gastroenterol Hepatol 2008;4(10): 737.
35. Csendes A, Becerra M, Rojas J, et al. Number and size of stones in patients with asymptomatic and symptomatic gallstones and gallbladder carcinoma: a prospective study of 592 cases. J Gastrointest Surg 2000;4(5):481–5.
36. Moerman C, Lagerwaard F, De Mesquita HB, et al. Gallstone size and the risk of gallbladder cancer. Scand J Gastroenterol 1993;28(6):482–6.
37. Lowenfels A, Walker A, Althaus D, et al. Gallstone growth, size, and risk of gallbladder cancer: an interracial study. Int J Epidemiol 1989;18(1):50–4.
38. Diehl AK. Gallstone size and the risk of gallbladder cancer. JAMA 1983;250(17): 2323–6.
39. Sheth S, Bedford A, Chopra S. Primary gallbladder cancer: recognition of risk factors and the role of prophylactic cholecystectomy. Am J Gastroenterol 2000;95(6):1402.
40. Mazeh H, Mizrahi I, Dior U, et al. Role of antibiotic therapy in mild acute calculus cholecystitis: a prospective randomized controlled trial. World J Surg 2012; 36(8):1750–9.
41. Kanafani ZA, Khalife N, Kanj SS, et al. Antibiotic use in acute cholecystitis: practice patterns in the absence of evidence-based guidelines. J Infect 2005;51(2): 128–34.
42. Solomkin JS, Mazuski JE, Bradley JS, et al. Diagnosis and management of complicated intra-abdominal infection in adults and children: guidelines by the Surgical Infection Society and the Infectious Diseases Society of America. Clin Infect Dis 2010;50(2):133–64.
43. Strasberg SM. Clinical practice. Acute calculous cholecystitis. N Engl J Med 2008;358(26):2804–11.
44. Fuks D, Cosse C, Regimbeau JM. Antibiotic therapy in acute calculous cholecystitis. J Visc Surg 2013;150(1):3–8.
45. Landau O, Kott I, Deutsch AA, et al. Multifactorial analysis of septic bile and septic complications in biliary surgery. World J Surg 1992;16(5):962–4 [discussion: 964–5].

46. Gomi H, Solomkin JS, Schlossberg D, et al. Tokyo Guidelines 2018: antimicrobial therapy for acute cholangitis and cholecystitis. J Hepatobiliary Pancreat Sci 2018;25(1):3–16.
47. Dolan JP, Diggs BS, Sheppard BC, et al. The national mortality burden and significant factors associated with open and laparoscopic cholecystectomy: 1997–2006. J Gastrointest Surg 2009;13(12):2292.
48. Livingston EH, Rege RV. A nationwide study of conversion from laparoscopic to open cholecystectomy. Am J Surg 2004;188(3):205–11.
49. Berger M, Olde Hartman T, Bohnen A. Abdominal symptoms: do they disappear after cholecystectomy? Surg Endosc 2003;17(11):1723–8.
50. Keus F, Gooszen H, Van Laarhoven C. Systematic review: open, small-incision or laparoscopic cholecystectomy for symptomatic cholecystolithiasis. Aliment Pharmacol Ther 2009;29(4):359–78.
51. Wolf AS, Nijsse BA, Sokal SM, et al. Surgical outcomes of open cholecystectomy in the laparoscopic era. Am J Surg 2009;197(6):781–4.
52. Kune GA. Bile duct injury during cholecystectomy: causes, prevention and surgical repair in 1979. Aust N Z J Surg 1979;49(1):35–40.
53. Hermann RE. A plea for a safer technique of cholecystectomy. Surgery 1976; 79(6):609–11.
54. Arnold DJ. 28,621 cholecystectomies in Ohio: results of a survey in Ohio hospitals by the Gallbladder Survey Committee, Ohio Chapter, American College of Surgeons. Am J Surg 1970;119(6):714–7.
55. Bredesen J, Jørgensen T, Andersen T, et al. Early postoperative mortality following cholecystectomy in the entire female population of Denmark, 1977–1981. World J Surg 1992;16(3):530–5.
56. McSHERRY CK, Glenn F. The incidence and causes of death following surgery for nonmalignant biliary tract disease. Ann Surg 1980;191(3):271.
57. Roslyn JJ, Binns GS, Hughes E, et al. Open cholecystectomy. A contemporary analysis of 42,474 patients. Ann Surg 1993;218(2):129.
58. Johansson M, Thune A, Nelvin L, et al. Randomized clinical trial of open versus laparoscopic cholecystectomy in the treatment of acute cholecystitis. Br J Surg 2005;92(1):44–9.
59. McMAHON AJ, Russell IT, Ramsay G, et al. Laparoscopic and minilaparotomy cholecystectomy: a randomized trial comparing postoperative pain and pulmonary function. Surgery 1994;115(5):533–9.
60. Soper NJ, Barteau JA, Clayman RV, et al. Comparison of early postoperative results for laparoscopic versus standard open cholecystectomy. Surg Gynecol Obstet 1992;174(2):114–8.
61. Trondsen E, Reiertsen O, Andersen O, et al. Laparoscopic and open cholecystectomy. A prospective, randomized study. Eur J Surg 1993;159(4):217–21.
62. Steiner CA, Bass EB, Talamini MA, et al. Surgical rates and operative mortality for open and laparoscopic cholecystectomy in Maryland. N Engl J Med 1994; 330(6):403–8.
63. MacFadyen B, Vecchio R, Ricardo A, et al. Bile duct injury after laparoscopic cholecystectomy. Surg Endosc 1998;12(4):315–21.
64. Moore MJ, Bennett CL. The learning curve for laparoscopic cholecystectomy. Am J Surg 1995;170(1):55–9.
65. Woods MS, Traverso LW, Kozarek RA, et al. Characteristics of biliary tract complications during laparoscopic cholecystectomy: a multi-institutional study. Am J Surg 1994;167(1):27–34.

66. Ludwig K, Bernhardt J, Steffen H, et al. Contribution of intraoperative cholangiography to incidence and outcome of common bile duct injuries during laparoscopic cholecystectomy. Surg Endosc 2002;16(7):1098–104.
67. Legorreta AP, Silber JH, Costantino GN, et al. Increased cholecystectomy rate after the introduction of laparoscopic cholecystectomy. JAMA 1993;270(12):1429–32.
68. Leveau P, Andersson E, Carlgren I, et al. Percutaneous cholecystostomy: a bridge to surgery or definite management of acute cholecystitis in high-risk patients? Scand J Gastroenterol 2008;43(5):593–6.
69. Macri A, Scuderi G, Saladino E, et al. Acute gallstone cholecystitis in the elderly. Surg Endosc 2006;20(1):88–91.
70. Itoi T, Coelho-Prabhu N, Baron TH. Endoscopic gallbladder drainage for management of acute cholecystitis. Gastrointest Endosc 2010;71(6):1038–45.
71. Zou Y-P, Du J-D, Li W-M, et al. Gallstone recurrence after successful percutaneous cholecystolithotomy: a 10-year follow-up of 439 cases. Hepatobiliary Pancreat Dis Int 2007;6(2):199–203.
72. Rassameehiran S, Tantrachoti P, Nugent K. Proc (Bayl Univ Med Cent) 2016;29:381–4.
73. Venara A, Carretier V, Lebigot J, et al. Technique and indications of percutaneous cholecystostomy in the management of cholecystitis in 2014. J Visc Surg 2014;151(6):435–9.
74. Feretis CB, Manouras A, Apostolidis N, et al. Endoscopic transpapillary drainage of gallbladder empyema. Gastrointest Endosc 1990;36(5):523–5.
75. McCarthy ST, Tujios S, Fontana RJ, et al. Endoscopic transpapillary gallbladder stent placement is safe and effective in high-risk patients without cirrhosis. Dig Dis Sci 2015;60(8):2516–22.
76. Maekawa S, Nomura R, Murase T, et al. Endoscopic gallbladder stenting for acute cholecystitis: a retrospective study of46 elderly patients aged 65 years or older. BMC Gastroenterol 2013;13(1):65.
77. Lee TH, Park DH, Lee SS, et al. Outcomes of endoscopic transpapillary gallbladder stenting for symptomatic gallbladder diseases: a multicenter prospective follow-up study. Endoscopy 2011;43(8):702–8.
78. Barkay O, Bucksot L, Sherman S. Endoscopic transpapillary gallbladder drainage with the SpyGlass cholangiopancreatoscopy system. Gastrointest Endosc 2009;70(5):1039–40.
79. Chen YK, Parsi MA, Binmoeller KF, et al. Peroral cholangioscopy (POC) using a disposable steerable single operator catheter for biliary stone therapy and assessment of indeterminate strictures-a multi-center experience using SPYGLASS. Gastrointest Endosc 2009;69(5):AB264–5.
80. Shin JU, Lee JK, Kim KM, et al. Endoscopic naso-gallbladder drainage by using cholangioscopy for acute cholecystitis combined with cholangitis or choledocholithiasis (with video). Gastrointest Endosc 2012;76(5):1052–5.
81. Kedia P, Kuo V, Tarnasky P. Digital cholangioscopy-assisted endoscopic gallbladder drainage. Gastrointest Endosc 2017;85(1):257–8.
82. Tyberg A, Zerbo S, Kahaleh M, et al. Digital cholangioscopy-assisted gallbladder drainage: seeing is accessing. Endoscopy 2015;47(Suppl 1 UCTN):E417.
83. Itoi T, Kawakami H, Katanuma A, et al. Endoscopic nasogallbladder tube or stent placement in acute cholecystitis: a preliminary prospective randomized trial in Japan (with videos). Gastrointest Endosc 2015;81(1):111–8.

84. Yang MJ, Yoo BM, Kim JH, et al. Endoscopic naso-gallbladder drainage versus gallbladder stenting before cholecystectomy in patients with acute cholecystitis and a high suspicion of choledocholithiasis: a prospective randomised preliminary study. Scand J Gastroenterol 2016;51(4):472–8.
85. Huibregtse K, van Amerongen R, van Deventer SJ. Drainage of the gallbladder in patients with acute acalculous cholecystitis by transpapillary endoscopic cholecystoxeransis. Gastrointest Endosc 1994;40(4):523.
86. Brugge WR, Friedman LS. A new endoscopic procedure provides insight into an old disease: acute acalculous cholecystitis. Gastroenterology 1994;106(6): 1718–20.
87. Inoue T, Okumura F, Kachi K, et al. Long-term outcomes of endoscopic gallbladder stenting in high-risk surgical patients with calculous cholecystitis (with videos). Gastrointest Endosc 2016;83(5):905–13.
88. Iino C, Shimoyama T, Igarashi T, et al. Comparable efficacy of endoscopic transpapillary gallbladder drainage and percutaneous transhepatic gallbladder drainage in acute cholecystitis. Endosc Int Open 2018;06(05):E594–601.
89. Baron TH, Topazian MD. Endoscopic transduodenal drainage of the gallbladder: implications for endoluminal treatment of gallbladder disease. Gastrointest Endosc 2007;65(4):735–7.
90. Jang JW, Lee SS, Song TJ, et al. Endoscopic ultrasound-guided transmural and percutaneous transhepatic gallbladder drainage are comparable for acute cholecystitis. Gastroenterology 2012;142(4):805–11.
91. Lee SS, Park DH, Hwang CY, et al. EUS-guided transmural cholecystostomy as rescue management for acute cholecystitis in elderly or high-risk patients: a prospective feasibility study. Gastrointest Endosc 2007;66(5):1008–12.
92. Peñas-Herrero I, de la Serna-Higuera C, Perez-Miranda M. Endoscopic ultrasound-guided gallbladder drainage for the management of acute cholecystitis (with video). J Hepatobiliary Pancreat Sci 2015;22(1):35–43.
93. Anderloni A, Buda A, Vieceli F, et al. Endoscopic ultrasound-guided transmural stenting for gallbladder drainage in high-risk patients with acute cholecystitis: a systematic review and pooled analysis. Surg Endosc 2016;30(12):5200–8.
94. Hikichi T, Irisawa A, Takagi T, et al. A case of transgastric gallbladder puncture as a complication during endoscopic ultrasound-guided drainage of a pancreatic pseudocyst. Fukushima J Med Sci 2007;53(1):11–8.
95. Widmer J, Singhal S, Gaidhane M, et al. Endoscopic ultrasound-guided endoluminal drainage of the gallbladder. Dig Endosc 2014;26(4):525–31.
96. Jang JW, Lee SS, Park DH, et al. Feasibility and safety of EUS-guided transgastric/transduodenal gallbladder drainage with single-step placement of a modified covered self-expandable metal stent in patients unsuitable for cholecystectomy. Gastrointest Endosc 2011;74(1):176–81.
97. Kwan V, Eisendrath P, Antaki F, et al. EUS-guided cholecystenterostomy: a new technique (with videos). Gastrointest Endosc 2007;66(3):582–6.
98. Song TJ, Park DH, Eum JB, et al. EUS-guided cholecystoenterostomy with single-step placement of a 7F double-pigtail plastic stent in patients who are unsuitable for cholecystectomy: a pilot study (with video). Gastrointest Endosc 2010;71(3):634–40.
99. Itoi T, Itokawa F, Kurihara T. Endoscopic ultrasonography-guided gallbladder drainage: actual technical presentations and review of the literature (with videos). J Hepatobiliary Pancreat Sci 2011;18(2):282–6.
100. Subtil JC, Betes M, Munoz-Navas M. Gallbladder drainage guided by endoscopic ultrasound. World J Gastrointest Endosc 2010;2(6):203–9.

101. Choi J-H, Lee SS, Choi JH, et al. Long-term outcomes after endoscopic ultrasonography-guided gallbladder drainage for acute cholecystitis. Endoscopy 2014;46(08):656–61.
102. Widmer J, Alvarez P, Gaidhane M, et al. Endoscopic ultrasonography-guided cholecystogastrostomy in patients with unresectable pancreatic cancer using anti-migratory metal stents: a new approach. Dig Endosc 2014;26(4):599–602.
103. Ogura T, Masuda D, Imoto A, et al. EUS-guided gallbladder drainage and hepaticogastrostomy for acute cholecystitis and obstructive jaundice (with video). Endoscopy 2014;46(S 01):E75–6.
104. Kamata K, Takenaka M, Kitano M, et al. Endoscopic ultrasound-guided gallbladder drainage for acute cholecystitis: Long-term outcomes after removal of a self-expandable metal stent. World J Gastroenterol 2017;23(4):661–7.
105. Garcia-Alonso FJ, Sanchez-Ocana R, Peñas-Herrero I, et al. Cumulative risks of stent migration and gastrointestinal bleeding in patients with lumen-apposing metal stents. Endoscopy 2018;50(04):386–95.
106. Moon JH, Choi HJ, Kim DC, et al. A newly designed fully covered metal stent for lumen apposition in EUS-guided drainage and access: a feasibility study (with videos). Gastrointest Endosc 2014;79(6):990–5.
107. Irani S, Kozarek RA. The buried lumen-apposing metal stent: Is this a stent problem, a location problem, or both? VideoGIE 2016;1(1):25–6.
108. Irani S, Baron TH, Grimm IS, et al. EUS-guided gallbladder drainage with a lumen-apposing metal stent (with video). Gastrointest Endosc 2015;82(6): 1110–5.
109. Walter D, Teoh AY, Itoi T, et al. EUS-guided gall bladder drainage with a lumen-apposing metal stent: a prospective long-term evaluation. Gut 2016;65(1):6–8.
110. de la Serna-Higuera C, Pérez-Miranda M, Gil-Simón P, et al. EUS-guided transenteric gallbladder drainage with a new fistula-forming, lumen-apposing metal stent. Gastrointest Endosc 2013;77(2):303.
111. Dollhopf M, Larghi A, Will U, et al. EUS-guided gallbladder drainage in patients with acute cholecystitis and high surgical risk using an electrocautery-enhanced lumen-apposing metal stent device. Gastrointest Endosc 2017;86(4):636–43.
112. Ligresti D, Cipolletta F, Amata M, et al. Buried lumen-apposing metal stent (LAMS) following endoscopic ultrasound-guided gallbladder drainage: the LAMS-in-LAMS rescue treatment. Endoscopy 2018;50(8):822–3.
113. Seerden TC, Vleggaar FP. Endoscopic removal of buried lumen-apposing metal stents used for cystogastrostomy and cholecystogastrostomy. Endoscopy 2016; 48(Suppl 1):E179.
114. Kedia P, Boumitri C, Sharaiha RZ, et al. Conversion of a percutaneous cholecystotomy tube into an internal cholecystogastrostomy by use of a novel anastomotic stent. Gastrointest Endosc 2015;81(1):228–9.
115. Itoi T, Binmoeller KF, Shah J, et al. Clinical evaluation of a novel lumen-apposing metal stent for endosonography-guided pancreatic pseudocyst and gallbladder drainage (with videos). Gastrointest Endosc 2012;75(4):870–6.
116. Teoh AYB, Binmoeller KF, Lau JYW. Single-step EUS-guided puncture and delivery of a lumen-apposing stent for gallbladder drainage using a novel cautery-tipped stent delivery system. Gastrointest Endosc 2014;80(6):1171.
117. Mönkemüller K, Zabielski M, Didowacz-Grollmann A, et al. Endoluminal transgastric endoscopic anastomosis of the gallbladder using an anchoring self-expanding metal stent. Endoscopy 2013;45(S 02):E164–6.
118. Teoh AY, Chan AW, Chiu PW, et al. In vivo appearances of gallbladder carcinoma under magnifying endoscopy and probe-based confocal laser

endomicroscopy after endosonographic gallbladder drainage. Endoscopy 2014;46(S 01):E13–4.
119. Binmoeller K, Shah J. A novel lumen-apposing stent for transluminal drainage of nonadherent extraintestinal fluid collections. Endoscopy 2011;43(04):337–42.
120. Takagi W, Ogura T, Sano T, et al. EUS-guided cholecystoduodenostomy for acute cholecystitis with an anti-stent migration and anti-food impaction system; a pilot study. Therap Adv Gastroenterol 2016;9(1):19–25.
121. Saumoy M, Novikov A, Kahaleh M. Long-term outcomes after EUS-guided gallbladder drainage. Endosc Ultrasound 2018;7(2):97.
122. Khan MA, Atiq O, Kubiliun N, et al. Efficacy and safety of endoscopic gallbladder drainage in acute cholecystitis: Is it better than percutaneous gallbladder drainage? Gastrointest Endosc 2017;85(1):76–87.e3.
123. Baron TH, Grimm IS, Gerber DA. Liver transplantation after endoscopic ultrasound–guided cholecystoduodenostomy for acute cholecystitis: a note of caution. Liver Transpl 2015;21(10):1322–3.
124. Baron TH, Zacks S, Grimm IS. Endoscopic ultrasound-guided cholecystoduodenostomy for acute cholecystitis in a patient with thrombocytopenia and end-stage liver disease awaiting transplantation. Clin Gastroenterol Hepatol 2015;13(2):e13–4.
125. Baron TH, Grimm IS, Swanstrom LL. Interventional approaches to gallbladder disease. N Engl J Med 2015;373(4):357–65.
126. Tsin DA, Sequeria RJ, Giannikas G. Culdolaparoscopic cholecystectomy during vaginal hysterectomy. JSLS 2003;7(2):171.
127. Dhillon KS, Awasthi D, Dhillon AS. Natural orifice transluminal endoscopic surgery (hybrid) cholecystectomy: the Dhillon technique. J Minim Access Surg 2017;13(3):176.
128. Zornig C, Siemssen L, Emmermann A, et al. NOTES cholecystectomy: matched-pair analysis comparing the transvaginal hybrid and conventional laparoscopic techniques in a series of 216 patients. Surg Endosc 2011;25(6):1822–6.
129. Zornig C, Mofid H, Emmermann A, et al. Scarless cholecystectomy with combined transvaginal and transumbilical approach in a series of 20 patients. Surg Endosc 2008;22(6):1427–9.
130. Bulian DR, Knuth J, Cerasani N, et al. Transvaginal/transumbilical hybrid—NOTES—versus 3-trocar needlescopic cholecystectomy: short-term results of a randomized clinical trial. Ann Surg 2015;261(3):451.
131. Brescia A, Masoni L, Gasparrini M, et al. Laparoscopic assisted transvaginal cholecystectomy: single centre preliminary experience. Surgeon 2013;11:S1–5.
132. Noguera JF, Cuadrado A, Dolz C, et al. Prospective randomized clinical trial comparing laparoscopic cholecystectomy and hybrid natural orifice transluminal endoscopic surgery (NOTES) (NCT00835250). Surg Endosc 2012;26(12):3435–41.
133. Borchert DH, Federlein M, Fritze-Buttner F, et al. Postoperative pain after transvaginal cholecystectomy: single-center, double-blind, randomized controlled trial. Surg Endosc 2014;28(6):1886–94.
134. Wood SG, Solomon D, Panait L, et al. Transvaginal cholecystectomy: effect on quality of life and female sexual function. JAMA Surg 2013;148(5):435–8.

Endoscopic Ultrasound-Guided Interventions for the Measurement and Treatment of Portal Hypertension

Jason B. Samarasena, MD, Kenneth J. Chang, MD*

KEYWORDS

- Endoscopic ultrasound • Portal pressure gradient • Hepatic venous portal gradient
- Portal vein sampling • Transhepatic intrahepatic portosystemic shunt • Portal vein

KEY POINTS

- Direct access of the portal vein can be more easily achieved by endoscopic ultrasound (EUS) than via a standard percutaneous approach, and as such there exists great potential for diagnostic and therapeutic applications.
- In animal studies, EUS-guided portal pressure gradient measurements were strongly correlated with values obtained through a percutaneous approach, with an excellent safety profile.
- In human studies EUS-guided portal pressure gradient measurement seems to be safe and correlates well with clinical and endoscopic parameters such as portal hypertensive gastropathy, the presence of esophageal varices, and thrombocytopenia.
- EUS-guided transhepatic intrahepatic portosystemic shunt was successfully performed in pigs without any reported serious postprocedural or intraprocedural complications.

INTRODUCTION

The number of endoscopic ultrasound (EUS)-guided interventions is rapidly growing within advanced endoscopy. Endoscopists with specialized training are now able to perform procedures traditionally performed by interventional radiologists and surgeons. EUS offers high-resolution imaging of mediastinal and intra-abdominal vasculature, which can be targeted for various interventions. As a result, a growing number of studies have explored EUS-guided vascular catheterization because of the relative proximity of the gastrointestinal tract to the major blood vessels of the mediastinum and abdomen. In

Disclosure Statement: Dr Chang is a consultant, Advisory Board - Cook Medical Jason Samarasena and Educational Grant - Cook Medical.
Division of Gastroenterology and Hepatology, University of California - Irvine, 333 The Boulevard West, Suite 400, Orange, CA 92868, USA
* Corresponding author.
E-mail address: kchang@uci.edu

Gastrointest Endoscopy Clin N Am 29 (2019) 311–320
https://doi.org/10.1016/j.giec.2018.12.004
giendo.theclinics.com
1052-5157/19/© 2018 Elsevier Inc. All rights reserved.

particular, EUS-guided access of the portal vein (PV) is especially favorable given the relative difficulty of PV access via standard percutaneous routes. Potential clinical applications of EUS-guided portal venous access include angiography, measurement of the portosystemic pressure gradient, EUS-guided transhepatic intrahepatic portosystemic shunt creation, and PV sampling for evaluation in gastrointestinal cancer. This review outlines the different devices and techniques used in these applications. Ease of access, safety, and important lessons learned from each approach are highlighted.

ENDOSCOPIC ULTRASOUND-GUIDED PORTAL VENOUS ANGIOGRAPHY

The PV is seen from the stomach and the duodenum during EUS and is in very close proximity to the tip of the echoendoscope, making this an ideal target for vascular access. Initial cases of successful in vivo EUS-guided PV catheterization were performed in porcine models. In 2004, Lai and colleagues[1] reported an EUS-guided transduodenal approach to access the extrahepatic PV in 21 swine with a 22-gauge (22G) fine-needle aspiration (FNA) needle. A small amount of contrast was injected through the needle for fluoroscopic confirmation of proper placement. This study proved the technical feasibility of EUS-guided PV access.

The first study assessing PV angiography was an animal study reported in 2007 by Magno and colleagues.[2] 19G, 22G, and 25G needles were inserted under EUS guidance into the celiac trunk, splenic artery, superior mesenteric artery, the thoracic and abdominal aorta, and the splenic vein, portal vein (PV), and hepatic vein (HV) of pigs. All vessels were successfully identified and punctured in 5 of 5 pigs. No signs of intraprocedural hemodynamic instability were observed. Immediate postprocedure necropsy showed no signs of injury with the 25G needle. The 22G needle left puncture marks without bleeding, and the 19G needle caused a vascular hematoma in large-caliber vessels with intra-abdominal bleeding in 1 of the 5 pigs. Injection of contrast provided good opacification of smaller vessels—the celiac trunk, splenic artery, and HV—with only transient opacification in larger-caliber vessels. As would be expected, the amount of resistance associated with instilling the iodinated contrast was inversely correlated with needle caliber.

Giday and colleagues[3] attempted EUS-guided PV access in 2007 using a transgastric, transhepatic approach with a 25G needle and a modified endoscopic retrograde cholangiopancreatography (ERCP) catheter. This protocol was again performed in 2008 as part of another PV catheterization study.[4] Angiography was achieved using both standard iodinated contrast and medical-grade carbon dioxide (CO_2). PV catheterization was achieved in 6 of 6 swine in 2007 and 6 of 6 swine in 2008, with no complications noted in either study. Necropsy showed no evidence of bleeding, hematoma formation, or liver injury. The transgastric, transhepatic approach is postulated to be safer than the transduodenal approach by allowing for natural tamponade of the needle track by liver parenchyma during withdrawal.[3,5] The use of CO_2 as a contrast medium allowed for better visualization of the PV and easier intravascular administration through the small-caliber FNA needle when compared with the viscous iodine-based contrast. These studies as a whole suggested that needle puncture of these vessels would not necessarily lead to intra-abdominal hemorrhage or vascular injury.

The safety of CO_2 use has been evaluated in both animals and humans. CO_2 is highly soluble and easily cleared by the lungs[6] and, unlike iodinated contrast, is not associated with nephrotoxicity or increased risk for hepatorenal syndrome.[7] The current data suggest that combining CO_2 with a 25G needle may allow for easier injection of contrast, adequate visualization of the portal circulation, and possibly decreased risk of needle-related and contrast-related complications.

ENDOSCOPIC ULTRASOUND-GUIDED PORTAL PRESSURE GRADIENT MEASUREMENT

Portal hypertension (PH), resulting from increased resistance of hepatic sinusoids to blood flow, is most commonly a complication of liver cirrhosis. The pathogenesis involves alteration of the liver vasculature caused by fibrosis as well as increased production of vasoconstrictive mediators relative to endogenous vasodilators. Complications of PH include esophageal varices, portal hypertensive gastropathy, ascites, and hepatorenal syndrome. Measurement of PH has been useful in determining the stage, progression, and prognosis of cirrhosis in individual patients. Portal pressure gradient (PPG) measurement of ≥10 mm Hg is associated with development of esophageal varices[8] and PPG of ≥12 mm Hg with variceal hemorrhage.[9] Reduction of PPG by 20% or to less than 12 mm Hg with pharmacotherapy has been found to decrease the risk of future bleeding or rebleeding episodes.[10,11]

In current practice, PPG values are obtained via a percutaneous approach. This evaluation of PH is an indirect measurement of the hepatic venous pressure gradient (HVPG). For this technique, a catheter is inserted into the HV percutaneously via either the jugular or femoral vein. The free hepatic venous pressure is recorded and subtracted from the wedged hepatic venous pressure to determine the HVPG. Both percutaneous PV catheterization and HVPG measurement are invasive procedures and require a high level of technical expertise. Direct PV catheterization has been associated with a high complication rate[12,13] and is not commonly performed. Despite the overall safety profile of HVPG measurement, it is only routinely performed at tertiary medical centers.[14,15] Furthermore, HVPG has been shown to correlate poorly with directly measured portal pressure in cases of presinusoidal PH, which may be seen in cases of noncirrhotic portal fibrosis and presinusoidal PH, including PV thrombosis and schistosomiasis.[4,16,17]

Animal Studies

Lai and colleagues[1] were the first to report EUS-guided PV pressure (PVP) measurement in a porcine model. In a cohort of 21 pigs, a PH model was generated in 14 animals using polyvinyl alcohol injection and a coagulopathy model generated in 7 animals with heparin administration. A transduodenal EUS approach was used to access the PV in 21 pigs with a 22G FNA needle and a transabdominal ultrasound (TAUS)-guided transhepatic approach in 14 of 21 pigs via a 22G needle. PVP measurements were obtained in 18 of 21 swine. Minor complications found at necropsy included small subserosal hematomas at the EUS puncture site in all 21 pigs and a 25-mL blood collection between the liver and duodenum in 1 of 7 anticoagulated pigs. Failure to measure pressures in 3 subjects may have occurred as a result of thrombosis within the FNA needle. There was a strong correlation between EUS-measured and transhepatically measured PVP ($r = 0.91$). The development of hematomas in this study suggests that a transduodenal approach that does not traverse the liver may increase risk of bleeding, and therefore an approach traversing through liver parenchyma may be favorable.

In 2007, Giday and colleagues[3] used a transgastric approach with a 19G needle and modified ERCP catheter to obtain continuous PVP measurement without an echoendoscope in place. Five of 5 pigs were successfully catheterized, and no hemorrhage or liver injury was noted on necropsy in all subjects despite use of a significantly larger-caliber needle. Two of 5 pigs survived for 2 weeks and showed no signs of adverse events before and after necropsy. In a later study, the same group used the same methods to measure fluctuations in PVP and inferior vena cava (IVC) pressures in pigs that underwent common endoscopic procedures: esophagogastroduodenoscopy (EGD), colonoscopy, and ERCP.[18] PV and IVC were accessed using a 19G

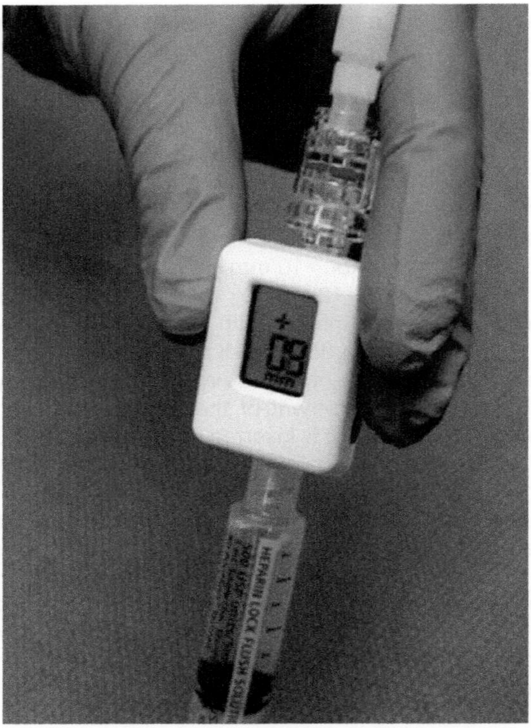

Fig. 1. Compact manometer used for EUS-guided portal pressure measurement. (*Courtesy of* Cook Medical, Bloomington, IN; with permission.)

needle and modified ERCP catheter. Access and pressure measurements of both vessels were achieved in 5 of 5 pigs. Necropsy showed no evidence of injury in all subjects. A 3-fold increase in PVP was noted between baseline and during ERCP. Values of IVC pressure, as well as of PVP for EGD and colonoscopy, were similar between baseline and procedure time.

Schulman and colleagues[19] demonstrated a novel method of measuring PVP in 2016 using an EUS-guided 22G needle through which a wire with a digital pressure sensor was passed. Conventional transjugular catheterization was performed as a control. Successful device placement and PVP measurement were achieved in 5 of 5 pigs with no hemorrhage or thrombosis noted on both EUS and postprocedural necropsy. Comparison of EUS-measured PVP with transjugular HVPG measurements showed a difference of within 1 mm Hg for all pigs. The study endoscopists rated the procedure as having overall low subjective workload. The authors used the same device to perform PVP measurement in 5 other pigs that then survived for 14 days before necropsy.[20] PVP was again measured on day 14. No signs of complications were observed during the 2-week survival period, and necropsy again showed no abnormalities. PVP values on day 0 and day 14 were similar for all 5 pigs.

Our group developed a method of EUS-guided portal pressure measurement using a 25G needle and simple transducer setup. The apparatus for PPG measurement included a linear echoendoscope, a 25G FNA needle, and a compact manometer (**Fig. 1**) with noncompressible tubing.[21] Before echoendoscope insertion, the manometer was zeroed at the midaxillary line. Measurements were conducted in the PV, HV, and the IVC. When the PV was targeted, manometry was performed via a transgastric, and less often a transduodenal, transhepatic approach and only the intrahepatic portion near the PV bifurcation was accessed. When evaluating the HV, the needle tip was placed 2 cm distal to the ostia when possible. Needle placement was meticulous to ensure consistency. One milliliter of heparinized saline was flushed through the needle before pressure measurement to clear the needle lumen and confirm intravascular placement. We also measured pressures in a swine model of PH induced by dextran-40 administration. Percutaneous measurements in the same vessels were obtained for comparison. All vessels were successfully accessed and pressures measured via EUS in all 3 pigs. Necropsy was not performed, but intraprocedural monitoring showed no signs of cardiorespiratory instability. Correlations between EUS-guided and percutaneous pressure measurements were very strong, with *r* values in all vessels greater than or equal to 0.985.

Human Studies

The first human single case of EUS-guided PVP measurement was reported by Fujii-Lau and colleagues[22] in 2014, in which a 22G FNA needle connected to an arterial pressure catheter was used to rule out PH in a 27-year-old man with arteriovenous malformations secondary to Noonan syndrome. The measured PPG was 1 mm Hg and correlated with the gradient obtained by interventional radiology at a prior procedure. There was no evidence of bleeding or hemodynamic instability after this procedure.

Our group performed the first prospective pilot study of PPG measurement in human patients with suspected or confirmed cirrhosis.[23] The setup used the simple transducer setup described in our animal study. The compact manometer was zeroed at the midaxillary line of each patient, and care was taken to consistently place the needle 2 cm distal to the HV ostia. Pressure readings were taken of the PV and either the HV or the IVC if anatomy was unfavorable for HV access. Needle placement was achieved and PPG measurement obtained in 28 of 28 patients, and no adverse events including bleeding, perforation, or infection were noted. The time required to obtain pressure measurements was short, less than 30 minutes per patient. PPG measurements correlated well with clinical and endoscopic parameters with significant differences in PPG noted in patients who were high-risk versus low-risk for cirrhosis and in patients with esophageal varices, portal hypertensive gastropathy, and thrombocytopenia relative to patients without these conditions. There were no complications in any of the 28 patients. In addition, most of the patients in this study underwent EUS-guided liver biopsies during the same procedure, suggesting that combining a PPG measurement and liver biopsy in the same session should be safe.

Recently, our prospective series has continued and data from 51 patients were recently presented.[24] These 51 patients underwent EUS-guided PPG measurement with 100% technical success and no adverse events. The PPG ranged from 0 to 27.3 mm Hg and was significantly higher in patients with clinical features of cirrhosis (11.26 versus 3.14 mm Hg, $P<.001$), endoscopic evidence of varices (14.94 versus 4.09 mm Hg, $P<.001$), or portal hypertensive gastropathy (14.37 versus 5.23 mm Hg, $P<.001$), and laboratory evidence of thrombocytopenia (10.91 versus 4.81 mm Hg, $P<0.001$). Minor discomfort was reported in 3 patients (6%), all of whom were managed with oral pain medication. No patients developed bleeding or infection, and none required admission to hospital as a result of the procedure.

ENDOSCOPIC ULTRASOUND-GUIDED PORTAL PRESSURE GRADIENT MEASUREMENT MEASUREMENT TECHNIQUE

The EUS manometry apparatus used in our human study is a simple setup that includes a 25G FNA needle, noncompressible tubing, a compact digital manometer, and heparinized saline. The tubing is connected by a luer lock to the distal port of the manometer while the heparinized saline is connected the proximal port. The end of the tubing is connected via a luer lock to the inlet of the 25G needle. The patient is positioned supine and during EUS-guided pressure measurement reading, the manometer is placed at the patient's midaxillary line (**Fig. 2**). We prefer monitored anesthesia care or general anesthesia for this procedure.

The HV measurement is conducted first. Of the HVs, the middle HV is targeted most commonly because of its larger caliber and better alignment with the needle trajectory on linear EUS (**Fig. 3**). Doppler flow is used to confirm the typical multiphasic waveform of hepatic venous flow (**Fig. 4**). Using the 25G FNA needle, a transgastric transhepatic approach is used to puncture the HV. Approximately 1 mL of heparinized saline is used to flush the needle, which is visible on EUS, confirming good position within the vessel. Following the flush, the pressure reading on the manometer will immediately increase and then decrease and equilibrate at a steady pressure, which is recorded. This measurement should be repeated a second and third time to minimize any error or fluctuation and to give a range of pressures from which to derive a mean pressure. The mean of the 3 pressures is then considered the HV pressure. The FNA needle is slowly withdrawn from the vein into the liver parenchyma and then back into the needle sheath with Doppler flow on to ensure there is no flow within the needle tract.

The PV measurement is conducted next and the umbilical portion of the left PV is targeted (**Fig. 5**). Doppler flow is used to confirm the typical venous hum of portal venous flow (**Fig. 6**). Using the 25G FNA needle, a transgastric transhepatic approach is used to puncture the PV. The procedure that follows is the same as that performed for the HV. Approximately 1 mL of heparinized saline is used to flush the needle, which is visible on EUS, confirming good position within the vessel. Following the flush, the

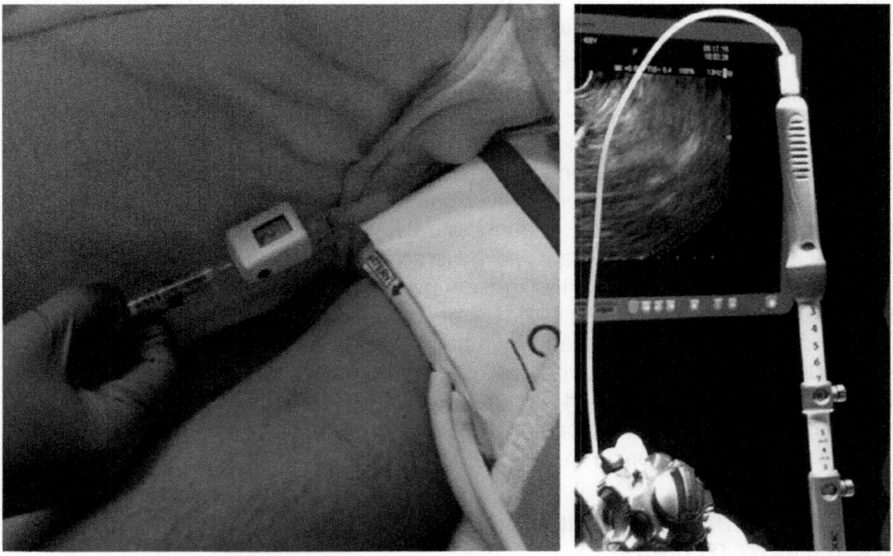

Fig. 2. EUS-guided portal pressure measurement apparatus showing noncompressible tubing attached to the FNA needle inlet (*right*) and compact manometer being placed at the midaxillary line of the patient (*left*).

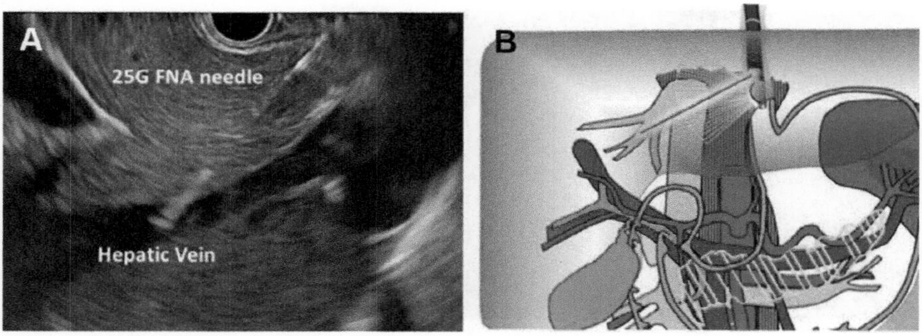

Fig. 3. EUS image (A) and schematic (B) of needle puncture of middle hepatic vein with 25-gauge FNA needle.

pressure reading on the manometer will immediately increase and then decrease and equilibrate at a steady pressure, which is recorded. This measurement should be repeated a second and third time. The mean of the 3 pressures is then considered the PV pressure. The FNA needle is slowly withdrawn from the vein into the liver parenchyma and then back into the needle sheath with Doppler flow on to ensure there is no flow within the needle tract.

The PPG is calculated by subtracting the mean PVP from the mean HV pressure. The patient is recovered in a manner similar to that used for routine diagnostic EUS with FNA. Postprocedural antibiotics are usually given for 3 to 5 days after the procedure.

ENDOSCOPIC ULTRASOUND-GUIDED TRANSHEPATIC INTRAHEPATIC PORTOSYSTEMIC SHUNT

Transhepatic intrahepatic portosystemic shunt (TIPSS) is an established treatment of PH and its complications, mainly for prevention of acute or recurrent esophageal and

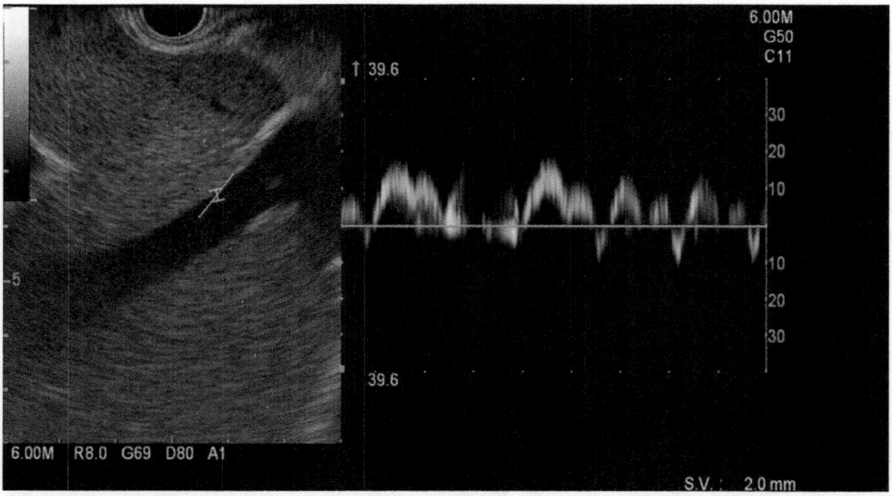

Fig. 4. EUS Doppler flow image of middle hepatic vein demonstrating multiphasic waveform.

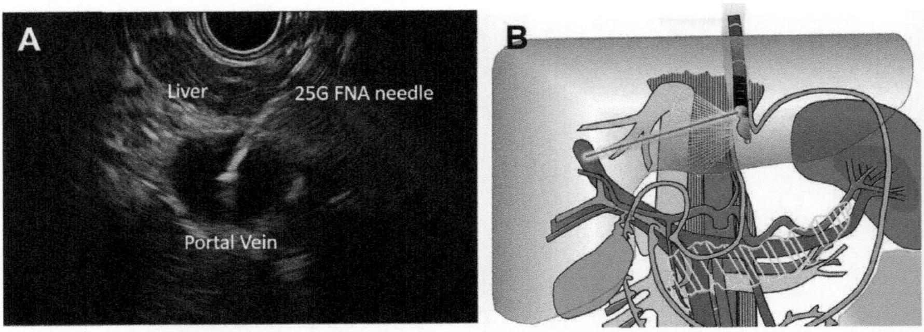

Fig. 5. EUS image (A) and schematic (B) of needle puncture of left portal vein with 25-gauge FNA needle.

gastric variceal bleeding and refractory ascites. Buscaglia and colleagues[25] described the first EUS-guided creation of an intrahepatic portosystemic shunt in a live porcine model. Under EUS guidance, the HV and PV were sequentially punctured and contrast was injected to confirm needle location within the PV, after which a guidewire was advanced through the needle to the PV. The needle was then removed, and a metal stent was inserted over the wire with its distal end in the PV and its proximal end in the HV. There were no complications in all 8 pigs, including a 2-week survival period in 2 pigs.

Binmoeller and Shah[26] used a similar technique to deploy a fully covered lumen-apposing metal stent in a porcine model. Necropsy confirmed successful stent placement between the PV and the HV with no tissue injury or hematomas. Schulman and colleagues[27] successfully deployed a lumen-apposing metal stent (LAMS) for creation of TIPSS in 5 pigs. The HV or IVC was identified using a linear-array echoendoscope and accessed with a 19G FNA needle preloaded with a digital pressure wire. Mean pressure was recorded. The needle was advanced into the PV, where pressure

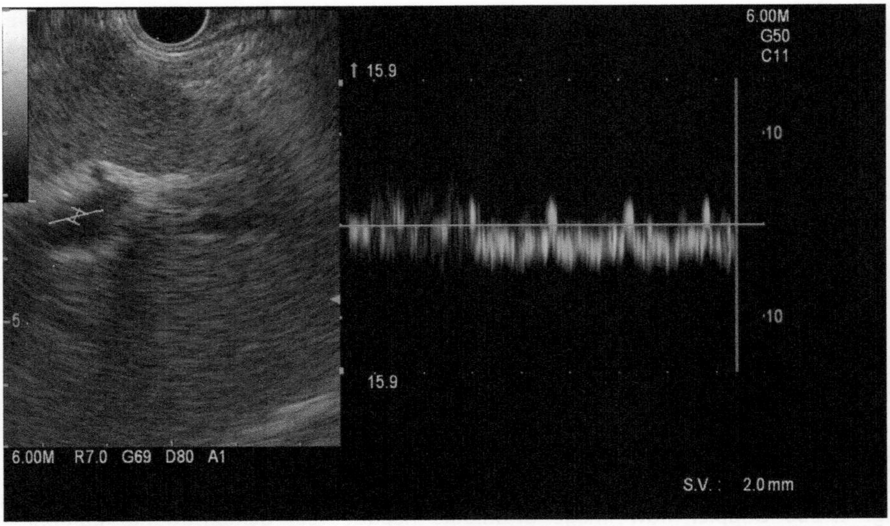

Fig. 6. EUS Doppler flow image of left portal vein demonstrating typical waveform.

measurements were again taken, and ultimately exchanged over a guidewire. A LAMS was deployed under EUS and fluoroscopic guidance, with distal and proximal ends positioned inside the PV and HV (IVC), respectively. Stent dilation was performed and pressure measurements repeated. Animals survived 2 weeks before necropsy. Placement of LAMS addressed the concern of stent migration. Technical success was 100%, with no bleeding on necropsy, but 2 pigs developed partial in-stent thrombosis. Further long-term studies, with refinements of devices and stents, are required before these procedures can be implemented in humans.

SUMMARY

Given the wide availability of EUS, an EUS-guided approach for the measurement of the PPG would be a great advance in endohepatology. The current literature including our expanded prospective series suggests that EUS-guided measurement of the PPG is safe and feasible. With further work in the area of EUS-specific vascular access technologies, the diagnostic and therapeutic opportunities with EUS-guided PV access will continue to expand and likely become a standard component in our current diagnostic evaluation.

REFERENCES

1. Lai L, Poneros J, Santilli J, et al. EUS-guided portal vein catheterization and pressure measurement in an animal model: a pilot study of feasibility. Gastrointest Endosc 2004;59(2):280–3.
2. Magno P, Ko CW, Buscaglia JM, et al. EUS-guided angiography: a novel approach to diagnostic and therapeutic interventions in the vascular system. Gastrointest Endosc 2007;66(3):587–91.
3. Giday SA, Ko CW, Clarke JO, et al. EUS-guided portal vein carbon dioxide angiography: a pilot study in a porcine model. Gastrointest Endosc 2007;66(4):814–9.
4. Giday SA, Clarke JO, Buscaglia JM, et al. EUS-guided portal vein catheterization: a promising novel approach for portal angiography and portal vein pressure measurements. Gastrointest Endosc 2008;67(2):338–42.
5. Brugge WR. EUS is an important new tool for accessing the portal vein. Gastrointest Endosc 2008;67(2):343–4.
6. Hawkins IF, Caridi JG. Carbon dioxide (CO_2) digital subtraction angiography: 26-year experience at the University of Florida. Eur Radiol 1998;8(3):391–402.
7. Liss P, Eklof H, Hellberg O, et al. Renal effects of CO_2 and iodinated contrast media in patients undergoing renovascular intervention: a prospective, randomized study. J Vasc Interv Radiol 2005;16(1):57–65.
8. Bosch J, Garcia-Pagan JC, Berzigotti A, et al. Measurement of portal pressure and its role in the management of chronic liver disease. Semin Liver Dis 2006; 26(4):348–62.
9. Groszmann RJ, Bosch J, Grace ND, et al. Hemodynamic events in a prospective randomized trial of propranolol versus placebo in the prevention of a first variceal hemorrhage. Gastroenterology 1990;99(5):1401–7.
10. Albillos A, Banares R, Gonzalez M, et al. Value of the hepatic venous pressure gradient to monitor drug therapy for portal hypertension: a meta-analysis. Am J Gastroenterol 2007;102(5):1116–26.
11. D'Amico G, Garcia-Pagan JC, Luca A, et al. Hepatic vein pressure gradient reduction and prevention of variceal bleeding in cirrhosis: a systematic review. Gastroenterology 2006;131(5):1611–24.

12. Perello A, Escorsell A, Bru C, et al. Wedged hepatic venous pressure adequately reflects portal pressure in hepatitis C virus-related cirrhosis. Hepatology 1999; 30(6):1393–7.
13. Tsushima Y, Koizumi J, Yokoyama H, et al. Evaluation of portal pressure by splenic perfusion measurement using dynamic CT. AJR Am J Roentgenol 1998;170(1):153–5.
14. Suk KT. Hepatic venous pressure gradient: clinical use in chronic liver disease. Clin Mol Hepatol 2014;20(1):6–14.
15. Thalheimer U, Bellis L, Puoti C, et al. Should we routinely measure portal pressure in patients with cirrhosis, using hepatic venous pressure gradient (HVPG) as a guide for prophylaxis and therapy of bleeding and rebleeding? No. Eur J Intern Med 2011;22(1):5–7.
16. Sarin SK, Khanna R. Non-cirrhotic portal hypertension. Clin Liver Dis 2014;18(2): 451–76.
17. Pomier-Layrargues G, Kusielewicz D, Willems B, et al. Presinusoidal portal hypertension in non-alcoholic cirrhosis. Hepatology 1985;5(3):415–8.
18. Buscaglia JM, Shin EJ, Clarke JO, et al. Endoscopic retrograde cholangiopancreatography, but not esophagogastroduodenoscopy or colonoscopy, significantly increases portal venous pressure: direct portal pressure measurements through endoscopic ultrasound-guided cannulation. Endoscopy 2008;40(8): 670–4.
19. Schulman AR, Thompson CC, Ryou M. EUS-guided portal pressure measurement using a digital pressure wire with real-time remote display: a novel, minimally invasive technique for direct measurement in an animal model. Gastrointest Endosc 2016;83(4):817–20.
20. Schulman AR, Thompson CC, Ryou M. endoscopic ultrasound-guided direct portal pressure measurement using a digital pressure wire with real-time remote display: a survival study. J Laparoendosc Adv Surg Tech A 2017;27(10):1051–4.
21. Huang JY, Samarasena JB, Tsujino T, et al. EUS-guided portal pressure gradient measurement with a novel 25-gauge needle device versus standard transjugular approach: a comparison animal study. Gastrointest Endosc 2016;84(2):358–62.
22. Fujii-Lau LL, Leise MD, Kamath PS, et al. Endoscopic ultrasound-guided portal-systemic pressure gradient measurement. Endoscopy 2014;46(Suppl 1 UCTN): E654–6.
23. Huang JY, Samarasena JB, Tsujino T, et al. EUS-guided portal pressure gradient measurement with a simple novel device: a human pilot study. Gastrointest Endosc 2017;85(5):996–1001.
24. Samarasena JB, Han J, Patel A, et al. EUS-guided portal pressure gradient measurement: a single center experience. Gastrointest Endosc 2018;87(6S):AB107.
25. Buscaglia JM, Dray X, Shin EJ, et al. A new alternative for a transjugular intrahepatic portosystemic shunt: EUS-guided creation of an intrahepatic portosystemic shunt (with video). Gastrointest Endosc 2009;69(4):941–7.
26. Binmoeller KF, Shah JN. Sa1428 EUS-guided transgastric intrahepatic portosystemic shunt using the axios stent. Gastrointest Endosc 2011;73(4):AB167.
27. Schulman AR, Ryou M, Aihara H, et al. EUS-guided intrahepatic portosystemic shunt with direct portal pressure measurements: a novel alternative to transjugular intrahepatic portosystemic shunting. Gastrointest Endosc 2017;85(1):243–7.

Endoscopic Management of Portal Hypertension–related Bleeding

Andrew Nett, MD*, Kenneth F. Binmoeller, MD

KEYWORDS

• Varices • Portal hypertension • GI bleed • Therapeutic endoscopy

KEY POINTS

- Portal hypertension–related bleeding can be catastrophic and fatal. Multidisciplinary management is necessary, potentially involving medical therapies, endoscopic intervention, and/or percutaneous or surgical portosystemic shunt creation.
- A wide variety of endoscopic and endosonographic therapies are available for hemostatic and prophylactic intervention. The appropriate therapy depends on the vascular lesion and its location.
- Endoscopic ultrasound (EUS) enhances the endoscopic management of gastric and ectopic varices. EUS-guided intravascular coil deployment may mitigate the risk of embolic complications associated with tissue adhesive injection.

INTRODUCTION

Gastrointestinal (GI) bleeding as a sequela of portal hypertension can be catastrophic and fatal. The overall approach to portal hypertension and related bleeding is multidisciplinary, potentially involving medical interventions and/or percutaneous or surgical portosystemic shunting for portal hypertension reduction. In addition, while doing nothing to correct underlying portal hypertension, endoscopic and endosonographic therapy plays a critical role in management—both for the achievement of hemostasis during active bleeding and for prevention of initial and recurrent bleeding.

PORTAL HYPERTENSION

Portal hypertension results from several disease states affecting the prehepatic, intrahepatic, or posthepatic circulation. In the Western world, sinusoidal hypertension from

Disclosure Statement: The authors have nothing to disclose.
Interventional Endoscopy Services, California Pacific Medical Center, 2351 Clay Street, 6th Floor Suite 600, San Francisco, CA 94115, USA
* Corresponding author.
E-mail address: Andrewnett83@Gmail.com

Gastrointest Endoscopy Clin N Am 29 (2019) 321–337
https://doi.org/10.1016/j.giec.2018.12.006
1052-5157/19/Published by Elsevier Inc.

cirrhosis is the most common cause of portal hypertension.[1] In cirrhosis, abnormal sinusoidal blood flow occurs due to structural aberrations, including scarring, regenerative nodules, and microvascular clotting, cause increased intrahepatic resistance and resultant portal hypertension.[2] Intrahepatic resistance is also elevated by increased vascular tone related to higher levels of local vasoconstrictors and reduced nitric oxide levels from endothelial dysfunction. Myofibroblasts form from hepatic stellate cells in response to inflammation and cytokine release induced by hepatocyte injury. These myofibroblasts also contract within the space of Disse, adding to increased intrahepatic resistance.[1]

When portal pressure in sufficiently elevated to be clinically significant (hepatic vein portal gradient [HPVG] >10 mm Hg), portosystemic collaterals develop. These collaterals arise with recannulation of embryonic vascular channels, reversal of flow within adult veins, or from neoangiogenesis.[3] Collateralization does not effectively relieve portal hypertension in cirrhotic patients, however. Increased splanchnic nitric oxide production results in splanchnic vasodilation and increased splanchnic blood flow, contributing to a persistent portal hypertensive state despite portosystemic collateral development. Back pressure caused by this portal hypertension thus transmits through these collaterals to perforating veins and the submucosal and subepithelial vessels they supply, which is where clinically significant varices may form. Esophageal and gastric varices are most common, but ectopic varices can develop anywhere in the GI tract.

ESOPHAGEAL VARICES

Esophageal varices are present in 30% to 40% of patients with compensated cirrhosis, but in up to 85% of those with decompensated cirrhosis.[2] The rate of variceal hemorrhage is approximately 10% to 15% per year with an associated 6-week mortality of 15% to 25%. Recurrent variceal hemorrhage occurs in 60% of patients without treatment.

The thoracic esophagus typically drains into the azygous and hemiazygos systemic venous systems.[3] In contrast, the abdominal esophagus typically drains to the portal system via the left gastric vein with lesser drainage to the systemic vascular system via superior and inferior phrenic veins into the inferior vena cava. With reversal of flow, it is the left gastric vein that usually acts as the afferent vessel supplying esophageal varices in cirrhotic patients.

Scenarios for Endoscopic Therapy

Primary prophylaxis

Endoscopic management may be appropriate for primary prophylaxis against bleeding of esophageal varices. The role for endoscopic intervention depends on the severity of underlying portal hypertension, variceal size, and whether or not decompensated cirrhosis is present. Patients with mild portal hypertension (HPVG >5 mm Hg but <10 mm Hg) do not develop varices.[2] Once clinically significant portal hypertension (HPVG >10 mm Hg) is present, however, variceal development may follow and there is potential for intervention prior to complication by variceal hemorrhage.

For this scenario—described as primary prophylaxis—intervention may be either medical or endoscopic. Endoscopic therapy is specifically considered in patients with evidence of increased risk of variceal bleed. This population includes all patients with decompensated cirrhosis and those with compensated cirrhosis with either medium to large varices (>5 mm). In patients with medium to large varices, endoscopic therapy with variceal ligation has been associated with decreased rates of variceal hemorrhage compared with medical therapy with a nonselective β-blocker.

Per the 2017 American Association for the Study of Liver Diseases guidance statement, small (<5 mm) but high-risk varices (small varices in decompensated patients or small varices with red wale signs) warrant nonselective β-blockers as preferential therapy over endoscopic intervention.

Secondary prophylaxis

For treatment of active variceal bleeding or for secondary prophylaxis after a variceal bleed, endoscopic intervention is indicated.

Technique/Method of Endoscopic Therapy

Endoscopic variceal ligation

The first-line endoscopic therapy for management of esophageal varices is endoscopic variceal ligation (EVL). EVL was introduced as a therapeutic option in 1986.[4] In EVL, a cap-assisted ligation device mounted on the scope is used to deploy an elastic ring ligature around a target varix suctioned into the cap. After suctioning of the varix into the cap, clockwise turning of a firing device attached at the external biopsy valve port results in ligature firing.

Particularly in the setting of scar tissue from prior therapy, adequate suctioning of the varix into the cap to ensure varix entrapment may be difficult. Prolonged, steady suctioning while gently torqueing the scope back and forth often induces more tissue into the cap. Release of suctioning prior to ligation deployment should generally be avoided, because this action may be enough to precipitate active bleeding. Once deployed successfully, the ligature entraps the mucosal and submucosal esophagus layers, causing varix strangulation for immediate hemostasis followed by intravascular thrombi formation, necrosis, and consequent fibrosis for variceal obliteration.

Active bleeding may be present that significantly impairs visualization. Water infusion can help obtain visualization of the bleeding source. If necessary, blind banding at the gastroesophageal (GE) junction may reduce bleeding enough for visualization and appropriate targeting of subsequent bands.

Ligature deployment for decompression along a variceal column should be performed distal to proximal because a caudal to rostral pressure gradient is typically present within the varix. In addition, the band-varix complex limits readvancement of the endoscope distally due to partial occlusion of the lumen and risk of band displacement. In the setting of acute variceal hemorrhage, banding should be preferentially targeted toward the culprit variceal column evidenced by stigmata of hemorrhage. In prophylactic EVL, red wale signs may also direct band placement. Generally, helical placement of bands moving distal to proximal allows application of the maximum number of bands while avoiding overlapping circumferential placement.[5]

Bands are typically placed along the distal 8 cm segment of the esophagus. This range is enough to target the palisade drainage and perforating zones. The palisade drainage zone (extending from the GE junction to 2–3 cm superiorly) is an azygous-portal watershed where veins in the proximal gastric submucosa penetrate through the muscularis mucosae at the GE junction and then course superficially within the lamina propria. The perforating zone extends from 3 cm to 5 cm from the GE junction, within which perforating veins extend from extrinsic paraesophageal venous plexuses, penetrate the muscularis propria, and supply intrinsic submucosal veins.[5–7] Due to their organization and response to portal hypertension, these areas are suggested critical areas of variceal development and rupture.[7] More proximal placement may have less efficacy and may serve only to exacerbate postligation retrosternal discomfort.

Multiple bands are typically placed until varices appear decompressed or until necessary placement becomes too proximal.

Efficacy of endoscopic variceal ligation

EVL is effective in immediate control of active variceal hemorrhage in approximately 90% of cases. Complications after EVL occur approximately 2% to 20% of the time and include transient dysphagia, retrosternal pain, esophageal stricture, ulcerations, perforation, and infection.[8] Rebleeding, sometimes massive, can also occur, either from recurrent variceal rupture or from postligation ulceration.

Ulcer management

After EVL, the ligature bands may stay in place for a range of 3 days to 7 days. An ulcer remains that heals within 2 weeks to 3 weeks.[9] If thrombus formation is incomplete when the ligature band sloughs off, postligation ulcer bleeding may occur. Overall the risk of post-EVL ulcer bleeding is 3.6% to 15%.[10] Such bleeding can often be managed conservatively with PPI therapy and supportive care. Nonendoscopic management with emergency transjugular intrahepatic portosystemic shunt (TIPS) or esophageal balloon tamponade may be pursued in cases of massive hemorrhage. Options for endoscopic treatment of postligation bleeding include repeat band ligation, endoscopic variceal obturation with cyanoacrylate injection, self-expandable metal stent placement, or hemostatic powder spray application.[10–12]

Interventions Other Than Endoscopic Variceal Ligation

Injection sclerotherapy

Prior to EVL, injection sclerotherapy was the first endoscopic treatment proved superior to balloon tamponade or vasoconstrictor administration in the management of esophageal varices. Unfortunately, complications occur in up to 40% of patients receiving sclerotherapy (esophageal ulceration, stricture, perforation, pulmonary thrombus, pleural effusion, hemothorax, mediastinitis, pericarditis, pneumothorax, renal dysfunction, and death).[8,13] Mortality related to this therapy occurs in 1% to 2%.[14]

Several studies have shown that band ligation is superior to endoscopic injection sclerotherapy. A 1995 meta-analysis of 7 randomized trials published in 2015 demonstrated EVL resulted in lower rebleeding, mortality, and complications as well as the need for fewer treatment sessions.[15] Similarly, Dai and colleagues[14] reported a meta-analysis of 14 studies involving 1236 patients treated for active esophageal variceal hemorrhage. EVL resulted in significantly lower rebleeding rates (27.7% vs 33.1%), higher eradication rates, lower complications, and no difference in mortality. A meta-analysis reviewing variceal band ligation alone versus band ligation plus sclerotherapy as therapy for secondary prophylaxis found that the addition of therapy did not improve rebleeding, the number of endoscopic sessions required for variceal obliteration, procedure-related complications, or mortality. Adding sclerotherapy to band ligation was associated, however, with higher rates of esophageal structuring.[16]

Despite its inferiority, injection sclerotherapy is still a potential option applied when EVL is technically difficult.[17] As discussed previously, significant active bleeding may impair visualization, complicating band ligation. Scar tissue may also prevent adequate suctioning of varices into a cap to achieve band ligation. Sclerosant injection is an option in such cases.

Agents with reported use consist of sodium tetradecyl sulfate (Food and Drug Administration approved), ethanolamine oleate, sodium morrhuate, polidocanol, or absolute alcohol. Intravariceal injection may be performed just distal to the site of bleeding or paravariceal injection may be performed immediately adjacent to a varix.

The sclerosant precipitates inflammation and thrombosis. After injection near the bleeding site, injections are performed starting at all varices at the GE junction, with proximal injections at 2-cm intervals, extending up to 5 cm to 6 cm from the GE junction.[8]

Metal stents

In cases of refractory or uncontrolled variceal bleeding, which occurs approximately 10% of the time despite EVL, balloon tamponade and TIPS are emergent salvage therapies. Balloon tamponade may be performed with placement of a Sengstaken-Blakemore tube. Although this method is helpful for hemostasis, it is only temporizing with a high risk of bleeding recurrence after deflation, which occurs in up to 50% of patients. There is also significant risk of other major complications including aspiration pneumonia and esophageal perforation (rate of up to 30%).[18] Covered self-expanding metal stent placement provides an endoscopic alternative to salvage therapy.

A specific stent system has been designed for treatment of acute variceal hemorrhage in which a 25-mm × 13.5-cm fully covered, self-expanding nitinol metal stent is used (SX-ELLA Danis Stent, Ella-CS, Hradec Králové, Czech Republic). This stent may be deployed without fluoroscopy or endoscopy although endoscopic guidance has been used in most reported cases.[18–20] The stent has atraumatic edges and is left in place for up to 14 days prior to removal. The stent thus can serve as bridge therapy for subsequent repeat EVL or TIPS.

A randomized controlled trial (RCT) comparing use of this stent versus balloon tamponade showed stenting resulted in significantly increased therapeutic success (66% vs 20%), decreased rebleeding at 15 days (77% vs 52%) and decreased adverse events (8% vs 52%) but no difference in 6-week survival.[21] In a 2017 meta-analysis examining 80 total cases in which esophageal stenting was performed for refractory variceal bleeding, a therapeutic success rate of 93.9% was reported with a 13.2% rebleed rate, no stent-related complications, and 21.6% stent migration rate. Mortality was 34.5% (only 12.6% died from uncontrolled bleeding).[20]

Argon plasma coagulation

A prospective, randomized trial compared EVL followed by argon plasma coagulation (APC) and EVL alone for esophageal variceal management. Significantly lower recurrence of esophageal varices was noted at 24 months after treatment when APC was also used (49.6% vs 74.2%). More recent RCTs examined a role for APC in secondary prophylaxis. Cipolletta and colleagues[22] in 2002 randomized 30 cirrhotics with a history of acute variceal hemorrhage and subsequent EVL eradication of varices to either observation versus APC. APC was applied to the entire circumferential mucosa spanning 4-cm to 5-cm proximal to the GE junction in 1 session to 3 sessions at weekly intervals. No significant complications were reported although APC did cause transient fever in 13 of 16 patients and 8 of 13 had dysphagia or retrosternal discomfort; 0% recurrence occurred in patients after APC therapy when followed with endoscopy for every 3 months for up to 28 months (9–28 mo). Meanwhile, recurrence occurred in 43% of the control group, with a 7% recurrent bleeding rate.

A 2017 meta-analysis by Li and colleagues[23] compared the safety and efficacy of EVL alone versus EVL + APC for secondary prophylaxis of esophageal variceal bleeding. Across 4 RCTs, combination therapy did show significantly lower variceal recurrence rates (relative risk 0.09). No difference in bleeding recurrence or mortality was present. Fever occurred more often after combination therapy. In addition, in 2012, 60 patients with large varices were randomized to primary prophylactic therapy with either EVL alone or EVL plus postvariceal obliteration APC for 1 session. In this study, APC did not result in any improvement in variceal recurrence at 7-month follow-up. Neither group had variceal bleeding.

Clipping and endoloops

Prospective studies have suggested either endoscopic clipping or endoloop ligation may achieve comparable rates of initial effective hemostasis and rebleeding compared with EVL.[24,25] Clipping resulted in a decreased number of treatment sessions until obliteration whereas endoloop ligation and EVL were comparable in this regard. Data for both techniques are limited, however, and both studies were non-randomized. With clipping, the risk of precipitating significant bleeding from variceal puncture by clip prongs exists and the cost of multiple clips seems exorbitant compared with that of the band ligation device.

Tissue adhesive injection

The injection of cyanoacrylate has been compared with EVL for the initial treatment of medium to large esophageal varices in an RCT published by Santos and colleagues.[26] The 2 therapies resulted in similar rates of variceal eradication, major complications, and mortality when followed over 6 months, but cyanoacrylate resulted in more minor complications and variceal recurrence (33% vs 57% recurrence).

Adhesive injection may also be performed for active variceal bleeding. Tissue adhesives used in acute variceal hemorrhage may achieve hemostasis in a high number of patients (94.2% in a study of 133 cirrhotic patients with 52 with active and 81 with recent bleeding).[27] In class C cirrhotic patients, Ribeiro and colleagues[28] reported in 2015 a retrospective study involving 63 patients admitted with acute esophageal variceal hemorrhage that *n*-butyl 2-cyanoacryle injection achieved hemostasis in approximately 75% of patients. Only 46% of patients were able to go 6 weeks after treatment without bleeding, however. In 2011, a small RCT compared EVL and injection of *n*-butyl cyanoacrylate in acute variceal bleeding.[29] Regardless of the initial therapy, follow-up EVL was performed within 2 weeks until varices were completely eradicated. Both interventions were comparable in achieving hemostasis. Although there was no difference in initial hemostasis, there was a suggestion of higher rebleeding in patients receiving *n*-butyl cyanoacrylate injection (although not statistically significant—13.6% vs 4.7%; $n = 0.60692$).

Overall, there is no definitive evidence supporting use of cyanoacrylate injection for management of bleeding varices or for variceal bleed prophylaxis. Tissue adhesive injection may be considered in lieu of or in conjunction with sclerotherapy, however, when EVL is technically challenging. Sclerotherapy is, of course, a second resort to EVL for treatment of bleeding esophageal varices, but an RCT did show *n*-butyl cyanoacrylate and sclerosant injection resulted in lower rebleeding and mortality compared with sclerotherapy alone.[30] Other studies have also shown combination sclerosant and *n*-butyl cyanoacrylate injection results in lower rebleeding, mortality, and minor complications compared with sclerotherapy alone.[31,32]

GASTRIC VARICES

Gastric varices are the second most common cause of GI bleeding in patients with portal hypertension. Gastric variceal bleeding, although less prevalent, has the propensity to be more severe, associated with higher transfusion requirement and with higher morbidity and mortality compared with esophageal variceal bleeding.[33,34] Afferent vessels supplying gastric varices typically consist of the left gastric, posterior gastric, and short gastric veins. Varices arising with left gastric supply develop in the cardia and those arising from the short and posterior gastric veins form in the fundus.

Gastric varices anastomose with the systemic circulation most commonly through esophageal varices into the superior vena cava. When gastric varices are isolated, they typically have afferent venous drainage through posterior or short gastric veins while efferent drainage is through a gastric—splenorenal shunt and the inferior vena cava via the inferior phrenic veins.

The Sarin classification system categorizes gastric varices based on whether or not they are contiguous with esophageal varices and their location in the stomach. Gastroesophageal varices type 1 (GOV1) and GOV2 varices are contiguous with esophageal varices extending either into the lesser curvature (GOV1) or the fundus along the greater curvature (GOV2).[3,6] These varices, also known as junctional varices, share the pathophysiology of esophageal varices, arising from the left gastric vein and originating in the lamina propria.[35]

Isolated Gastric Varices type 1 (IGV1) and IGV2 varices are fundal-type varices distinct from esophageal varices formed in the cardia (IGV1) or outside of the cardia and fundus, usually around the antrum or pylorus (IGV2).[3,6] They arise from the short and posterior gastric veins, originating in the submucosa. Bleeding risk is significantly higher for fundal varices (IGV1 77% and GOV2 55%) than either GOV1 or ectopic varices (10%).[36] Extrahepatic portal vein obstruction more commonly results in IGV1 varices whereas cirrhotic-related portal hypertension more commonly results in GOV2 varices.[34]

The Sarin classification system aligns with therapeutic distinctions. Specifically, GOV1 varices may be managed the same as esophageal varices. In this scenario, obliteration of esophageal varices with EVL frequently results in disappearance of the gastric varices as well in approximately 60% of patients.[36]

Sclerotherapy

Endoscopic sclerosant injection is not a good option in management of gastric varices due to association with high rates of complication including gastric ulceration, perforation, and rebleeding (37%–53%).[36,37] Furthermore, in patients with IGV1 varices, it is associated with low rates of variceal obliteration (41%) and high rates of rebleeding may occur (37% to 89%).[38,39] In 2002, Sarin and colleagues[40] performed an RCT comparing cyanoacrylate injection versus alcohol-based sclerotherapy in 37 patients with isolated fundal gastric varices (17 of 37 presented with active bleeding). Cyanoacrylate was more efficacious than alcohol in immediate hemostasis (89% vs 62%) and variceal obliteration (100% vs 44%), achieving obliteration significantly quicker (2 weeks vs 4.7 weeks).

Endoscopic Variceal Ligation Versus Tissue Adhesive Injection

As discussed previously, GOV1 varices specifically may be managed the same as esophageal varices. For other varix types, however, EVL can result in severe bleeding and is not advised for patients with IGV varices, which arise in the submucosa. The presence of thicker overlying mucosa within the stomach and the larger size of IGVs both make it difficult to fully entrap a gastric varix with suctioning into the banding ligation cap. If a band ligature does not fully capture the deeper gastric variceal wall, thrombotic obliteration of the lumen may not occur and postligation ulceration with sloughing of the ligature can result in severe hemorrhage.[2,41] Instead of band ligation, the current worldwide standard for treatment of IGVs is glue injection. Several studies support this practice.

Soehendra and colleagues[42] first reported the use of *n*-2-butyl-cyanoacrylate for endoscopic injection of gastric varices in 1986. This method is capable of achieving 58% to 100% hemostasis, with a rebleed rate ranging from 0% to 40%.[43] In 2013, Tantau and colleagues[44] prospectively compared *n*-butyl 2-cyanoacrylate injection with EVL in acute gastric variceal bleeding. Both treatments obtained initial hemostasis in a high percentage of patients. Rebleeding, however, was significantly more frequent after EVL (72% vs 32%; $P = .03$) and the rebleeding-free period was larger after glue injection ($P = .006$).

Subsequent RCTs have buttressed the superiority of cyanoacrylate injection. A meta-analysis reviewing treatment of acute gastric variceal bleeding compared cyanoacrylate injection versus other endoscopic intervention. Analysis of 3 RCTs showed that EVL and cyanoacrylate injection achieve comparable rates of initial hemostasis, but EVL therapy carries a significantly higher risk of rebleeding.[41] Treatments were similar in bleeding control, complications, and bleeding-related mortality although cyanoacrylate injection was found superior to EVL in prevention of rebleeding. The largest RCT included in this meta-analysis examined only GOV1 varices, expected to overestimate the efficacy of EVL applied to cardiofundal varices (IGV1/GOV2).[45]

Endoscopic ultrasound–Guided Tissue Adhesive Injection

Endoscopic ultrasound (EUS) can enhance endoscopic management of gastric varices in several regards.[46] EUS has been shown to increase the detection rate of gastric varices 6-fold in cirrhotic patients (79% vs 12.5%).[47] Due to their deeper intramural location, gastric varices may be overlooked as gastric folds on direct endoscopy. After therapy, Doppler assessment is valuable in confirming obliteration of vascular flow through a variceal complex, which is important because residual flow has prognostic implications regarding rebleeding risk.[48] In cases of significant hemorrhage, torrential active bleeding or large clots can prevent adequate visualization for identification of a culprit gastric varix and subsequent cyanoacrylate injection. EUS enables guidance of therapy without direct endoscopic visualization.[46] EUS may also direct therapy more precisely into a perforating vessel with preceding contrast injection showing whether the feeding vessel is efferent or afferent, potentially reducing embolization risk by enabling use of a smaller volume of cyanoacrylate.[49] If endoscopic therapy fails, EUS provides additional information regarding portal vein and splenic vein patency, helping to assess candidacy for TIPS versus balloon-occluded retrograde transvenous obliteration.

Complications of tissue adhesive injection

Technical complications that may arise during cyanoacrylate injection include adhesive-related endoscope damage or needle entrapment in a varix with adhesive curation/hardening. Clinical complications from cyanoacrylate injection typically involve the risk of adhesive systemic embolization with primary concern for pulmonary embolism or paradoxic embolic events, such as cerebral embolism in patients with a patent foramen ovale. Coronary and splenic artery embolism also may occur as well as splenic and renal vein thrombosis. Sepsis has also resulted after glue embolization with the embolus serving as a nidus of infection. Visceral fistulization from the stomach into the pleura or mediastinum also may occur after unintentional paravariceal injection.[50]

Embolization with cyanoacrylate injection actually may be alarmingly common although fortunately typically inconsequential. Routine CT imaging after *n*-butyl 2-cyanoacrylate diluted with 1:1 lipidiol injection shows that asymptomatic glue embolization may occur in approximately 50%.[51] Clinically significant embolization, in contrast, is fairly rare but when embolization is substantial, complications may be catastrophic with resultant death.[52] Embolization risk may be enhanced with excessively rapid cyanoacrylate injection, large-volume glue injection, rapid variceal flow rate, or overdilution of *n*-butyl 2-cyanoacrylate with lipidiol, which prolongs hardening.[41]

Tissue adhesive selection

Although most studies involving cyanoacrylate injection of gastric varies use *n*-butyl 2-cyanoacrylate, several cyanoacrylate monomers are available. *n*-Butyl 2-cyanoacrylate has a rapid polymerization time. Therefore, it is typically diluted with lipidiol to avoid premature intraneedle hardening or needle entrapment within the varix.[41] Water and not saline should be flushed through the needle, because saline accelerates polymerization. 2-Octyl cyanoacrylate, in contrast, has a slower polymerization time limiting risk of premature hardening and obviating need for lipidiol dilution, which complicates injection due to its viscosity. The needle can also be flushed with saline when 2-octyl-cyanoacrylate is used. Of course, 2-octyl-cyanoacrylate may augment the risk of distant embolization if rapid injection is performed.

Glue-coil Embolization

In further efforts to mitigate potentially devastating embolic complications after cyanoacrylate injection, Binmoeller and colleagues[39] first performed ex vivo analysis of the utility of concomitant local coil and glue injection in the treatment of gastric varices. Initial deployment of intravascular coils provides a scaffold for glue polymerization and fixation to prevent inadvertent glue embolization. To test this hypothesis, in ex vivo study, a coil was deployed into a container of heparinized blood; 1 mL of cyanoacrylate was then injected with immediate adherence of the glue to the coil's synthetic fibers. The coil and its adherent glue were then removed from the container and no free glue remained (**Fig. 1**).

Pioneering this combined injection technique in humans, Binmoeller and colleagues[53] first reported EUS-guided glue-coil embolization in a case involving massive hemorrhage refractory to standard cyanoacrylate injection. Subsequently, Binmoeller and colleagues reported a series of 30 patients with large gastric varices with active or

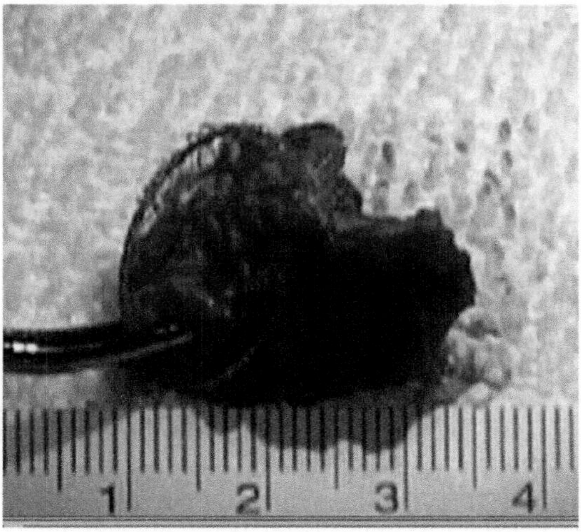

Fig. 1. Glue fixated to coil scaffolding after injection into container of heparinized blood. (*From* Weilert F, Binmoeller KF. Endoscopic management of gastric variceal bleeding. Gastroenterol Clin North Am 2014;43(4):812; with permission.)

recent (<1 week) bleeding and poor candidacy for TIPS. After endosonographic visualization of the gastric varices, transesophageal, transcrural deployment of a coil into a gastric variceal lumen was performed using the 19-gauge echoendoscope followed by injection of 1 mL of 2-octyl cyanoacrylate. Observation with color Doppler effect was then performed to confirm hemostasis. If necessary, an additional 1 mL of cyanoacrylate was injected (**Fig. 2**).

Therapeutic success was 100% with no procedure-related complications. In follow-up, 24 patients had repeat endoscopy by the time of study publication with complete obliteration of gastric varices after a single session of therapy achieved in 95.8%, as confirmed by color Doppler analysis showing no residual vascular flow. One patient had recurrent bleeding from gastric varices at 21 days post-treatment treated successfully with additional coil and cyanoacrylate injection. No surgical or percutaneous shunts were required for salvage therapy. After treatment, the natural anticipated behavior of coils is eventual extrusion into the GI lumen.

In 2016, Our centre published an expanded series involving 152 patients with extended follow-up over a mean of 436 days.[54] Among these patients, 5% received EUS-guided glue-coil injection for active bleeding; 69% received therapy for recent bleeding and 26% for primary prophylaxis; 143 patients had IGV1 varices; and the other 9 had GOV2 varices. Therapeutic success was 99% using either a transgastric or transcrural approach. In the 1 technical failure, treatment of a gastric varix with adherent clot was performed after the patient presented with hematemesis. Persistent bleeding was present despite treatment with a 15 mm diameter coil and injection of 6 mL of 2-octyl cyanoacrylate requiring referral for emergent TIPS.

Follow-up EUS was performed in 100 of 152 patients with a rate of complete gastric variceal obliteration of 93% (79% single session, 10% 2 sessions, 2% 3 sessions, and 2% 4 sessions). Only 3% of patients had gastric variceal bleeding during the follow-up period after initial obliteration was achieved. On average, bleeding occurred at 146 weeks after initial glue-coil therapy. Minor delayed bleeding related to coil

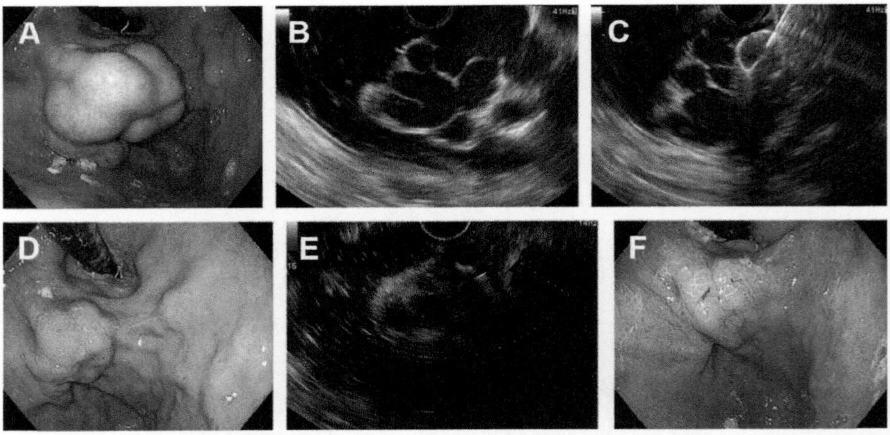

Fig. 2. (*A*) IGV1 varices. (*B*) Endosonography of same IGV1 varices. (*C*) EUS-guided glue coil embolization. (*D*) One month post-treatment. (*E*) Persistent obliteration of flow through variceal complex at 1 month. (*F*) Nine-month follow-up showing variceal eradication. (*From* Bhat YM, Weilert F, Fredrick RT, et al. EUS-guided treatment of gastric fundal varices with combined injection of coils and cyanoacrylate glue: a large U.S. experience over 6 years (with video). Gastrointest Endosc 2016;83(6):1166; with permission.)

extrusion occurred in additional 3% of patients whereas 3% had mild postprocedure pain and 1% (1 patient) has evidence of pulmonary embolism. The pulmonary embolism did not present until 1 week after treatment after having been discharged home postprocedure with no chest pain or dyspnea and no hypoxia or other signs of acute embolism. The rate of symptomatic embolism in this study 0.7% (1/152) was lower than that previously reported with EUS-guided cyanoacrylate injection without coils (2/19; 10.5%).[51]

Coil Injection Alone

Levy and colleagues[55] reported sole injection of embolization coils without cyanoacrylate for therapy for ectopic variceal bleeding. Refractory bleeding from choledochojejunal anastomosis varices was treated with injection of an embolization coil through a 22-gauge needle using a linear echoendoscope. Three coils were used with obliteration of flow observed after 10 minutes. Rebleeding occurred with repeat EUS performed. There was persistent absence of flow in the previously treated varices but injection of 2 additional coils in untreated varices was performed.

EUS-guided coil embolization therapy was reported for gastric varices by Romero-Castro and colleagues[56] in 2010. EUS-guided coil embolization has been compared retrospectively to EUS-guided cyanoacrylate injection for therapy for gastric varices.[51] Eleven patients were treated with coils (coiled diameter ranging from 8 mm to 20 mm), with coil size chosen approximately 20% larger than the variceal lumen diameter. Obliteration was achieved with coil injection in 90.9% of patients. Complications were significantly lower in the coil group versus the cyanoacrylate injection group (58% vs 9%; $P<.01$). Symptomatic pulmonary embolism occurred in 2 of 19 patients after cyanoacrylate injection whereas only 1 of 11 patients after coil injection had an adverse event. As discussed previously, however, CT imaging showed that 11 of 19 patients actually had evidence of pulmonary embolization after cyanoacrylate injection.

Occasionally, the authors have noted patients suffering suspected gastric variceal bleeding with only small diameter gastric varices present. In such cases, sole coil embolization therapy without cyanoacrylate injection can be effective and allows avoidance of extravascular glue injection into the submucosal space, which otherwise can rapidly compress and obfuscate the endosonographic view of target vessels. Typically, the authors deploy 1 or more 10-mm–diameter × 7-cm–length coils for therapy in this instance until obliteration of flow is achieved.

Gastric Varices Primary Prophylaxis

Although gastric variceal bleeding occurs less commonly than esophageal variceal bleeding, the potential lethality of a gastric variceal bleed remains alarming. In examination of the role of primary prophylactic therapy, an RCT involving 89 patients with either GOV2 varices with eradicated esophageal varices or IGV1 varices greater than 1 cm without prior bleeding were managed with either cyanoacrylate injection, medical intervention with nonselective β-blockers, or observation.[57] Cyanoacrylate injection resulted in lower rates of hemorrhage (10%) compared with either nonselective β-blockers (38%) or observation (53%) strategies. Cyanoacrylate management group survival was statistically equivalent to the nonselective β-blockers group (93% vs 83%) but higher compared with that of the observation group (74%).

Review of bleeding events showed that a large-size (varix >20 mm), high Model for End-Stage Liver Disease score greater than 16, and presence of portal gastropathy all were predictive high-risk factors for bleeding. Based on this trial, prophylactic intervention should be considered when large or high-risk gastric varices are present for reduction of bleeding and mortality. In the series of 152 patients treated with EUS-guided glue coil embolization, 40 received therapy for primary prophylaxis, with complete obliteration rate of 96% with no procedure-related complications. Based on these outcomes, the authors propose routine prophylactic therapy for IGV1 and GOV2 varices larger than 2 cm in size.[54]

PORTAL GASTROPATHY

Limited effective endoscopic options exist for the management of portal hypertensive gastropathy (PHG) bleeding. In PHG, ectatic mucosal capillaries and venules develop, which may result in diffuse and recurrent bleeding presenting acutely or as chronic occult blood loss. APC has been evaluated for treatment of PHG with suggestion that, in combination with nonselective β-blocker therapy, it can reduce rates of blood transfusion and ICU admission and improve hemoglobin levels.[58] Spray application of a hemostatic agent is also an option for treatment of active PHG bleeding. Although this therapy achieves no long-term control of PHG, it may be used as an effective method of acute hemostasis until nonselective β-blocker therapy, TIPS, or correction of coagulopathy is pursued.[59]

RECTAL VARICES

Rectal varices develop from submucosal portosystemic connections between the midrectum and anorectal junction.[60] They exist between approximately 40% and 55% of patients with cirrhosis and between approximately 60% to 90% of patients with extrahepatic portal vein hypertension.[6] Bleeding occurs from rectal varices in approximately 0.5% to 5% of patients who develop them. They are the source of ectopic variceal bleeding in approximately 8% of cases of ectopic bleeding. Most rectal varices are supplied by the inferior mesenteric vein or the superior rectal vein, a branch of the inferior mesenteric vein, that feeds into the intrinsic rectal venous plexus spanning along the lateral rectal wall. Systemic system outflow from this plexus occurs into the middle and inferior rectal veins or the internal iliac vein. Rectal varices should not be confused with internal hemorrhoids, which arise from submucosal arteriovenous connections at the anorectal vascular plexus without communication with major vessels of the portal venous system. Rectal varices do not extend to the anal columns and dentate line. Although frequently detected with endoscopic examination, endosonography provides a superior means of diagnosis.[61]

No consensus exists for a standard endoscopic (or overall) management approach to rectal varices. Options for endoscopic therapy include sclerosant injection, cyanoacrylate glue injection, glue-coil embolization, and band ligation. If band ligation is performed, EUS characterization first may help to direct banding by enabling localization of inflowing vessels supplied by the superior rectal vein as they penetrate through the rectal wall. Banding of rectal varices can then be performed at the site of these penetrating vessels and proceed distally toward the anorectal junction.[60] Band ligation of rectal varices has been associated with high recurrence rates, however. Comparison with sclerotherapy has shown reduced bleeding recurrence after sclerotherapy versus band ligation—33.3% versus 55.6%.[62] For complete obliteration, sclerosant injection into rectal varices may require use of large volumes compared with cyanoacrylate. Thus, cyanoacrylate use, with injection of smaller volumes, may at least theoretically reduce risk of systemic embolization. As with gastric varices, use of an EUS-guided injection of an embolization coil followed by cyanoacrylate may be used to act as a scaffolding for cyanoacrylate fixation for further reduction of distant embolization risk (**Fig. 3**).[63]

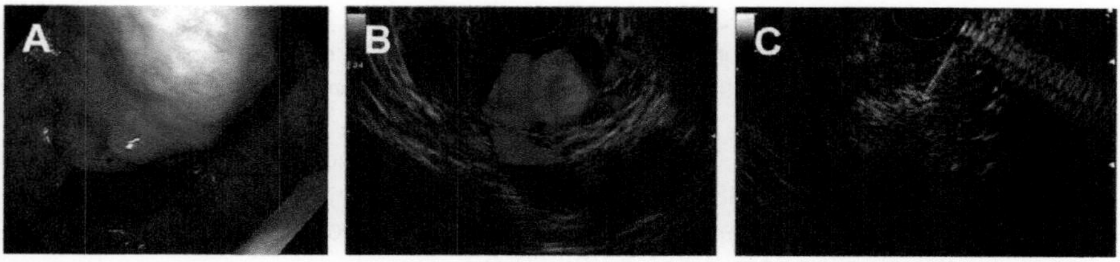

Fig. 3. (*A*) Endoscopic view of rectal varix *Black arrow* shows nipple sign at gastric varix. (*B*) EUS visualization. (*C*) Status post–glue-coil embolization with no residual flow. (*From* Weilert F, Shah JN, Marson FP, et al. EUS-guided coil and glue for bleeding rectal varix. Gastrointest Endosc 2012;76(4):915–6; with permission.)

OTHER ECTOPIC VARICES

Ectopic varices are a rare cause of bleeding in patients with portal hypertension, accounting for only 2% to 5% of variceal bleeding cases.[64] They may be more common in patients with prehepatic etiologies of portal hypertension rather than cirrhosis, occurring in 27% to 40% of patients with splanchnic vein thromboses.[65] Bleeding from ectopic varices also seems rarer but more severe than esophageal variceal bleeding, with mortality rates of up to 40%.[64,66] In a retrospective case series of 169 patients, peristomal, duodenal, and jejunoileal varices were the most common sites of ectopic variceal bleeding.[67] Biliary tract, colonic, periumbilical, and peritoneal varices may occur as well.[68]

No standardized treatment exists for ectopic varices, but endoscopic treatment options include those treatments used for varices in the stomach and esophagus—band ligation, EUS-guided coil embolization, and/or cyanoacrylate injection.[2] Band ligation should be pursued with caution if the diameter of the varix is too large to fully entrap within a ligature. Hemostatic clip placement has been reported as well for ectopic variceal therapy though failure of obliteration and rebleeding may be anticipated.[64] APC in conjunction with band ligation may be considered for prevention of variceal occurrence, as has been reported in the treatment of ileocolonic anastomotic varices.[68] Endoscopic therapy may be complicated by postligation ulcer bleeding, pyelephlebitis, and portal biliopathy. Given the overall dearth of data supporting endoscopic obliteration and long-term control, the role of percutaneous embolization and shunting and surgical interventions should always be considered for ectopic variceal management.

SUMMARY

The management of portal hypertension related bleeding requires a multidisciplinary approach involving hepatology, interventional radiology, surgery, and luminal and interventional gastroenterology. For hemostasis and prophylaxis against initial and recurrent bleeding, endoscopic therapy is a critical modality. A variety of techniques, including band ligation, sclerosant injection, tissue adhesive injection, and coil embolization, are available for endoscopic therapy. When injection therapy is used, endosonography can enhance the therapeutic value of intervention.

REFERENCES

1. Bloom S, Kemp W, Lubel J. Portal hypertension: pathophysiology, diagnosis and management. Intern Med J 2015;45(1):16–26.

2. Garcia-Tsao G, Abraldes JG, Berzigotti A, et al. Portal hypertensive bleeding in cirrhosis: Risk stratification, diagnosis, and management: 2016 practice guidance by the American Association for the study of liver diseases. Hepatology 2017;65(1):310–35.
3. Sharma M, Rameshbabu CS. Collateral pathways in portal hypertension. J Clin Exp Hepatol 2012;2(4):338–52.
4. Van Stiegmann G, Cambre T, Sun JH. A new endoscopic elastic band ligating device. Gastrointest Endosc 1986;32(3):230–3.
5. Poza Cordon J, Froilan Torres C, Burgos García A, et al. Endoscopic management of esophageal varices. World J Gastrointest Endosc 2012;4(7):312–22.
6. Philips CA, Augustine P. Endoscopic ultrasound-guided management of bleeding rectal varices. ACG Case Rep J 2017;4:e101.
7. Vianna A, Hayes PC, Moscoso G, et al. Normal venous circulation of the gastroesophageal junction. A route to understanding varices. Gastroenterology 1987; 93(4):876–89.
8. Kapoor A, Dharel N, Sanyal AJ. Endoscopic diagnosis and therapy in gastroesophageal variceal bleeding. Gastrointest Endosc Clin N Am 2015;25(3): 491–507.
9. Nijhawan S, Rai RR, Nepalia S, et al. Natural history of postligation ulcers. Am J Gastroenterol 1994;89(12):2281–2.
10. Cho E, Jun CH, Cho SB, et al. Endoscopic variceal ligation-induced ulcer bleeding: what are the risk factors and treatment strategies? Medicine (Baltimore) 2017;96(24):e7157.
11. Sanglodkar UA, Jothimani D, Rela M. Hemospray for recurrent esophageal band ulcer bleeding. Clin Exp Hepatol 2018;4(1):46–8.
12. Tierney A, Toriz BE, Mian S, et al. Interventions and outcomes of treatment of postbanding ulcer hemorrhage after endoscopic band ligation: a single-center case series. Gastrointest Endosc 2013;77(1):136–40.e1.
13. Ochiai T, Nakade Y, Kitano R, et al. Hemothorax following uncomplicated endoscopic variceal sclerotherapy and ligation for esophageal varices. Case Rep Gastroenterol 2017;11(3):531–8.
14. Dai C, Liu WX, Jiang M, et al. Endoscopic variceal ligation compared with endoscopic injection sclerotherapy for treatment of esophageal variceal hemorrhage: a meta-analysis. World J Gastroenterol 2015;21(8):2534–41.
15. Laine L, Cook D. Endoscopic ligation compared with sclerotherapy for treatment of esophageal variceal bleeding. A meta-analysis. Ann Intern Med 1995;123(4): 280–7.
16. Karsan HA, Morton SC, Shekelle PG, et al. Combination endoscopic band ligation and sclerotherapy compared with endoscopic band ligation alone for the secondary prophylaxis of esophageal variceal hemorrhage: a meta-analysis. Dig Dis Sci 2005;50(2):399–406.
17. de Franchis R, Baveno VIF. Expanding consensus in portal hypertension: report of the baveno VI consensus workshop: stratifying risk and individualizing care for portal hypertension. J Hepatol 2015;63(3):743–52.
18. Cardenas A, Fernandez-Simon A, Escorcell A. Endoscopic band ligation and esophageal stents for acute variceal bleeding. Clin Liver Dis 2014;18(4):793–808.
19. McCarty TR, Njei B. Self-expanding metal stents for acute refractory esophageal variceal bleeding: a systematic review and meta-analysis. Dig Endosc 2016; 28(5):539–47.
20. Shao XD, Qi XS, Guo XZ. Esophageal stent for refractory variceal bleeding: a systemic review and meta-analysis. Biomed Res Int 2016;2016:4054513.

21. Escorsell A, Pavel O, Cárdenas A, et al. Esophageal balloon tamponade versus esophageal stent in controlling acute refractory variceal bleeding: a multicenter randomized, controlled trial. Hepatology 2016;63(6):1957–67.
22. Cipolletta L, Bianco MA, Rotondano G, et al. Argon plasma coagulation prevents variceal recurrence after band ligation of esophageal varices: preliminary results of a prospective randomized trial. Gastrointest Endosc 2002;56(4):467–71.
23. Li X, Jiang T, Gao J. Endoscopic variceal ligation combined with argon plasma coagulation versus ligation alone for the secondary prophylaxis of variceal bleeding: a systematic review and meta-analysis. Eur J Gastroenterol Hepatol 2017;29(6):621–8.
24. Yol S, Belviranli M, Toprak S, et al. Endoscopic clipping versus band ligation in the management of bleeding esophageal varices. Surg Endosc 2003;17(1): 38–42.
25. Naga MI, Okasha HH, Foda AR, et al. Detachable endoloop vs. elastic band ligation for bleeding esophageal varices. Gastrointest Endosc 2004;59(7):804–9.
26. Santos MM, Tolentino LH, Rodrigues RA, et al. Endoscopic treatment of esophageal varices in advanced liver disease patients: band ligation versus cyanoacrylate injection. Eur J Gastroenterol Hepatol 2011;23(1):60–5.
27. Cipolletta L, Zambelli A, Bianco MA, et al. Acrylate glue injection for acutely bleeding oesophageal varices: a prospective cohort study. Dig Liver Dis 2009; 41(10):729–34.
28. Ribeiro JP, Matuguma SE, Cheng S, et al. Results of treatment of esophageal variceal hemorrhage with endoscopic injection of n-butyl-2-cyanoacrylate in patients with Child-Pugh class C cirrhosis. Endosc Int Open. 3(6):E584–589.
29. Ljubicic N, Bisćanin A, Nikolić M, et al. A randomized-controlled trial of endoscopic treatment of acute esophageal variceal hemorrhage: N-butyl-2-cyanoacrylate injection vs. variceal ligation. Hepatogastroenterology 2011;58(106): 438–43.
30. Maluf-Filho F, Sakai P, Ishioka S, et al. Endoscopic sclerosis versus cyanoacrylate endoscopic injection for the first episode of variceal bleeding: a prospective, controlled, and randomized study in Child-Pugh class C patients. Endoscopy 2001;33(5):421–7.
31. Feretis C, Dimopoulos C, Benakis P, et al. N-butyl-2-cyanoacrylate (Histoacryl) plus sclerotherapy versus sclerotherapy alone in the treatment of bleeding esophageal varices: a randomized prospective study. Endoscopy 1995;27(5): 355–7.
32. Thakeb F, Salama Z, Salama H, et al. The value of combined use of N-butyl-2-cyanoacrylate and ethanolamine oleate in the management of bleeding esophagogastric varices. Endoscopy 1995;27(5):358–64.
33. Al-Osaimi FR, Bennamoun M, Mian A. Spatially optimized data-level fusion of texture and shape for face recognition. IEEE Trans Image Process 2012;21(2): 859–72.
34. Sharma BC, Varakanahalli S, Singh JP, et al. Gastric varices in cirrhosis vs. extrahepatic portal venous obstruction and response to endoscopic N-butyl-2-cyanoacrylate injection. J Clin Exp Hepatol 2017;7(2):97–101.
35. Binmoeller KF. Endoscopic ultrasound-guided coil and glue injection for gastric variceal bleeding. Gastroenterol Hepatol (N Y) 2018;14(2):123–6.
36. Sarin SK, Lahoti D, Saxena SP, et al. Prevalence, classification and natural history of gastric varices: a long-term follow-up study in 568 portal hypertension patients. Hepatology 1992;16(6):1343–9.

37. Trudeau W, Prindiville T. Endoscopic injection sclerosis in bleeding gastric varices. Gastrointest Endosc 1986;32(4):264–8.
38. Sarin SK. Long-term follow-up of gastric variceal sclerotherapy: an eleven-year experience. Gastrointest Endosc 1997;46(1):8–14.
39. Weilert F, Binmoeller KF. Endoscopic management of gastric variceal bleeding. Gastroenterol Clin North Am 2014;43(4):807–18.
40. Sarin SK, Jain AK, Jain M et al. A randomized controlled trial of cyanoacrylate versus alcohol injection in patients with isolated fundic varices. Am J Gastroenterol. 97(4):1010–1015
41. Rios Castellanos E, Seron P, Gisbert JP, et al. Endoscopic injection of cyanoacrylate glue versus other endoscopic procedures for acute bleeding gastric varices in people with portal hypertension. Cochrane Database Syst Rev 2015;(5):CD010180.
42. Soehendra N, Nam VC, Grimm H, et al. Endoscopic obliteration of large esophagogastric varices with bucrylate. Endoscopy 1986;18(1):25–6.
43. de Franchis R, Primignani M. Endoscopic treatments for portal hypertension. Semin Liver Dis 1999;19(4):439–55.
44. Tantau M, Crisan D, Popa D, et al. Band ligation vs. N-Butyl-2-cyanoacrylate injection in acute gastric variceal bleeding: a prospective follow-up study. Ann Hepatol 2013;13(1):75–83.
45. El Amin H, Abdel Baky L, Sayed Z, et al. A randomized trial of endoscopic variceal ligation versus cyanoacrylate injection for treatment of bleeding junctional varices. Trop Gastroenterol 2010;31(4):279–84.
46. Levy I, Binmoeller KF. EUS-guided vascular interventions. Endosc Ultrasound 2018;7(4):228–35.
47. Boustiere C, Dumas O, Jouffre C, et al. Endoscopic ultrasonography classification of gastric varices in patients with cirrhosis. Comparison with endoscopic findings. J Hepatol 1993;19(2):268–72.
48. Iwase H, Suga S, Morise K, et al. Color Doppler endoscopic ultrasonography for the evaluation of gastric varices and endoscopic obliteration with cyanoacrylate glue. Gastrointest Endosc 1995;41(2):150–4.
49. Romero-Castro R, Pellicer-Bautista FJ, Jimenez-Saenz M, et al. EUS-guided injection of cyanoacrylate in perforating feeding veins in gastric varices: results in 5 cases. Gastrointest Endosc 2007;66(2):402–7.
50. Battaglia G, Morbin T, Patarnello E, et al. Visceral fistula as a complication of endoscopic treatment of esophageal and gastric varices using isobutyl-2-cyanoacrylate: report of two cases. Gastrointest Endosc 2000;52(2):267–70.
51. Romero-Castro R, Ellrichmann M, Ortiz-Moyano C, et al. EUS-guided coil versus cyanoacrylate therapy for the treatment of gastric varices: a multicenter study (with videos). Gastrointest Endosc 2013;78(5):711–21.
52. Burke MP, O'Donnell C, Baber Y. Death from pulmonary embolism of cyanoacrylate glue following gastric varix endoscopic injection. Forensic Sci Med Pathol 2017;13(1):82–5.
53. Binmoeller KF, Weilert F, Shah JN, et al. EUS-guided transesophageal treatment of gastric fundal varices with combined coiling and cyanoacrylate glue injection (with videos). Gastrointest Endosc 2011;74(5):1019–25.
54. Bhat YM, Weilert F, Fredrick RT, et al. EUS-guided treatment of gastric fundal varices with combined injection of coils and cyanoacrylate glue: a large U.S. experience over 6 years (with video). Gastrointest Endosc 2016;83(6):1164–72.

55. Levy MJ, Wong Kee Song LM, Kendrick ML, et al. EUS-guided coil embolization for refractory ectopic variceal bleeding (with videos). Gastrointest Endosc 2008; 67(3):572–4.
56. Romero-Castro R, Pellicer-Bautista F, Giovannini M, et al. Endoscopic ultrasound (EUS)-guided coil embolization therapy in gastric varices. Endoscopy 2010; 42(Suppl 2):E35–6.
57. Mishra SR, Sharma BC, Kumar A, et al. Primary prophylaxis of gastric variceal bleeding comparing cyanoacrylate injection and beta-blockers: a randomized controlled trial. J Hepatol 2011;54(6):1161–7.
58. Hanafy AS, El Hawary AT. Efficacy of argon plasma coagulation in the management of portal hypertensive gastropathy. Endosc Int Open 2016;4(10):E1057–62.
59. Smith LA, Morris AJ, Stanley AJ. The use of hemospray in portal hypertensive bleeding; a case series. J Hepatol 2014;60(2):457–60.
60. Sharma M, Rai P, Bansal R. EUS-assisted evaluation of rectal varices before banding. Gastroenterol Res Pract 2013;2013:619187.
61. Al Khalloufi K, Laiyemo AO. Management of rectal varices in portal hypertension. World J Hepatol 2015;7(30):2992–8.
62. Sato T, Yamazaki K, Akaike J, et al. Retrospective analysis of endoscopic injection sclerotherapy for rectal varices compared with band ligation. Clin Exp Gastroenterol 2010;3:159–63.
63. Weilert F, Shah JN, Marson FP, et al. EUS-guided coil and glue for bleeding rectal varix. Gastrointest Endosc 2012;76(4):915–6.
64. Park SW, Cho E, Jun CH, et al. Upper gastrointestinal ectopic variceal bleeding treated with various endoscopic modalities: case reports and literature review. Medicine (Baltimore) 2017;96(1):e5860.
65. Henry Z, Uppal D, Saad W, et al. Gastric and ectopic varices. Clin Liver Dis 2014; 18(2):371–88.
66. Orr DW, Harrison PM, Devlin J, et al. Chronic mesenteric venous thrombosis: evaluation and determinants of survival during long-term follow-up. Clin Gastroenterol Hepatol 2007;5(1):80–6.
67. Norton ID, Andrews JC, Kamath PS. Management of ectopic varices. Hepatology 1998;28(4):1154–8.
68. Helmy A, Al Kahtani K, Al Fadda M. Updates in the pathogenesis, diagnosis and management of ectopic varices. Hepatol Int 2008;2(3):322–34.

Endoscopic Ultrasound for the Diagnosis and Staging of Liver Tumors

Andrew Lange, MD[a], Thiruvengadam Muniraj, MD[b], Harry R. Aslanian, MD[c,*]

KEYWORDS

- Endoscopic ultrasound • Focal liver lesion • Hepatocellular carcinoma

KEY POINTS

- Endoscopic ultrasound examination with fine needle aspiration has a role in diagnosing suspicious hepatic lesions and peri-hepatic nodes found to be 1 to 2 cm on conventional imaging.
- Endoscopic ultrasound examination with fine needle aspiration is useful in sampling portal vein thrombosis in the setting of hepatocellular carcinoma.
- Endoscopic ultrasound examination with fine needle aspiration is useful in staging liver lesions that are not classified as advanced stage by a validated staging tool.
- Novel modalities of endoscopic ultrasound examination will likely expand its use in the coming years.

INTRODUCTION

The use of endoscopic ultrasound (EUS) examination in the diagnosis and management of gastrointestinal tumors has evolved since its inception in the 1980s.[1–4] In the late 1990s, the safety and efficacy of EUS examination with fine needle aspiration (FNA) for the detection of small focal liver lesions undetected on conventional computed tomography (CT) scanning was established.[5–7] Over the next decade, the usefulness of EUS-guided FNA as a staging tool for a variety of solid liver lesions, including hepatocellular carcinoma (HCC), was demonstrated.[8] In this review, we present an overview of the diagnostic approach to liver tumors, and the role of EUS

Disclosure Statement: The authors have no conflicts of interest to disclose.
[a] Department of Internal Medicine, Yale University School of Medicine, Yale Primary Care Center, 789 Howard Avenue, New Haven, CT 06511, USA; [b] Section of Digestive Diseases, Laboratory for Medicine and Pediatrics, Yale University School of Medicine, 15 York Street, New Haven, CT 06510, USA; [c] Section of Digestive Diseases, Yale University School of Medicine, PO Box 208056, 333 Cedar Street, New Haven, CT 06520, USA
* Corresponding author:
E-mail address: harry.aslanian@yale.edu

Gastrointest Endoscopy Clin N Am 29 (2019) 339–350
https://doi.org/10.1016/j.giec.2018.12.005 giendo.theclinics.com
1052-5157/19/© 2018 Elsevier Inc. All rights reserved.

examination in diagnosis and staging of liver tumors, as well as newly developed imaging modalities for assessment of liver tumors.

OVERVIEW OF PRIMARY LIVER TUMORS

Liver tumors can be either benign or malignant.[9] The diagnosis and subsequent management of solid liver lesions relies on building an appropriate differential diagnosis based on history, risk factors, laboratory findings, and imaging studies.[10] Important historical clues that may suggest the etiology of primary liver lesions include the presence of cirrhosis and hepatitis B, the absence of extrahepatic malignancy, the lesion size, and the use of oral contraceptive medications.[11,12] If the history suggests a particular diagnosis, the American College of Gastroenterology advises imaging with triphasic contrast-enhanced (CE) CT scanning or MRI, over conventional US examination of the liver, owing to improved performance characteristics.[13,14] The need for CT scans with late arterial, portal, and delayed phases (triple phase) emphasizes the significance of vascular patterns in the diagnosis of focal liver lesions. This is particularly useful in primary liver neoplasms, where triple phase CT or MRI scanning alone has a greater than 90% diagnostic accuracy in lesions greater than 2 cm.[15] When imaging results are not confirmatory in making a diagnosis, a biopsy should be considered.

LIMITATIONS OF CONVENTIONAL IMAGING

Cross-sectional imaging has some limitations in the accurate detection of both primary and metastatic liver lesions[16] and EUS-guided FNA may provide beneficial complementary information. Nguyen and colleagues[6] demonstrated the superiority of EUS-guided FNA over CT scanning in the detection of primary liver lesions that were less than 1 cm. Awad and colleagues[17] identified management changes in 67% of patients who underwent EUS-guided FNA as compared with conventional CT scanning for the workup of primary liver lesions. EUS-guided FNA may have an important role in the diagnosis and management of secondary liver lesions as well (**Fig. 1**). A retrospective study in 2004 by Prasad and colleagues[18] found that 2.3% of metastatic liver lesions were not identified with conventional cross-sectional

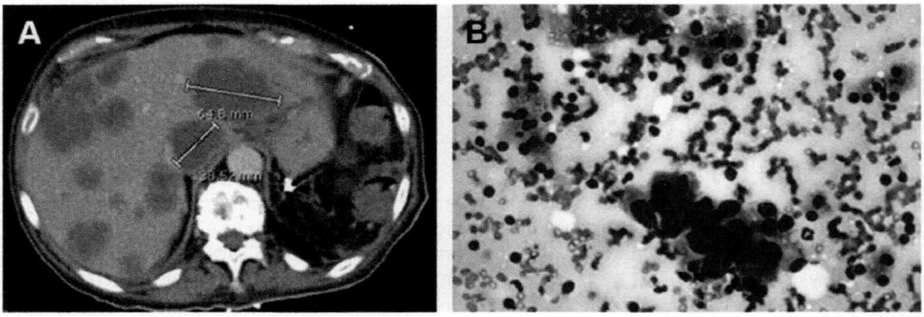

Fig. 1. (*A*) Computed tomography scan of the abdomen showing multiple low-attenuating metastatic lesions in the right and left hepatic lobes in a patient with pancreas adenocarcinoma. (*B*) Fine needle aspiration sample from the liver lesion shows single and loose cohesive clusters of tumor cells with moderate amount of vacuolated cytoplasm pleomorphic nuclei with irregular nuclear contours, and small nucleolus, characteristic of adenocarcinoma. A few small clusters of benign hepatocytes are present (stain: Diff-Quik stain; original magnification ×400).

imaging. A prospective cohort study by Singh and colleagues[19] in 2009 found that EUS examination detected a significantly higher number of malignant lesions when compared with conventional CT scanning. EUS-guided FNA was able to accurately determine the nature of the liver lesion in 88% of cases. Studies have not reassessed the role of EUS examination relative to current cross-sectional imaging technology following the significant advances in CT scanning, MRI, and contrast enhancement over the past decade. In current clinical practice, standard imaging EUS has a limited role in the detection of hepatic lesions not seen by CE CT scanning or MRI.

ENDOSCOPIC ULTRASOUND IMAGING IN THE DIAGNOSIS OF HEPATOCELLULAR CARCINOMA

HCC is the most common primary liver cancer, and the third most common cause of cancer death worldwide.[20,21] Recent data shows an incidence of 10.8 per 100,000 men and 3.2 per 100,000 women in 2012 (slightly increasing in 2013), with a 5-year survival rate of 17.6% in most patients.[22,23] The high incidence and mortality rate of HCC reflects the underlying aggressive nature of the disease, diagnostic challenges, and the strong correlation with underlying liver disease.[24] Differentiating the sequelae of chronic liver disease and HCC is challenging, with many organizations suggesting specific screening algorithms. Currently, guidelines suggest routine screening every 6 months using abdominal US imaging with or without serum alpha-fetoprotein levels in patients with chronic liver disease.[25] The regenerative potential of hepatocytes in the setting of chronic inflammation—whether it is due to viral hepatitis, chronic alcohol intake, nonalcoholic steatohepatitis, or other etiologies—leads to challenges in meaningfully differentiating liver nodules related to chronic liver disease. As such, the American Association for the Study of Liver Disease recommends monitoring nodules less than 1 cm found on screening, and further cross-sectional imaging using either triphasic CT scan or MRI for those greater than 1 cm.[25] For lesions greater than 2 cm, the American Association for the Study of Liver Disease and Barcelona Convention on HCC recommends a formal diagnosis of HCC if 2 separate imaging modalities confirm a lesion is larger than 2 cm in a patient with risk factors. For lesions between 1 and 2 cm without pathognomonic signs on cross-sectional imaging associated with a serum alpha-fetoprotein level of less than 200 ng/mL, further workup with a biopsy is recommended. EUS imaging may have the greatest impact on the diagnosis of primary HCC in the evaluation of indeterminate lesions.[26]

Although the American Association for the Study of Liver Disease guidelines do not comment on the role of EUS imaging in the diagnosis of liver tumors, a number of retrospective and prospective studies support its use.[27] Crowe and colleagues[28] compared 6 years of CT-guided biopsy results in the late 1990s with 2.5 years of EUS-guided biopsy, finding similar levels of diagnostic usefulness in sampling liver lesions. A 2003 study by DeWitt and associates[29] demonstrated positive EUS-guided FNA results in 41% of patients with previous cross-sectional imaging (CT scans) not suggesting a liver malignancy. This information impacted management in more than 80% of patients. In addition, EUS-guided FNA also provided the primary diagnosis and upstaged HCC in approximately 20% of patients, thereby avoiding unneeded surgical intervention. A single-center retrospective study of 23 liver masses amenable to EUS-guided FNA reported a sensitivity, specificity, and positive predictive value for malignancy of 94%, 100%, and 100%, respectively.[30] A prospective study of more than 50 patients demonstrated the effectiveness of EUS-guided FNA for the detection of HCC metastases to locoregional lymph nodes, obviating the need for surgical intervention[31] (**Fig. 2**). Additionally, a recent multicenter experience confirmed no statistical

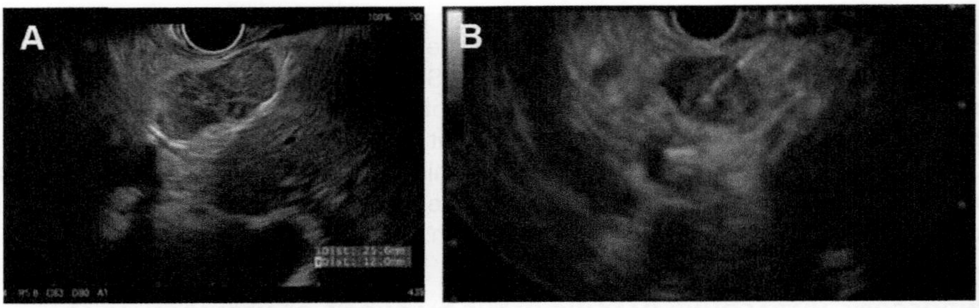

Fig. 2. *A*) A cluster of rounded, hypoechoic nodes in the gastrohepatic region measuring up to 2 cm in a patient with hepatocellular carcinoma. (*B*) A 22G fine needle biopsy needle was used to sample the gastrohepatic node, with malignant cells seen onsite.

difference between bilobar, right, or left lobe EUS-guided liver biopsies.[32] However, although EUS is an effective tool, it cannot visualize the entire right lobe of the liver, leaving many areas of the right lobe better suited for percutaneous biopsy.

Despite the paucity of data investigating the usefulness of EUS-guided FNA for indeterminate lesions requiring further evaluation per HCC screening algorithms, recent research suggests its safety and efficacy.[33] Singh and colleagues[34] evaluated 5 lesions less than 2 cm in a small number of patients. EUS-guided FNA determined 3 lesions to be malignant and 2 benign, allowing for early intervention.[35] Larger, prospective studies are needed to define the role of EUS in the diagnosis of primary liver tumors. Additionally, owing to the limitations of right lobe visualization, we do not recommend its use as a screening modality for liver lesions. We do recommend considering the use of EUS-guided FNA for lesions located in the left lobe of the liver adjacent to the stomach or right lobe near the duodenal bulb in patients with risk factors that are between 1 and 2 cm, or lesions greater than 2 cm without classic cross-sectional imaging findings to suggest HCC.

ENDOSCOPIC ULTRASOUND IMAGING AS A TOOL FOR DIAGNOSTIC SAMPLING OF PORTAL VEIN THROMBOSES

EUS-guided FNA is well-suited for the evaluation and diagnosis of portal vein thrombosis and the diagnosis of metastatic HCC to the portal vein,[27] as first reported by Lai and colleagues[36] in 2004. Additional case reports demonstrate the usefulness of EUS-guided FNA to detect malignant cells within tumor thrombus of the portal vein.[37,38]

Transabdominal US-guided biopsy of portal vein thromboses is well-described (**Fig. 3**).[39,40] Limitations of transabdominal US imaging include challenges in obese patients and a risk of bile duct or vascular injury.[41] Complications have not been encountered in the small number of EUS-guided biopsies reported. The diagnosis of malignant portal vein thrombus may have an impact on management, because this would preclude liver transplantation.[42] Kantsevoy and Thuluvath[43] detail additional considerations for EUS-guided FNA sampling of portal vein thromboses to include avoidance of the surrounding vasculature and associated risk of bleeding, potential concerns for tumor seeding through the FNA tract, and confounding of biopsy results owing to the presence of cells from the gastric and duodenal wall. Although experience in a greater numbers of patients would be beneficial, EUS-guided FNA seems to have an important role in the diagnosis of malignant portal vein thrombosis. Although not evaluated in the setting of HCC, direct portal venous sampling of blood has been shown to identify a greater number of circulating

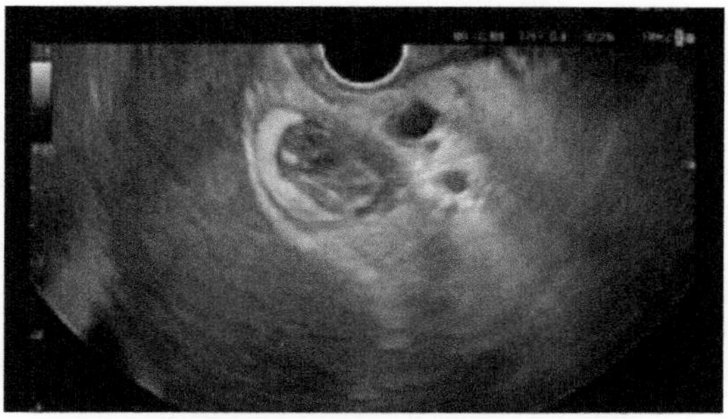

Fig. 3. Endoscopic ultrasound image revealing a partial thrombosis of the portal vein with limited Doppler flow seen around the heterogeneous clot.

pancreas adenocarcinoma cells in comparison with peripheral blood.[44,45] A pilot study has also demonstrated the capability to perform EUS-guided portal pressure measurements.[46] It is our recommendation that, when a portal vein thrombosis is identified without definitive evidence of metastatic HCC, biopsy via EUS-guided FNA should be considered.

ENDOSCOPIC ULTRASOUND IMAGING AND THE STAGING OF PRIMARY LIVER TUMORS

Many staging systems for primary liver tumors exist, and there is significant disagreement regarding which imaging and biochemical tests best reflect accurate staging of primary liver tumors.[27,47–49] Most staging schema focus their criteria on HCC, because it is by far the most common primary liver tumor.[20] The American Joint Committee on Cancer (AJCC) TNM (tumor, nodes, metastases) staging system uses tumor size, locoregional lymph nodes, and metastases as indictors for survival.[50] The AJCC uses a cutoff of a 2-cm tumor size combined with vascular invasion to differentiate stage I and II tumors. In addition, 2 cm is the size required on cross-sectional imaging to definitively diagnose HCC. Any regional lymph nodes or distant metastases place tumors into stage IV, which has a dismal prognosis.[51] Vascular invasion is also critical to the staging of HCC in the AJCC TNM model. Currently, triphasic CT or MRI scans are used to evaluate vascular invasion, with good efficacy,[52] yet as discussed elsewhere in this article, there remains concern over the malignant potential of portal venous thromboses. Additionally, the AJCCs TNM model does not take into consideration hepatic performance metrics when staging HCC, a pitfall that other staging systems attempt to mitigate.

The Barcelona Clinic Liver Cancer (BCLC) staging system is an alternative to the AJCC TNM staging model. This model incorporates hepatic performance status in addition to the size of the primary lesion, vascular/extrahepatic spread, constitutional symptoms, and Okuda stage.[53] BCLC also uses the 2-cm cutoff between stage 0 and stage A, along with the performance status of the patient. That the BCLC incorporates the Child-Pugh system of liver function sets it apart from the AJCC TNM model. The Child-Pugh liver classification uses biochemical markers such as bilirubin, albumin, and prothrombin time as evidence of hepatic synthetic performance.[54] Stage A requires Child-Pugh class A, and stages B and C require Child-Pugh class A or B. It is only BCLC stage D that requires patients to be in Child-Pugh class C. The BCLC staging system has been shown to outperform the AJCC TNM system in studies, despite significant criticism of its algorithmic approach.[55,56] The ability of EUS imaging to accurately evaluate the regional lymph nodes and vascular invasion, particularly in indeterminate liver lesions or portal vein thromboses, supports its usefulness.

The Cancer Liver Italian Program (CLIP) staging system is the most recent model developed to assess HCC.[57] This system combines Child-Pugh stage, tumor morphology, alpha-fetoprotein, and portal vein thrombosis status into an aggregate prognostic score, ranging from 0 to 6. Advancing CLIP stage reflects median survival of patients, ranging from 36 months for CLIP stage 0 to 3 months for CLIP stage 6. The CLIP system outperformed the AJCC TNM, BCLC, and Child-Pugh classifications in some studies, but was more useful in patients who did not require surgical intervention.[58] However, it does rank first among the HCC staging systems in its ability to predict survival.[59] The use of EUS examination in this system to more accurately evaluate tumor morphology and portal vein thromboses could potentially improve the prognostic value of this staging system, although further study is required.

Another commonly used HCC staging system is the Okuda system.[60] This system uses tumor size (>50% of tumor invasion of the liver), clinical presences of ascites, albumin (<3 mg/dL), and total serum bilirubin (>3 mg/dL). One of the major drawbacks to the Okuda system is that it does not incorporate lymph node involvement or vascular invasion. Additionally, it lacks the ability to identify less advanced patients.[48] As such, the application of EUS to this staging system is limited. Based on their ease of use and the Okuda system's lack of sensitivity to important tumor factors, it has been suggested that CLIP and other systems may by superior.[61]

There is no consensus on the preferred liver staging system. The usefulness of EUS-guided FNA to evaluate and diagnose small liver lesions, malignant portal vein thromboses, and locoregional lymph nodes could influence staging with all of the criteria mentioned herein. This is particularly true in early stage HCC and other primary liver tumors, where early intervention by transplantation, resection, or tumor ablation may lead to curative results. Additionally, EUS-guided FNA plays a role in the diagnosis and staging of later stage primary liver tumors, potentially obviating the need for inappropriate surgical intervention. Thus, we recommend considering the use of EUS-guided FNA to stage liver lesions that are not classified as advanced stage by a validated staging tool.

CONTRAST-ENHANCED ULTRASOUND EXAMINATION FOR THE DIAGNOSIS OF PRIMARY AND SECONDARY LIVER LESIONS

The recent approval by the US Food and Drug Administration of CE-US examination of the liver has been a welcome addition to the toolbox for imaging primary hepatic lesions.[62] CE-US imaging uses stabilized gas bubbles injected into the patient to provide higher levels of resolution, while deploying a transabdominal probe for the assessment of anatomic structures.[62,63] Studies indicate benefits of CE-US imaging over conventional methods of liver imaging. CE-US imaging can differentiate down to the level of the capillaries (100 microns), which allows for the quantification of tissue perfusion,[64] including an assessment of arterial and venous phases of blood flow to a liver lesion, which is critical in determining its etiology.[65] Additionally, similar to EUS imaging, there is no radiation exposure when using CE-US imaging. Seitz and colleagues[66] demonstrated a 95% sensitivity and 94% specificity in the characterization of focal liver lesions using CE-US imaging, which was noninferior to MRI. CU-EUS imaging is currently only approved for use in Europe. We anticipate that CE-EUS imaging will have further enhance the evaluation of liver lesions as it has for transabdominal US imaging. A recent study of 30 patients with metastatic liver lesions found 22 lesions visible with standard EUS imaging and 29 visible with the addition of CE-EUS imaging. EUS sampling was performed in all cases with a diagnostic accuracy of 87%.[67]

ENDOSCOPIC ULTRASOUND IMAGING AND THE APPLICATION OF ELASTOGRAPHY FOR THE EVALUATION OF LIVER LESIONS

Elastography is a noninvasive quantitative evaluation tool used to assess the stiffness of tissues. Although the physics of elastography are better explained elsewhere, US imaging produces 2 types of sound waves, longitudinal and shear, that interact with tissues depending largely on tissue density.[68] Using this phenomenon, an operator can evaluate liver lesions based on their density, under the assumption that malignant liver lesions may have a higher density than benign lesions[68,69] EUS elastography has been suggested as a useful tool for the evaluation of liver lesions.[70,71] A 2014 metaanalysis by Ma and colleagues[72] demonstrated clinical usefulness in differentiating benign and malignant liver lesions using EUS elastography. They reported an 85%, 84%, and 5.69 sensitivity, specificity, and positive likelihood ratio for tumor differentiation when compared with the gold standard of histology. A 2015 study found similar sensitivities and specificities (74% and 84%, respectively) for the differentiation of benign and malignant liver lesions.

These results, however, have not been consistently reproducible. Frulio and colleagues[73] did not find a significant difference between benign and malignant lesions using EUS elastography, nor did Heide and colleagues,[74] using acoustic radiation force elastography. This is likely due to the inherent heterogeneity in tissue density found in a range of normal and pathologic liver lesions. Hepatic venous congestion, steatohepatitis, and ongoing inflammation from external toxins such as alcohol influence the stiffness of the liver, and may confound the ability of EUS-elastography to accurately characterize focal lesions. Further research and technical improvements in EUS elastography are needed to support routine application.

ENDOSCOPIC ULTRASOUND IMAGING AND THE EVALUATION OF METASTATIC LIVER DISEASE

EUS imaging may have an important adjunctive role in the evaluation and management of metastatic liver disease.[75] Metastases to the liver are the most common form of hepatic neoplasm in the United States.[76] In 2016, de Ridder and colleagues[77] detailed the incidence and origin of more than 23,000 patients with histologically confirmed hepatic metastases. The majority of hepatic metastases were from adenocarcinoma not otherwise specified, followed by adenocarcinoma of the colorectum, pancreas, and breast. Melanoma and lung tumors were also common primary sources. The appearance of the metastatic lesion tends to mirror that of the primary tumor, which can be helpful when assessing vascularity and necrosis on radiographic imaging. The gold standard for radiographic imaging is CE CT scan, MRI, or transabdominal US imaging.[78,79] However, these modalities may underrepresent subcentimeter metastatic lesions. EUS provides a useful adjunctive tool in the diagnosis of these subcentimeter lesions, because it may identify and allow sampling of small hepatic lesions that are indeterminate on conventional cross-sectional imaging. EUS evaluation and biopsy of a suspected primary lesion, such as a pancreas mass, will typically include examination for metastatic lymphadenopathy in the subcarinal, celiac, and portal regions, along with evaluation of the liver. The identification of metastatic disease may significantly alter subsequent management.

To optimize EUS imaging of the liver, we have found the following technique to be helpful. Owing to the frequent subtlety of hepatic metastases, repeated back-and-forth scanning through the liver by torqueing the EUS probe is advised. While scanning, evaluation for hypoechoic or hyperechoic, often circular structures, which lead to disrupted normal liver parenchyma, vascular, and/or biliary ductular patterns is critical. When a suspicious lesion is found, FNA of the most accessible lesion (typically closest to the probe) may be performed. When possible, avoid subscapular lesions owing to the higher risk of hemorrhage. Hepatic metastases are typically very cellular, allowing for a 25G needle to be effectively used for a diagnostic sample.[75] If a cell block is required and the primary mass lesion has limited cellularity, repeated FNA sampling or fine needle biopsy of larger hepatic lesions may be pursued.

SUMMARY

EUS imaging may provide complementary information to cross-sectional imaging to characterize lesions in the liver, portal vein, and surrounding lymph nodes. Coupled with FNA, EUS imaging is a powerful tool for the frequently nuanced diagnosis of focal liver lesions including HCC. EUS-guided FNA has usefulness in the evaluation of indeterminate liver lesions, where a biopsy may help to guide early intervention. EUS imaging may influence hepatocellular cancer staging and EUS-guided FNA of locoregional nodes and portal vein thromboses has been shown to alter management. CE EUS imaging and EUS elastography are likely to expand the usefulness of EUS imaging in the evaluation of liver malignancy with continued technologic improvements.

REFERENCES

1. Dimagno EP, Buxton JL, Regan PT, et al. Ultrasonic endoscope. Lancet 1980;1(8169):629–31.
2. Godfrey EM, Rushbrook SM, Carroll NR. Endoscopic ultrasound: a review of current diagnostic and therapeutic applications. Postgrad Med J 2010;86(1016):346–53.
3. Jenssen C, Dietrich CF. Endoscopic ultrasound-guided fine-needle aspiration biopsy and trucut biopsy in gastroenterology - an overview. Best Pract Res Clin Gastroenterol 2009;23(5):743–59.
4. Wiersema MJ, Hawes RH, Tao LC, et al. Endoscopic ultrasonography as an adjunct to fine needle aspiration cytology of the upper and lower gastrointestinal tract. Gastrointest Endosc 1992;38:35–9.
5. Wiersema MJ, Wiersema LM, Khusro Q, et al. Combined endosonography and fine-needle aspiration cytology in the evaluation of gastrointestinal lesions. Gastrointest Endosc 1994;40(2 Pt 1):199–206.
6. Nguyen P, Feng JC, Chang KJ. Endoscopic ultrasound (EUS) and EUS-guided fine-needle aspiration (FNA) of liver lesions. Gastrointest Endosc 1999;50(3):357–61.
7. Bhutani MS, Logrono R. Endoscopic ultrasound-guided fine-needle aspiration cytology for diagnosis above and below the diaphragm. J Clin Ultrasound 2005;33(8):401–11.
8. Parekh PJ, Majithia R, Diehl DL, et al. Endoscopy ultrasound-guided liver biopsy. Endosc Ultrasound 2015;4(2):85–91.
9. Bonder A, Afdhal N. Evaluation of liver lesions. Clin Liver Dis 2012;16:271.
10. Reddy KR, Schiff ER. Approach to a liver mass. Semin Liver Dis 1993;13:423.
11. Torzilli G, Minagawa M, Takayama T, et al. Accurate preoperative evaluation of liver mass lesions without fine-needle biopsy. Hepatology 1999;30:889.
12. Rooks JB, Ory HW, Ishak KG, et al. Epidemiology of hepatocellular adenoma. The role of oral contraceptive use. JAMA 1979;242:644.

13. Marrero J, Ahn J, Reddy K, AGC Clinical Guideline. The diagnosis and management of focal liver lesions. Am J Gastroenterol 2014;109:1328–47.
14. Ros PR, Mortele KJ. Hepatic imaging: an overview. Clin Liver Dis 2002;6:1–16.
15. Di Martino M, De Filippis G, De Santis A, et al. Hepatocellular carcinoma in cirrhotic patients: prospective comparison of US CT and MR imaging. Eur Radiol 2013;23:887–96.
16. Glover C, Douse P, Kane P, et al. Accuracy of investigations for asymptomatic colorectal liver metastases. Dis Colon Rectum 2002;45:476–84.
17. Awad SS, Fagan S, Abudayyeh S, et al. Preoperative evaluation of hepatic lesions for the staging of hepatocellular and metastatic liver carcinoma using endoscopic ultrasonography. Am J Surg 2002;184(6):601–4.
18. Prasad P, Schmulewitz N, Patel A, et al. Detection of occult liver metastases during EUS for staging of malignancies. Gastrointest Endosc 2004;59:49–53.
19. Singh P, Mukhopadhyay P, Bhatt B, et al. Endoscopic ultrasound versus CT scan for detection of metastases to the liver. J Clin Gastroenterol 2009;43(4):367–73.
20. Bruix J, Sherman M. Management of hepatocellular carcinoma: an update. Hepatology 2011;53:1020–2.
21. Center for Disease Control and Prevention (CDC). Hepatocellular carcinoma-United States 2001–2006. MMWR Morb Mortal Wkly Rep 2010;59(17):517–20.
22. Hashem EB, Hernaez R. How we approach it: treatment options for hepatocellular carcinoma. Am J Gastroenterol 2018;113(6):791–4.
23. Altekruse S, McGlynn K, Reichman M, et al. Hepatocellular carcinoma incidence, mortality, and survival trends in the United States from 1975 to 2005. J Clin Oncol 2009;27(9):1485–91.
24. Balogh J, Victor D, Asham EH, et al. Hepatocellular carcinoma: a review. J Hepatocell Carcinoma 2016;3:41–53.
25. Heimbach J, Kulik L, Finn R, et al. AASLD guidelines for the treatment of hepatocellular carcinoma. Hepatology 2018;67(1):358–80.
26. Burak KW, Kneteman NM. An evidence-based multidisciplinary approach to the management of hepatocellular carcinoma (HCC): the Alberta HCC algorithm. Can J Gastroenterol 2010;24:643–50.
27. Girotra M, Soota K, Dhaliwal A, et al. Utility of endoscopic ultrasound and endoscopy in diagnosis and management of hepatocellular carcinoma and its complications: what does endoscopic ultrasonography offer above and beyond conventional cross-sectional imaging? World J Gastrointest Endosc 2018;10(2):56–68.
28. Crowe D, Eloubeidi M, Chhieng D, et al. Fine needle aspiration biopsy of hepatic lesions: computerized tomographic-guided versus endoscopic ultrasound-guided FNA. Cancer 2006;108(3):180–5.
29. DeWitt J, LeBlanc J, McHenry L, et al. Endoscopic ultrasound guided fine needle aspiration cytology of solid liver lesions: a large single-center experience. Am J Gastroenterol 2003;98(9):1976–81.
30. Anand D, Barroeta JE, Gupta PK, et al. Endoscopic ultrasound guided fine needle aspiration of non-pancreatic lesions: an institutional experience. J Clin Pathol 2007;60(11):1254–62.
31. Choudhary NS, Puri R, Saigal S, et al. Impact of endoscopic ultrasound-guided fine-needle aspiration in prospective liver transplant recipients with hepatocellular carcinoma and lymphadenopathy. Indian J Gastroenterol 2016;35:465–8.
32. Diehl D, Johal A, Khara H, et al. Endoscopic ultrasound-guided liver biopsy: a multiple center experience. Endosc Int Open 2015;3(3):E210–5.

33. Tellez-Avila FI, Duarte-Medrano G, Gallardo VE, et al. Diagnostic yield of endoscopic ultrasound-guided fine needle aspiration cytology of solid liver lesions in a single center. Gastrointestinal Endoscopy. Conference: Digestive Diseases Week, DDW 2016 ASGE. San Diego, CA, United States.
34. Singh P, Erickson RA, Mukhopadhyay P, et al. EUS for detection of the hepatocellular carcinoma: results of a prospective study. Gastrointest Endosc 2007;66: 265–73.
35. Fujii-Lau LL, Abu Dayyeh BK, Bruno MJ, et al. EUS-derived criteria for distinguishing benign from malignant metastatic solid hepatic masses. Gastrointest Endosc 2015;81:1188–96.
36. Lai R, Stephens V, Bardales R. Diagnosis and staging of hepatocellular carcinoma by EUS-FNA of a portal vein thrombus. Gastrointest Endosc 2004;59: 574–7.
37. Storch I, Gomez C, Contreras F, et al. Hepatocellular carcinoma (HCC) with portal vein invasion, masquerading as pancreatic mass, diagnosed by endoscopic ultrasound-guided fine needle aspiration (EUS-FNA). Dig Dis Sci 2007;52: 789–91.
38. Michael H, Lenza C, Gupta M, et al. Endoscopic ultrasound -guided fine-needle aspiration of a portal vein thrombus to aid in the diagnosis and staging of hepatocellular carcinoma. Gastroenterol Hepatol (NY) 2011;7:124–9.
39. Dusenbery D, Dodd GD III, Carr BI. Percutaneous fine-needle aspiration of portal vein thrombi as a staging technique for hepatocellular carcinoma. Cytologic findings of 46 patients. Cancer 1995;75:2057–62.
40. Cedrone A, Rapaccini GL, Pompili M, et al. Portal vein thrombosis complicating hepatocellular carcinoma. Value of ultrasound-guided fine-needle biopsy of the thrombus in the therapeutic management. Liver 1996;16:94–8.
41. Dodd GD III, Carr BI. Percutaneous biopsy of portal vein thrombus: a new staging technique for hepatocellular carcinoma. AJR Am J Roentgenol 1993;161:229–33.
42. Vilana R, Bru C, Bruix J, et al. Fine-needle aspiration biopsy of portal vein thrombus: value in detecting malignant thrombosis. AJR Am J Roentgenol 1993;160:1285–7.
43. Kantsevoy S, Thuluvath P. Utility and safety of EUS-guided portal vein FNA. Gastroenterol Hepatol (NY) 2011;7:129–31.
44. Catenacci DV, Chapman CG, Xu P, et al. Acquisition of portal venous circulating tumor cells from patients with pancreaticobiliary cancers by endoscopic ultrasound. Gastroenterology 2015;149:1794–803.
45. Muniraj T, Aslanian HR. New developments in endoscopic ultrasound tissue acquisition. Gastrointest Endosc Clin N Am 2017;27(4):585–99.
46. Huang JY, Samarasena JB, Tsujino T, et al. EUS—guided portal pressure gradient measurement with a novel 25-guage needle device versus standard transjugular approach: a comparison animal study. Gastrointest Endosc 2016;84(2):358–62.
47. Pons F, Varela M, Llovet J. Staging systems in hepatocellular carcinoma. HPB (Oxford) 2005;7(1):35–41.
48. Adhoute X, Penaranda G, Raoul J, et al. Usefulness of staging systems and prognostic scores for hepatocellular carcinoma treatments d. J Hepatol 2016;8(17): 703–15.
49. Koduru P, Rei S, Lakhtakia S, et al. Role of endoscopic ultrasound in diagnosis and management of hepatocellular carcinoma. J Hepatocell Carcinoma 2015;2: 143–9.
50. Abou-Alfa GK, Pawlik SJ, et al. AJCC cancer staging manual. 8th edition. Chicago: AJCC; 2017. p. 287.

51. Greten T, Papendorf F, Bleck J, et al. Survival rate in patients with hepatocellular carcinoma: a retrospective analysis of 389 patients. Br J Cancer 2005;92(10): 1862–8.
52. Mathieu D, Grenier P, Larde D, et al. Portal vein involvement in hepatocellular carcinoma: dynamic CT features. Radiology 1984;152:127–32.
53. Llovet JM, Brú C, Bruix J. Prognosis of hepatocellular carcinoma: the BCLC staging classification. Semin Liver Dis 1999;19:329.
54. Pugh RN, Murray-Lyon IM, Dawson JL, et al. Transection of the oesophagus for bleeding oesophageal varices. Br J Surg 1973;60:646–9.
55. Marrero JA, Fontana RJ, Barrat A, et al. Prognosis of hepatocellular carcinoma: comparison of 7 staging systems in an American cohort. Hepatology 2005;41: 707.
56. Yu SJ. A concise review of updated guidelines regarding the management of hepatocellular carcinoma around the world: 2010-2016. Clin Mol Hepatol 2016;22:7.
57. The Cancer of the Liver Italian Program (CLIP) Investigators. A new prognostic system for hepatocellular carcinoma: a retrospective study of 435 patients. Hepatology 1998;28:751–5.
58. Okuda K, Ohtsuki T, Obata H, et al. Natural history of hepatocellular carcinoma and prognosis in relation to treatment. Study of 850 patients. Cancer 1985;56: 918.
59. Liu PH, Hsu CY, Hsia CY, et al. Prognosis of hepatocellular carcinoma: assessment of eleven staging systems. J Hepatol 2016;64:601–8.
60. Farinati F, Rinaldi M, Gianni S, et al. How should patients with hepatocellular carcinoma be staged? Validation of a new prognostic system. Cancer 2000;89:2266.
61. Levy I, Sherman M, Liver Cancer Study Group of the University of Toronto. Staging of hepatocellular carcinoma: assessment of the CLIP, Okuda, and Child-Pugh staging systems in a cohort of 257 patients in Toronto. Gut 2002;50(6):881–5.
62. Claudon M, Dietrich CF, Choi BI, et al. Guidelines and good clinical practice recommendations for Contrast Enhanced Ultrasound (CEUS) in the liver - update 2012: a WFUMB-EFSUMB initiative in cooperation with representatives of AFSUMB, AIUM, ASUM, FLAUS and ICUS. Ultrasound Med Biol 2013;39:187.
63. Albrecht T, Blomley M, Bolondi L, et al. Guidelines for the use of contrast agents in ultrasound. Ultraschall Med 2004;25:249.
64. Schinkel AF, Krueger CG, Tellez A, et al. Contrast-enhanced ultrasound for imaging vasa vasorum: comparison with histopathology in a swine model of atherosclerosis. Eur J Echocardiogr 2010;11:659.
65. Wilson SR, Burns PN. An algorithm for the diagnosis of focal liver masses using microbubble contrast-enhanced pulse-inversion sonography. AJR Am J Roentgenol 2006;186:1401.
66. Seitz K, Bernatik T, Strobel D, et al. Contrast-enhanced ultrasound (CEUS) for the characterization of focal liver lesions in clinical practice (DEGUM Multicenter Trial): CEUS vs. MRI–a prospective comparison in 269 patients. Ultraschall Med 2010;31:492.
67. Oh D, Seo DW, Hong SM, et al. The usefulness of contrast-enhanced harmonic EUS-fine needle aspiration for the evaluation of hepatic lesions (with video). Gastrointest Endosc 2018;88:495–501.
68. Shiina T, Nightingale KR, Palmeri ML, et al. WFUMB guidelines and recommendations for clinical use of ultrasound elastography: part 1: basic principles and terminology. Ultrasound Med Biol 2015;41:1126–47.
69. Kamaya A, Machtaler S, Safari Sanjani S, et al. New technologies in clinical ultrasound. Semin Roentgenol 2013;48:214–23.

70. Gennisson JL, Deffieux T, Fink M, et al. Ultrasound elastography: principles and techniques. Diagn Interv Imaging 2013;94(5):487–95.
71. Cui X, Chang J, Kan Q, et al. Endoscopic ultrasound elastography: current status and future perspectives. World J Gastroenterol 2015;21(47):13212–24.
72. Ma X, Zhan W, Zhang B, et al. Elastography for the differentiation of benign and malignant liver lesions: a meta-analysis. Tumour Biol 2014;35(5):4489–97.
73. Frulio N, Laumonier H, Carteret T, et al. Evaluation of liver tumors using acoustic radiation force impulse elastography and correlation with histologic data. J Ultrasound Med 2013;32:121–30.
74. Heide R, Strobel D, Bernatik T, et al. Characterization of focal liver lesions (FLL) with acoustic radiation force impulse (ARFI) elastometry. Ultraschall Med 2010; 31(4):405–9.
75. Yousaf M, Cai G, Aslanian HR. EUS evaluation of liver lesions. VideoGIE 2017; 3(1):31–3.
76. Sheth KR, Clary BM. Management of hepatic metastases from colorectal cancer. Clin Colon Rectal Surg 2005;18:215–23.
77. de Ridder J, de Wilt J, Simmer F, et al. Incidence and origin of histologically confirmed liver metastases: an explorative case-study of 23,154 patients. Oncotarget 2016;7(34):55368–76.
78. Oliva MR, Saini S. Liver cancer imaging: role of CT, MRI, US and PET. Cancer Imaging 2004;4:S42–6.
79. Jenssen C, Siebert C, Gottschalk U. The role of endoscopic ultrasound in m-staging of gastrointestinal and pancreaticobiliary cancer. Video Journal and Encyclopedia of GI Endoscopy 2013;1:105–9.

Endoscopic Retrograde Cholangiopancreatography-Guided Ablation for Cholangiocarcinoma

Ross C.D. Buerlein, MD, Andrew Y. Wang, MD*

KEYWORDS

- Cholangiocarcinoma • Radiofrequency ablation • RFA • Photodynamic therapy
- Brachytherapy • Biliary stenting • Endoscopic retrograde cholangiopancreatography
- ERCP

KEY POINTS

- Perihilar cholangiocarcinoma is associated with significant morbidity and mortality, which often presents with poor biliary drainage from tumor obstruction.
- Endoscopically administered photodynamic therapy, radiofrequency ablation, and intraluminal brachytherapy are palliative options in the management of unresectable cholangiocarcinoma.
- Few comparative data exist for photodynamic therapy, radiofrequency ablation, and intraluminal brachytherapy, and comparative prospective studies are needed to better elucidate the optimal treatment approach.

INTRODUCTION

Cholangiocarcinoma (CCA) is a malignancy of biliary epithelial cells. Although it can arise anywhere along the intrahepatic or extrahepatic biliary tree, the majority (60%–70%) develop at the hepatic duct confluence in the perihilar region (also known as a Klatskin tumor). The diagnosis and management of this cancer is challenging, which has resulted in 60% to 80% of patients being considered as having unresectable disease at the time of diagnosis. Patients with unresectable disease have a poor 5-year survival of 5% to 10%, with a median survival duration of 3 to 9 months.[1–5] Surgical resection offers the best treatment option for patients with perihilar CCA and

Disclosure Statement: Dr A.Y. Wang has received research support from Cook Medical on the topic of metal biliary stents. Dr R.C.D. Buerlein has nothing to disclose.
Division of Gastroenterology and Hepatology, University of Virginia, PO Box 800708, Charlottesville, VA 22908, USA
* Corresponding author.
E-mail address: ayw7d@virginia.edu

Gastrointest Endoscopy Clin N Am 29 (2019) 351–367
https://doi.org/10.1016/j.giec.2018.11.006 giendo.theclinics.com
1052-5157/19/© 2018 Elsevier Inc. All rights reserved.

is associated with a 5-year survival as high as 67%.[6] Unfortunately, surgical resection is not an option for most patients at the time of diagnosis.[1,7] Palliative attempts at chemoradiation and transarterial chemoembolization have proven to be of limited benefit, and the goal of treatment is mainly focused on the relief of malignant biliary obstruction. Percutaneous or endoscopic biliary stenting are options, although the long-term efficacy of these treatment modalities are often compromised by stent occlusion, migration, dysfunction, or tumor ingrowth.[1,7] Additionally, although biliary stenting alone in patients with unresectable CCA has been shown to improve quality of life and help in the treatment of cholangitis, it does not improve survival.[8,9] As a result, endoscopically directed ablative therapies, including photodynamic therapy (PDT), radiofrequency ablation (RFA), or intraluminal brachytherapy (ILBT) for local tumor control, have been used in attempts to improve stent patency, reduce the recurrence of biliary obstruction, and extend overall survival.

ENDOSCOPIC RETROGRADE CHOLANGIOPANCREATOGRAPHY-GUIDED PHOTODYNAMIC THERAPY

PDT is a method of ablative local tumor control that has been used in the management of various malignancies.[10] PDT requires an intravenously administered photosensitizing agent that concentrates inside of target cells and becomes activated by exposure to light of a specific wavelength. Absorption of the photosensitizer results in the generation of reactive oxygen species that cause photoperoxidation of cellular membranes, leading to loss of membrane fluidity, direct DNA damage with simultaneous inhibition of DNA repair mechanisms, destruction of the mitochondrial activity, damage to lysosomes and nuclei, and, ultimately, activation of cellular apoptosis. Inflammatory cascades and antiangiogenic pathways are also activated by PDT, which are believed to assist in additional local tumor control.[10–12] Finally, the activating laser light used in PDT is capable of refracting within bile, resulting in delivery of PDT to malignant tissue that is not in immediate proximity to the laser fiber.[13]

Several photosensitizing agents have been used in PDT for CCA, although none is approved by the US Food and Drug Administration for this use. Porfimer sodium (Photofrin, Pinnacle Biologics, Bannockburn, IL) is the most commonly used photosensitizer, although others like metatetrahydroxyphenyl chlorine (Foscan, Biolitec Pharma, Dublin, Ireland), hematoporphyrin derivatives like Photogem (TimTec, Russia/Newark, DE), Photoscan-3 (Seehof Laboratorium, Wesselburenerkoog, Germany), and meso-tetrahydroxyphenylchlorin (Temoporfin, Biolitec Pharma, Dublin, Ireland) have been used.[11]

Porfimer sodium is intravenously administered at a dose of 2 mg/kg of body weight for PDT. Although studies have shown this agent is absorbed by cells of numerous tissues in a nonspecific manner, it is highly concentrated in malignant biliary epithelial cells. Approximately 48 hours (and up to 72 hours) after administration of porfimer sodium, the patient undergoes endoscopic retrograde cholangiopancreatography (ERCP) with cholangiogram, and in some cases cholangioscopy, to identify tumor margins and the extent of the biliary obstruction. A fiber with a cylindrical diffuser at the distal-most end is then inserted endoscopically into the biliary tree to the targeted level (**Fig. 1**). Photoactivation is performed using a diode laser system (InGaAIP, Laser Diode; Diomed Inc., Andover, MA, USA) that delivers light with a wavelength of 630 nm, fluence of 0.250 W/cm^2, with a light dose of 180 to 200 J/cm^2 for a treatment time of 750 seconds.[11,14,15]

Destruction of tumor cells causes tissue inflammation and edema, which can lead to post-PDT biliary obstruction and result in cholangitis in some cases. Therefore, it is

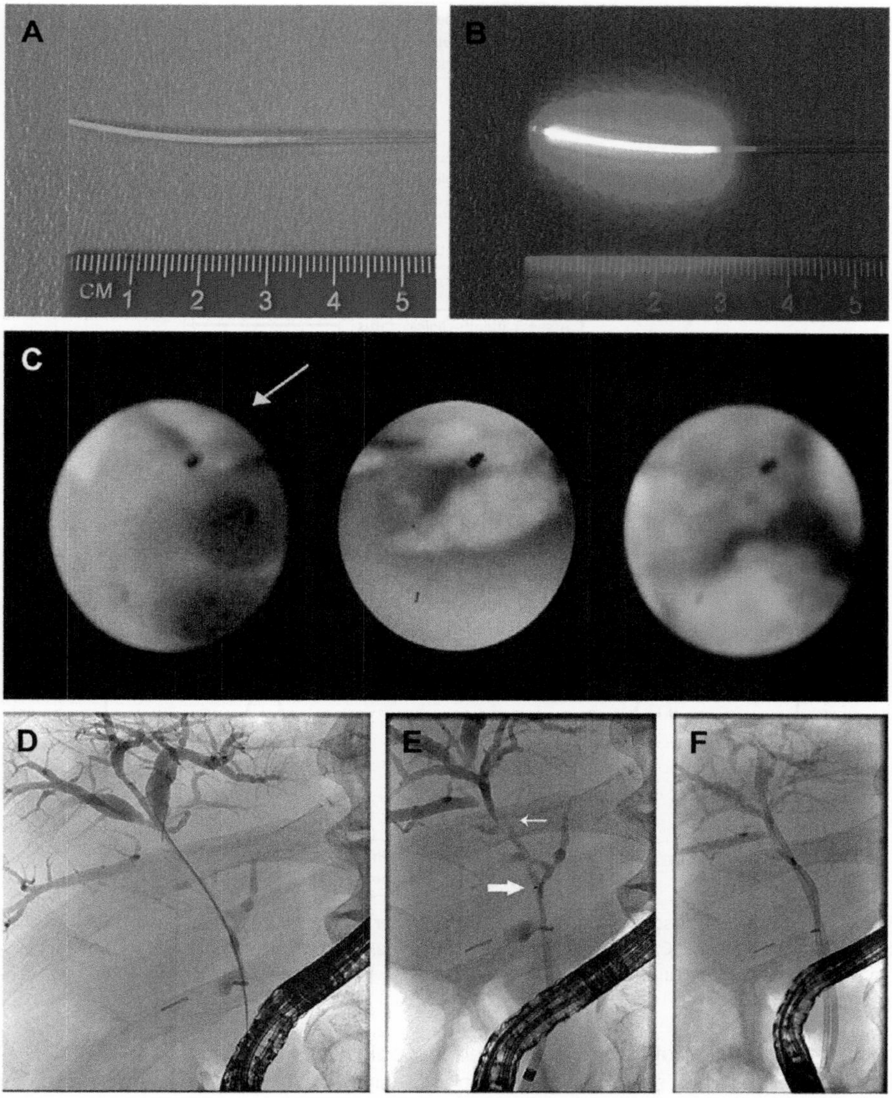

Fig. 1. Endoscopic retrograde cholangiopancreatography (ERCP)-directed photodynamic therapy (PDT) followed by plastic biliary stenting. A laser fiber with a 2.5-cm diffuser (Pioneer Optics, Windsor Locks, CT) that is used to perform endobiliary PDT is displayed (*A*). A diode laser system is used to deliver activating light (at 630 nm for 750 seconds, with a light dose of 180 J/cm^2) via the laser fiber, which is now shown activated (*B*). ERCP was performed in a patient with unresectable perihilar (Bismuth IIIA) cholangiocarcinoma who had a history of primary sclerosing cholangitis, cirrhosis, and ulcerative colitis. On the initial ERCP, choledochoscopy demonstrated polypoid, friable tissue consistent with biliary neoplasia arising from a right hepatic duct (*yellow arrow* on the left, in a trifurcated biliary confluence) that progressed as the single-operator choledochoscope traveled proximally into the right hepatic duct (images go from left to right; *C*). A cholangiogram during a subsequent ERCP demonstrated intrahepatic biliary dilation proximal to a long right hepatic duct stricture, and a guidewire was directed across the stricture (*D*). A 10F bougie catheter

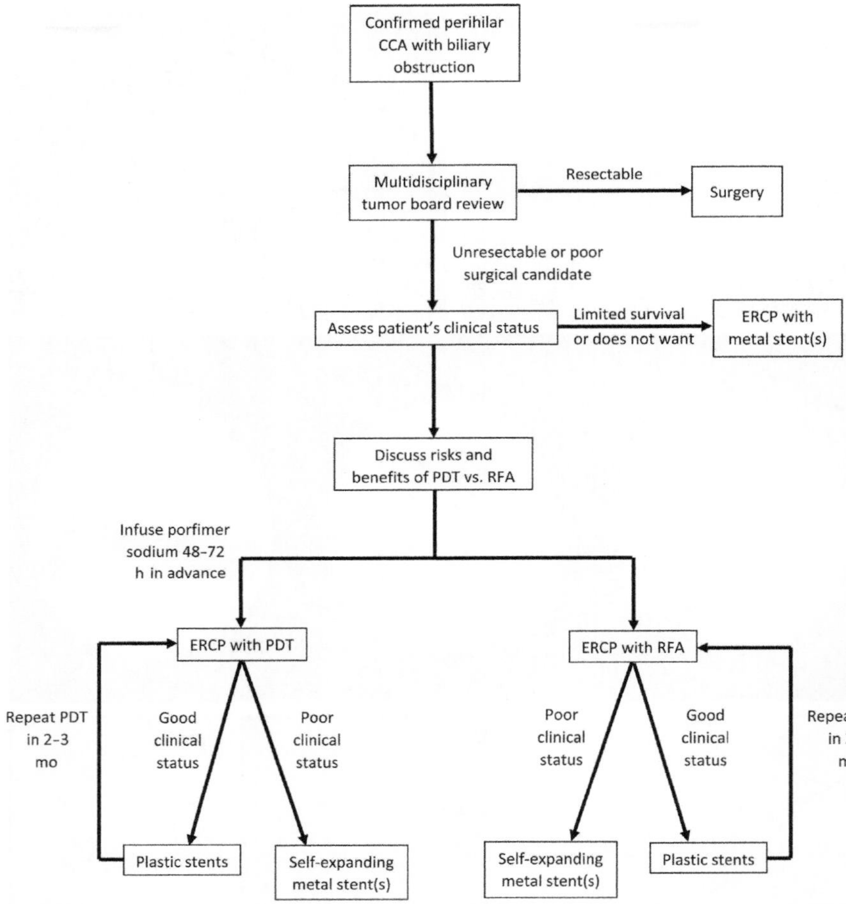

Fig. 2. Proposed endoscopic treatment strategy for patients with unresectable perihilar cholangiocarcinoma (CCA), with a focus on palliative endoscopic retrograde cholangiopancreatography (ERCP)-guided ablative therapies. PDT, photodynamic therapy; RFA, radiofrequency ablation.

considered standard of care to perform endoscopic biliary stenting following PDT.[11,15] The number of biliary segments treated per session and the frequency of treatments are at the discretion of the endoscopist, because high-quality evidence in this area is lacking. Although uncovered metal stenting can be pursued in patients with good functional status, we recommend that plastic biliary stents are placed and then PDT can be repeat at the time of stent exchange 2 to 3 months later, if needed (**Fig. 2**).[15]

was introduced over the wire, which was then removed. The laser fiber was passed through the bougie and across the right hepatic duct stricture and PDT was performed (the *thick arrow* pointing right denotes the radiopaque dot at the distal end of the diffuser; the *thin arrow* pointing left shows the nearly invisible proximal end of the diffuser on the laser fiber; *E*). A total of 2 plastic biliary stents were deployed across the malignant perihilar stricture after the application of PDT (*F*). (*From* Uppal DS, Wang AY. Cholangiocarcinoma: endoscopic therapies. Tech Gastrointest Endosc 2016;18(2):86; with permission.)

The first case report using endoscopic PDT in the management of CCA was published in 1991 by McCaughan and coworkers.[16] Since that time, numerous studies including several metaanalyses have been published showing improvement in overall survival, stent patency, relief of biliary obstruction, and serum bilirubin levels in patients with unresectable CCA who underwent endoscopically administered PDT (see **Fig. 1**).

Leggett and colleagues[17] published a metaanalysis that included 6 randomized studies that compared 170 patients who had PDT plus biliary stenting with 157 patients who had biliary stenting alone. Using a weighted mean difference (WMD) and relative risk for dichotomous outcomes, they found that patients undergoing PDT plus biliary stenting had statistically significant improvements in length of survival (WMD, 265 days; 95% confidence interval [CI], 154–376; *P* = .01) and improved quality of life as measured by increased Karnofsky Index (WMD, 7.74; 95% CI, 3.73–11.76; *P* = .01). There was a trend in reduction in the risk of death in the PDT plus biliary stenting group (relative risk, 0.90; 95% CI, 0.80–1.0; *P* = .05), but there was no difference in the reduction of serum bilirubin levels or rates of biliary sepsis between the 2 groups.

Lu and colleagues[8] performed a metaanalysis comparing a total of 266 patients with PDT plus stenting to 336 patients with biliary stenting alone. They used a hazard ratio (HR) model and showed a statistically significant improvement in survival in patients undergoing PDT plus stenting (HR, 0.49; 95% CI, 0.33–0.73; *P* = .0005), although there was marked heterogeneity between the 2 groups. Of the 8 trials included in their metaanalysis, 4 assessed the effect of PDT on bilirubin levels. Two of these trials showed a statistically significant decrease in serum bilirubin levels, whereas the other 2 trials showed only a trend toward a significant decrease.

The most recently published metaanalysis assessing PDT plus stenting (n = 256) versus stenting alone (n = 146) was performed by Moole and colleagues.[18] Of the 10 studies included in this metaanalysis, 1 study used PDT delivered percutaneously and 3 used PDT delivered via endoscopic or percutaneous routes; additionally, all studies included at least some patients who had percutaneous biliary stenting rather than endoscopic biliary stenting alone. Therefore, as it pertains to purely endoscopic management of CCA, the results of this metaanalysis are difficult to interpret. However, this study did report a statistically significant improvement in survival in patients undergoing PDT plus stenting (413.04 days; 95% CI, 349.54–476.54) compared with stenting alone (183.41 days; 95% CI, 136.81–230.02). A summary of the studies comparing endoscopically administered PDT plus stenting to stenting alone can be found in **Table 1**.

Lee and colleagues[19] specifically compared the patency of metal stents in patients with unresectable CCA who were treated with PDT compared with those treated with biliary stenting alone. In this retrospective analysis, 18 patients were treated with PDT followed by insertion of uncovered metal stents and were compared with 15 patients treated with uncovered metal stents alone. The PDT group was found to have statistically significant longer stent patency compared with the stent only group (median 244 $\pm$ 66 days vs 177 $\pm$ 45 days; *P* = .002) and longer survival (median 356 $\pm$ 213 days vs 230 $\pm$ 73 days; *P* = .006).

In an attempt to identify factors that might predict which patients with unresectable CCA would benefit most from PDT, Prasad and colleagues[20] studied 25 patients with unresectable CCA who underwent PDT (20 patients had endoscopically administered PDT while 5 had percutaneously administered PDT) plus stenting between 1991 and 2004. The median survival time after PDT in this patient population was 214 days. When assessing time from diagnosis to PDT, univariate analysis indicated that shorter time intervals were associated with higher survival rates (HR, 1.11; 95% CI, 1.002–1.23; *P* = .046) and that lower pre-PDT albumin levels were associated with worse survival (HR, 0.35; 95% CI, 0.12–0.97; *P* = .041). Multivariate analysis found that the

Table 1
Summary of studies assessing survival in endoscopically administered PDT plus stenting versus stenting alone

Study	Mean Difference in Survival (d)	Lower Limit (d)	Upper Limit (d)	*P* Value	PDT Population Size (n)	Control Population Size (n)	Randomized Controlled Trial
Zoepf et al,[50] 2005	420	296.94	543.06	.01	16	16	Yes
Ortner et al,[51] 2003	395	172.07	617.93	<.0001	20	19	Yes
Dumoulin et al,[52] 2003	129	2.29	255.71	.05	24	20	No
Witzigmann et al,[53] 2006	168	45.69	290.31	.01	68	56	No
Kahaleh et al,[54] 2008	264	11.41	516.59	.04	19	29	No
Quyn et al,[55] 2009	256	59.81	452.19	.01	23	17	No
Cheon et al,[56] 2012	66	NR	NR	.038	72	71	No
Lee et al,[19] 2012	126	NR	NR	.006	18	15	No

Abbreviations: NR, not reported; PDT, photodynamic therapy.

presence of a mass on imaging (HR, 3.55; 95% CI, 1.21–10.38; *P* = .021), lower serum albumin (HR, 0.16; 95% CI, 0.04–0.59; *P* = .005), and longer time between diagnosis and undergoing PDT (HR, 1.13; 95% CI, 1.02–1.25; *P* = .029) were associated with increased mortality.

To improve the poor survival associated with unresectable perihilar CCA,[21] the use of PDT in combination with the chemotherapy has been studied. Hong and colleagues[3] assessed the effect of systemic chemotherapy (gemcitabine with or without cisplatin) with PDT in 16 patients compared with PDT alone in 58 patients. In this study, PDT was administered either percutaneously or via ERCP. All patients treated with PDT subsequently underwent insertion of a 10F plastic biliary stent. The overall median survival in the chemotherapy plus PDT group was 17.9 months compared with 11.1 months in the PDT-alone group (*P* = .05). However, this survival benefit was lost after 1 year. In a similar study, Park and colleagues[22] performed a prospective, randomized, phase II trial comparing the efficacy of adding oral fluoropyrimidine S-1 with PDT in patients with unresectable CCA. They showed that 21 patients receiving fluoropyrimidine S-1 plus PDT had a longer overall survival (median, 17 months) compared with the 22 patients receiving PDT alone (median, 8 months; *P* = .005) and that the fluoropyrimidine S-1 plus PDT group had prolonged progression-free survival (median, 10 months) compared with the PDT-alone group (median, 2 months; *P* = .009). In a retrospective study of patients with unresectable CCA, Wentrup and colleagues[23] compared 33 patients who underwent chemotherapy plus PDT with 35 matched patients who underwent PDT alone (all patients underwent prophylactic biliary stenting after PDT). The chemotherapy regimens used in this study varied slightly, but all included gemcitabine either alone or in combination with cisplatin, oxaliplatin, capecitabine, irinotecan, or 5-fluorouracil. These investigators showed an improved overall survival in the chemotherapy plus PDT group compared with the PDT-alone group (520 days vs 374 days, respectively; *P* = .021).

Furthermore, PDT has been used in a small study to downstage what was considered to be unresectable CCA in the hopes of eventual operative resection. A study by Wagner and colleagues[24] described in a small study the long-term outcomes (>15 years) of 7 patients who were initially deemed to have unresectable disease owing to local tumor extension but underwent PDT followed by surgical resection within 30 to 72 days after PDT. When compared with a similar historical cohort of 35 patients who underwent surgical resection without prior PDT, there was no difference in overall survival.

Another potential use for PDT to augment locoregional control alongside neoadjuvant chemoradiation in selected patients with unresectable CCA who are candidates for liver transplantation. Darwish Murad and colleagues[25] reported in a retrospective study of 287 patients with unresectable perihilar CCA who underwent neoadjuvant chemoradiation followed by liver transplantation a 5-year survival rate of 53% and a 65% posttransplant disease-free survival. On subgroup analysis, recurrence-free survival for patients who had received brachytherapy was similar to those who did not (HR, 1.05; 95% CI, 0.60–1.85).[25] To provide an alternative to brachytherapy in this patient population, the substitution of neoadjuvant PDT in place of brachytherapy before liver transplantation was reported by Cosgrove and colleagues[26] in 4 patients, in a proof-of-principle study. At a mean follow-up time of 28.1 months, there was a 75% disease-free survival in this intention-to-treat analysis.

The use of PDT is not without its complications and downsides. Side effects of PDT are typically minimal, with the most common being phototoxicity. Because absorption of the photosensitizer occurs in tissues apart from the malignant biliary epithelial cells, patients are advised to avoid direct sunlight for 4 to 6 weeks after PDT. Failure to do so has resulted in pruritus, diffuse pain, skin erythema, and even blistering.[11] A phototoxic reaction was seen in 11% of patients in a metaanalysis by Lu and colleagues,[8] which included 266 patients undergoing PDT. Because PDT is used as a palliative therapy in patients with incurable perihilar CCA, who often have limited life expectancy, the need to avoid sunlight for up to 6 weeks after PDT can negatively affect patients' quality of life and should be carefully discussed with patients considering treatment. Studies on newer photosensitizers at lower dosages are being performed and may result in a decreased likelihood of developing systemic phototoxicity.[27,28]

Other side effects from PDT include localized tissue edema, which can result in biliary obstruction. Although studies have shown that PDT might not result in an increased risk of biliary sepsis.[17] However, as discussed elsewhere in this article, endoscopic biliary stenting after PDT is recommended.[11] Last, the expense of ERCP-directed PDT can be a major drawback. In 2017, the average wholesale cost of a single 75-mg vial of porfimer sodium was USD $24,512, with a typical 75-kg patient requiring 2 vials.[13,26,29] However, Medicare and most private insurers will cover the cost of this medication for the palliation of patients with unresectable CCA.[26]

Overall, endoscopically directed PDT for patients with unresectable CCA has been shown to improve survival and stent patency, but the ideal number of sessions, time between sessions, and whether bilateral PDT is preferred over unilateral treatment in cases of Bismuth IV CCA remain unanswered.[13] A proposed treatment algorithm is provided in **Fig. 2**.

ENDOSCOPIC RETROGRADE CHOLANGIOPANCREATOGRAPHY-GUIDED RADIOFREQUENCY ABLATION

Endobiliary RFA via ERCP is another modality being used with increasing frequency in the management of perihilar CCA. RFA uses alternating current to create electromagnetic wave frequencies in the range of 10^4 to 3×10^{12} Hz, which when applied to human tissue results in molecular friction and heating.[30] Heat generation via electric current has been used for medical purposes since the early 1900s when physicist William T. Bovie and surgeon Harvey Cushing developed the radiofrequency generator, which has been adapted for modern electrocautery. Since that time, RFA has been greatly improved and specialized for a large variety of medical indications. When using RFA for the treatment of CCA or for tumor in-growth into a stent, the goal is heat generation to result in local tissue coagulative necrosis.

ERCP-directed RFA is performed with a therapeutic duodenoscope and typically requires a prior biliary sphincterotomy. The RFA catheter is passed over a guidewire to the desired location within the biliary system via fluoroscopic guidance (**Fig. 3**).[11] As opposed to PDT, RFA requires direct tissue contact to result in tissue destruction.

There are 2 endobiliary RFA probe systems available worldwide. The ELRA Endobiliary RFA System (TaeWoong Medical, South Korea) is a 7F, 1.75-m-long catheter with multiple bipolar electrodes spanning a distance of either 18 or 33 mm. This system must be connected to a VIVA Combo generator (TaeWoong Medical). The system that is available commercially in the United States is the Habib EndoHBP (formerly manufactured by EMcision, London, UK, and now produced by Boston Scientific, Marlborough, MA), which is an 8F, 1.8-m-long catheter with 2 bipolar electrodes at the distal tip, each separated by 8 mm to create a 2.5-cm-long ablative field.[11,13] This catheter is connected to a bipolar radiofrequency generator or to a commercially available electrosurgical generator that can be programmed to deliver 7 to 10 W for 120 seconds (7 W has been recommended for RFA of the perihilar and intrahepatic bile ducts to decrease the risk of thermal injury to nearby vessels and pseudoaneurysm formation). Endobiliary RFA using this system is delivered over two 90-second intervals with a 1-minute intervening rest period. As of August 2018, the price for the Boston Scientific endobiliary RFA catheter ranges from USD $1595 to $2895, which represents a significant cost saving when considering the marked expense of a laser fiber and porfimer sodium required for performing PDT.

There are 2 electrosurgical generators that can be programmed for use with the RFA probe that is commercially available in the United States—the VIO 300D (ERBE, Marietta, GA) and the ESG-100 (Olympus America, Center Valley, PA).[13] After RFA of the malignant biliary tissue, the bile duct is swept by using a retrieval balloon to remove any necrotic debris. For long malignant biliary strictures, multiple overlapping applications of RFA can be applied sequentially to treat the entire length of the stricture.[31] The optimal number of applications of RFA per procedure is left to the discretion of the endoscopist and has not been well studied. Endoscopic biliary stenting is indicated after RFA to maintain biliary patency. Plastic stents are used if future RFA sessions are anticipated, whereas metal stents are recommended if only a single RFA session is planned.[11,32] Please refer to **Fig. 2** for our proposed treatment algorithm.

The first reported use of endoscopically delivered RFA in the treatment of unresectable malignant biliary obstruction was by Steel and colleagues,[33] in 2011. In this open-label pilot study, 22 patients (16 with pancreatic cancer and 6 with CCA) were enrolled for RFA followed by metal stent placement. RFA was delivered in 21 of these patients and all but 1 had successful biliary decompression that persisted to 30 days; 16 patients maintained biliary patency at 90 days. There have been several studies that have assessed the efficacy and safety of RFA for malignant biliary obstruction since this initial study, although the generalizability of these results have been hindered by small sample sizes, lack of randomization, and study heterogeneity (such as by the inclusion of both pancreatic- and CCA-induced biliary strictures as well as by inclusion of both percutaneously and endoscopically applied RFA).

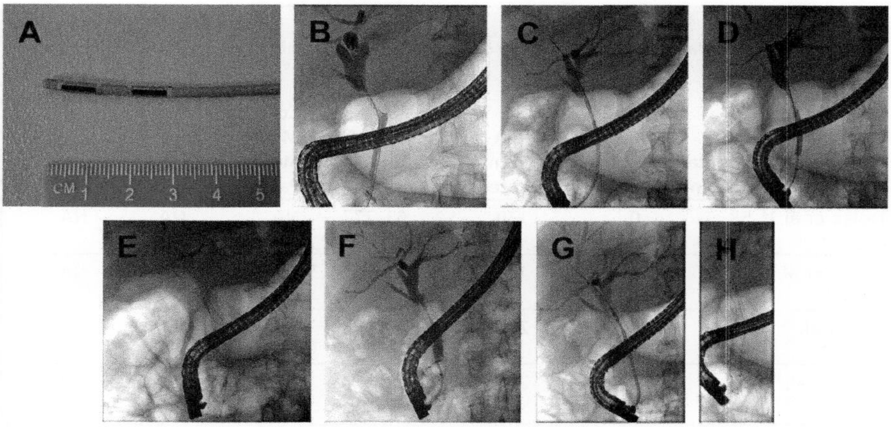

Fig. 3. Endoscopic retrograde cholangiopancreatography (ERCP)-directed radiofrequency ablation (RFA) followed by metal stenting. An 8F endobiliary RFA catheter with 2 electrodes spaced 8 mm apart that produces a treatment field 2.5-cm in length (Habib EndoHPB; formerly EMcision, London, UK; now Boston Scientific, Marlborough, MA) is displayed (*A*). ERCP was performed in a patient with unresectable perihilar (Bismuth I) cholangiocarcinoma in the setting of liver metastases. A cholangiogram demonstrated a stricture that involved the common hepatic duct with upstream intrahepatic biliary ductal dilation, and a guidewire was directed across the stricture (*B*). Over the wire, the RFA catheter was deployed directly into the bile duct and across the malignant stricture and RFA was applied (*C*). After RFA, a retrieval balloon sweep to remove ablated tumor debris demonstrated improved patency across the biliary stricture (*D*). A 10 mm $\times$ 8 cm, uncovered, metal stent was placed across the treated malignant stricture (*E*). After 13 months, the patient presented with biliary obstruction, and a repeat ERCP demonstrated progression of the malignant stricture with associated tumor ingrowth through the uncovered metal stent (*F*). ERCP-directed RFA was applied through the previously placed metal stent to ablate the tumor ingrowth (*G*). After RFA, a second, overlapping, 10 mm $\times$ 8 cm, uncovered, metal stent was deployed within the existing metal stent with good effect (*H*). (*From* Uppal DS, Wang AY. Cholangiocarcinoma: endoscopic therapies. Tech Gastrointest Endosc 2016;18(2):87; with permission.)

A metaanalysis by Zheng and colleagues[34] in 2016 included 9 studies with 263 patients who underwent endoscopically delivered RFA for malignant biliary obstruction secondary to CCA (65.8%), pancreatic cancer (29.3%), metastatic cancer (1.5%), or other cancer types (4.9%). They showed that RFA led to a significant improvement in bile duct diameter at the site of the stricture, with an average increase from 1.189 mm before the procedure to 4.635 mm after the procedure, indicating an average increase of 3.446 mm owing to RFA. When assessing stent patency, they found the median duration of post-RFA stent patency was 7.6 months (95% CI, 6.9–8.4 months). This study also demonstrated that the 30-day, 90-day, and 2-year mortality was 2% (95% CI, 0.5%–5.9%), 21% (95% CI, 5%–37%), and 48% (95% CI, 37%–59%), respectively.

Most studies using ERCP-guided RFA in the treatment of CCA assessed improvements in stent patency duration and luminal diameter. Pozsár and colleagues[35] in 2011 assessed the efficacy of RFA for treating metal stents occluded by tumor ingrowth or overgrowth in 5 patients. They showed significant increases in biliary lumen diameter and improved duration of stent patency after RFA, without any complications attributable to RFA. Kadayifci and colleagues[36] similarly assessed the efficacy of RFA in the management of biliary metal stent occlusion owing to malignancy and

Table 2
Summary of studies assessing the efficacy of endoscopically administered biliary RFA on stent patency

Study	RFA Population Size (n)	Control Population Size (n)	RFA Median Stent Patency (d)	95% CI for RFA (d)	Control Median Stent Patency (d)	95% CI for Control Group (d)	*P* Value
Dolak et al,[32] 2014	58	0	170	63–277	NA	NA	NA
Wang et al,[57] 2016	11	0	125	94.7–155.3	NA	NA	NA
Alis et al,[58] 2013	9	0	270	180–450	NA	NA	NA
Yang et al,[39] 2018	32	33	204	108–246	102	72–195	.02

Abbreviations: CI, confidence interval; NA, not applicable; RFA, radiofrequency ablation.

demonstrated improved stent patency time in 25 patients undergoing RFA plus stenting when compared with 25 patients undergoing stenting alone (119.5 vs 65.3 days; $P = .03$). Other studies[37] have also shown improvements in the duration of stent patency and biliary lumen diameter after RFA, as summarized in **Tables 2** and **3**.

Assessing the survival benefits of endoscopically administered RFA in the treatment of CCA has been studied, although the data are not as robust as the data for PDT. Sharaiha and colleagues[38] prospectively studied 66 patients with biliary obstruction from either CCA or pancreatic cancer, with 26 patients treated by RFA and 40 matched controls who underwent stenting alone. They found no significant difference in survival between the 2 groups (median survival, 5.9 months; $P = .87$). However, using a multivariate Cox proportional hazard model, they suggested that RFA was a predictor of survival (HR, 0.29; 95% CI, 0.11–0.76; $P = .012$), as was chemotherapy and younger age. Yang and colleagues[39] reported on an important trial in 2018 that enrolled 65 patients with unresectable CCA (excluding Bismuth Type III and IV cases) and randomized them into 2 groups: RFA plus stenting (with an 8.5F biliary stent) versus stenting alone. They found that RFA plus stenting compared with stenting alone had significantly improved survival (13.2 $\pm$ 0.6 months vs 8.3 $\pm$ 0.5 months; $P<.001$) and mean stent patency (6.8 vs 3.4 months; $P = .02$), without any significant

Table 3
Summary of studies assessing the efficacy of endoscopically administered RFA on biliary lumen diameter

Study	Number of Patients	Mean Difference (mm)	*P* Value	Pre-RFA Mean (mm)	Pre-RFA 95% CI (mm)	Post-RFA Mean (mm)	Post-RFA 95% CI (mm)
Figueroa-Barojas et al,[59] 2013	20	3.5	<.0001	1.7	0.5–3.4	5.2	2.6–9
Alis et al,[58] 2013	17	3.5	NR	1.5	1.5–2	5	4–7
Steel et al,[33] 2011	22	4	NR	0	0–1	4	3–6
Pozsár et al,[35] 2011	5	2.7	<.05	2	NR	4.7	NR

Abbreviations: CI, confidence interval; NA, not applicable; RFA, radiofrequency ablation.

increase in postprocedural adverse event rates (6.3% vs 9.1%; P = .67). On Cox regression analysis, they showed that RFA was a significant protective factor in overall survival (HR, 0.182; 95% CI, 0.08–0.322; P<.001).

The most recent metaanalysis assessing RFA plus stenting versus stenting alone was conducted by Sofi and colleagues[40] in 2018. This study included 505 patients with malignant biliary obstruction, 239 of whom had RFA that was either performed endoscopically or percutaneously. They found a significant increase in stent patency duration in the RFA group with a WMD of 50.6 days (95% CI, 32.83–68.48; P = .02). However, in a subgroup analysis of studies of patients with biliary obstruction secondary to CCA, the difference in stent patency was no longer significant (WMD of 42.7 days; 95% CI, 17.19–68.19; P = .11). These investigators also demonstrated a significant survival benefit in patients undergoing RFA plus stenting (285 days; 95% CI, 270–309 days) compared with stenting alone (248 days; 95% CI, 188–272 days; P<.001). One concern about this study was the significantly larger number of patients who underwent chemotherapy in the stent-only group, although one might have expected this to have a positive impact on survival benefit, which was not the case. A summary of studies of the effect of ERCP-guided RFA for malignant biliary obstruction can found in **Tables 4** and **5**.

RFA is typically a well-tolerated procedure, and RFA-associated adverse events are uncommon. However, RFA has been associated with a few side effects aside from the potential complications attributable to ERCP and biliary cannulation. The metaanalysis by Zheng and colleagues[34] that included 9 studies with 263 patients undergoing endoscopically delivered RFA for malignant biliary obstruction found a pooled adverse event rate of 17%. Post-RFA abdominal pain is the most common adverse event (estimated at 11%–13%),[34,40] although this symptom typically resolves in a short time period. Hemobilia has been reported, and Tal and colleagues[41] observed hemobilia 4 to 6 weeks after RFA in 3 of 12 cases, and 2 of these patients died. Other studies report the risk of hemobilia to be closer to 2% and have not shown this more frequently in patients after RFA compared with stenting alone without RFA.[40,42] Cholangitis or bacterial translocation resulting in sepsis have been reported as well (estimated at 2%–8%),[40,42] although most studies also indicate that the frequency of these events is not increased compared with patients who underwent stenting alone. Cholecystitis requiring percutaneous drainage has rarely been reported after endoscopically administered RFA (estimated to be 2%–4%[40,42]), which seems to be significantly higher than

Table 4
Summary of comparative studies assessing the effect of ERCP-guided RFA for malignant biliary obstruction on survival

Study	Survival Difference	RFA Group Mean Survival	Control Group Mean Survival	*P* value	RFA Group (n)	Control Group (n)
Sharaiha et al,[38] 2014[a]	5.9 mo (median)	NR	NR	.87	26	40
Yang et al,[39] 2018	4.9 mo (mean)	13.2 mo	8.3 mo	<.001	32	33
Sofi et al,[40] 2018	37 d (mean)	285 d	248 d	<.001	239	266

Abbreviations: ERCP, endoscopic retrograde cholangiopancreatography; NR, not reported; RFA, radiofrequency ablation.

[a] Sharaiha and collagues[38] did not publish separate survival rates for the 2 groups.

Table 5
Summary of noncontrolled studies assessing the effect of endoscopically administered RFA for malignant biliary obstruction on survival

Study	Number of Patients	Median Survival (mo)	95% CI, Lower Limit (mo)	95% CI, Upper Limit (mo)
Tal et al,[41] 2014	12	6.4	0.05	12.7
Dolak et al,[32] 2014	58	10.6	6.9	14.4
Laquiere et al,[43] 2016	12	12.3	3	32
Wang et al,[57] 2016	12	7.7	3.1	12.3
Strand et al,[1] 2014	16	9.6	5.1	11.7

Abbreviations: CI, confidence interval; RFA, radiofrequency ablation.

in patients who underwent stenting alone.[13,31,34,41,43] Although biliary fistulas have been reported after RFA administered via open surgery or by interventional radiology techniques, no such complication has been reported after endoscopic delivery of RFA.[11]

COMPARISON OF RADIOFREQUENCY ABLATION AND PHOTODYNAMIC THERAPY

Few data exist comparing endoscopically administered PDT with RFA. In 2014, Strand and colleagues[1] performed a retrospective cohort study to compare the effect of PDT (n = 32 patients) and RFA (n = 16) on overall survival in patients with malignant biliary obstruction from CCA. In this study, no significant difference in survival was found between the 2 treatment modalities (7.5 months; 95% CI, 4.3–16 months vs 9.6 months; 95% CI, 5.1–11.7 months; $P = .799$). However, in patients undergoing RFA, these investigators did note a statistically significant increase in the rate of both stent occlusion ($P = .008$) and cholangitis ($P = .008$).

INTRALUMINAL BRACHYTHERAPY

ILBT is another treatment modality that can be used for the endoscopic ablation of unresectable CCA.[21] ILBT brings logistical challenges including the technical aspects of handling, storing, and delivering radioactive material that has a relatively short half-life. This technique uses the insertion of iridium-192 (^{192}Ir) or iodine-125 (^{125}I) seeds within a ribbon or an impregnated wire into the biliary lumen either via a percutaneous transhepatic approach or through ERCP to allow localized delivery of high-dose radiation resulting in direct DNA damage, inhibition of cellular replication, and induction of apoptosis of the tumor cells.[44,45]

The use of ILBT was first reported by Benjamin and colleagues[46] in 1981. Since that time, there have been additional studies assessing the efficacy of this treatment modality in improving overall survival and stent patency in patients with CCA. However, many of these studies did not contain control groups, and their small patient populations were heterogeneous owing to prior treatment approaches and biliary stenting modalities as well as different types of cancer causing malignant biliary obstruction. As a result, the technical aspects of the procedures often vary between studies and it remains unclear if low- or high-dose rate ILBT is ideal, although most studies support the combination of ILBT with external beam radiation with or without chemotherapy for prolonged survival.[47] The use of high-dose rate systems for ILBT has been advocated because it allows the radiation treatment to be administered to a patient alone in a shielded room, which limits radiation exposure to the medical staff.[13,48] In patients with unresectable CCA undergoing neoadjuvant chemotherapy with the goal of liver transplantation, Mukewar and colleagues,[48] at the Mayo Clinic, reported using a combination of external radiation and high-dose rate ILBT (using 930–1600 cGy in 1–4 fractions delivered over 1–2 days) that was administered via an endoscopically placed 8.5F or 10F nasobiliary tube through which the brachytherapy catheter was subsequently loaded.

Chen and colleagues[49] compared ILBT delivered through percutaneous transhepatic biliary drainage on stent patency and overall survival in patients with CCA. Twenty patients (9 with CCA) with malignant biliary obstruction underwent percutaneous transhepatic biliary drainage without ILBT and 14 patients (7 with CCA) underwent ILBT plus stenting. These investigators found a significant increase in stent patency in the ILBT group compared with the control group (12.6 months vs 8.3 months; $P<.05$) but no statistically significant difference in overall mean survival (9.4 months vs 6.0 months). Xu and colleagues[44] performed a metaanalysis comparing outcomes in patients with malignant biliary obstruction treated with stenting alone (301 patients) versus ILBT with stenting (340 patients, who had either ERCP or percutaneous transhepatic biliary drainage). Twelve studies, 7 of which were nonrandomized, were included. Pooled analysis showed lower rates of stent occlusion (odds ratio, 0.19; 95% CI, 0.13–0.28; $P<.00001$) and prolonged mean survival (mean difference, 3.15 months; 95% CI, 2.64–3.66 months; $P<.0001$) in patients undergoing ILBT compared with biliary stenting/drainage alone. There was no difference in rates of complications or reduction in serum bilirubin levels.

ILBT has been associated with adverse events including cholangitis, hemobilia, and biliary obstruction. Additionally, delayed complications such as gastrointestinal bleeding, duodenal stenosis, and again hemobilia have been reported as a result of radiation damage to nearby structures and organs.[45]

SUMMARY

Over the past 2 decades, several options for the endoscopic ablation and management of unresectable CCA have emerged. Commercially available devices and platforms now enable ERCP-guided RFA, PDT, and ILBT for the palliation of incurable malignant perihilar biliary obstruction. Endobiliary ablative therapy has been used as neoadjuvant therapy in the hopes of fostering locoregional control of perihilar CCA in patients awaiting protocol liver transplantation. Appropriately powered studies are required to further elucidate the benefits and risks associated with the various endobiliary ablative treatments compared with stenting alone. Additional studies that directly compare the efficacy and safety of the 3 ERCP-guided ablative therapies are also required. Despite differences in methods of delivery, action, and varying levels of clinical evidence, ERCP-guided PDT, RFA, and ILBT are important palliative options in patients with inoperable perihilar CCA, which offer the potential for increased survival and prolonged stent patency.

REFERENCES

1. Strand DS, Cosgrove ND, Patrie JT, et al. ERCP-directed radiofrequency ablation and photodynamic therapy are associated with comparable survival in the treatment of unresectable cholangiocarcinoma. Gastrointest Endosc 2014;80(5):794–804.
2. Anderson CD, Pinson CW, Berlin J, et al. Diagnosis and treatment of cholangiocarcinoma. Oncologist 2004;9(1):43–57.

3. Hong MJ, Cheon YK, Lee EJ, et al. Long-term outcome of photodynamic therapy with systemic chemotherapy compared to photodynamic therapy alone in patients with advanced hilar cholangiocarcinoma. Gut Liver 2014;8(3):318–23.
4. Razumilava N, Gores GJ. Cholangiocarcinoma. Lancet 2014;383(9935):2168–79.
5. Rerknimitr R, Angsuwatcharakon P, Ratanachu-ek T, et al. Asia-Pacific consensus recommendations for endoscopic and interventional management of hilar cholangiocarcinoma. J Gastroenterol Hepatol 2013;28(4):593–607.
6. Nagino M, Ebata T, Yokoyama Y, et al. Evolution of surgical treatment for perihilar cholangiocarcinoma: a single-center 34-year review of 574 consecutive resections. Ann Surg 2013;258(1):129–40.
7. Boulay BR, Birg A. Malignant biliary obstruction: from palliation to treatment. World J Gastrointest Oncol 2016;8(6):498–508.
8. Lu Y, Liu L, Wu JC, et al. Efficacy and safety of photodynamic therapy for unresectable cholangiocarcinoma: a meta-analysis. Clin Res Hepatol Gastroenterol 2015;39(6):718–24.
9. Kaassis M, Boyer J, Dumas R, et al. Plastic or metal stents for malignant stricture of the common bile duct? Results of a randomized prospective study. Gastrointest Endosc 2003;57(2):178–82.
10. Skupin-Mrugalska P, Sobotta L, Kucinska M, et al. Cellular changes, molecular pathways and the immune system following photodynamic treatment. Curr Med Chem 2014;21(35):4059–73.
11. Patel J, Rizk N, Kahaleh M. Role of photodynamic therapy and intraductal radiofrequency ablation in cholangiocarcinoma. Best Pract Res Clin Gastroenterol 2015;29(2):309–18.
12. Henderson BW, Dougherty TJ. How does photodynamic therapy work? Photochem Photobiol 1992;55(1):145–57.
13. Uppal DS, Wang AY. Cholangiocarcinoma: endoscopic therapies. Tech Gastrointest Endosc 2016;18(2):83–90.
14. Talreja JP, Degaetani M, Ellen K, et al. Photodynamic therapy in unresectable cholangiocarcinoma: not for the uncommitted. Clin Endosc 2013;46(4):390–4.
15. Talreja JP, Kahaleh M. Photodynamic therapy for cholangiocarcinoma. Gut Liver 2010;4(Suppl 1):S62–6.
16. McCaughan JS Jr, Mertens BF, Cho C, et al. Photodynamic therapy to treat tumors of the extrahepatic biliary ducts. A case report. Arch Surg 1991;126(1):111–3.
17. Leggett CL, Gorospe EC, Murad MH, et al. Photodynamic therapy for unresectable cholangiocarcinoma: a comparative effectiveness systematic review and meta-analyses. Photodiagnosis Photodyn Ther 2012;9(3):189–95.
18. Moole H, Tathireddy H, Dharmapuri S, et al. Success of photodynamic therapy in palliating patients with nonresectable cholangiocarcinoma: a systematic review and meta-analysis. World J Gastroenterol 2017;23(7):1278–88.
19. Lee TY, Cheon YK, Shim CS, et al. Photodynamic therapy prolongs metal stent patency in patients with unresectable hilar cholangiocarcinoma. World J Gastroenterol 2012;18(39):5589–94.
20. Prasad GA, Wang KK, Baron TH, et al. Factors associated with increased survival after photodynamic therapy for cholangiocarcinoma. Clin Gastroenterol Hepatol 2007;5(6):743–8.
21. Chan SY, Poon RT, Ng KK, et al. Long-term survival after intraluminal brachytherapy for inoperable hilar cholangiocarcinoma: a case report. World J Gastroenterol 2005;11(20):3161–4.

22. Park DH, Lee SS, Park SE, et al. Randomised phase II trial of photodynamic therapy plus oral fluoropyrimidine, S-1, versus photodynamic therapy alone for unresectable hilar cholangiocarcinoma. Eur J Cancer 2014;50(7):1259–68.
23. Wentrup R, Winkelmann N, Mitroshkin A, et al. Photodynamic therapy plus chemotherapy compared with photodynamic therapy alone in hilar nonresectable cholangiocarcinoma. Gut Liver 2016;10(3):470–5.
24. Wagner A, Wiedmann M, Tannapfel A, et al. Neoadjuvant down-sizing of hilar cholangiocarcinoma with photodynamic therapy–long-term outcome of a phase II pilot study. Int J Mol Sci 2015;16(11):26619–28.
25. Darwish Murad S, Kim WR, Harnois DM, et al. Efficacy of neoadjuvant chemoradiation, followed by liver transplantation, for perihilar cholangiocarcinoma at 12 US centers. Gastroenterology 2012;143(1):88–98.e3 [quiz: e14].
26. Cosgrove ND, Al-Osaimi AM, Sanoff HK, et al. Photodynamic therapy provides local control of cholangiocarcinoma in patients awaiting liver transplantation. Am J Transplant 2014;14(2):466–71.
27. Gao F, Bai Y, Ma SR, et al. Systematic review: photodynamic therapy for unresectable cholangiocarcinoma. J Hepatobiliary Pancreat Sci 2010;17(2):125–31.
28. Kniebuhler G, Pongratz T, Betz CS, et al. Photodynamic therapy for cholangiocarcinoma using low dose mTHPC (Foscan((R))). Photodiagnosis Photodyn Ther 2013;10(3):220–8.
29. Wang AY, Yachimski PS. Endoscopic management of pancreatobiliary neoplasms. Gastroenterology 2018;154(7):1947–63.
30. Ni Y, Mulier S, Miao Y, et al. A review of the general aspects of radiofrequency ablation. Abdom Imaging 2005;30(4):381–400.
31. Mensah ET, Martin J, Topazian M. Radiofrequency ablation for biliary malignancies. Curr Opin Gastroenterol 2016;32(3):238–43.
32. Dolak W, Schreiber F, Schwaighofer H, et al. Endoscopic radiofrequency ablation for malignant biliary obstruction: a nationwide retrospective study of 84 consecutive applications. Surg Endosc 2014;28(3):854–60.
33. Steel AW, Postgate AJ, Khorsandi S, et al. Endoscopically applied radiofrequency ablation appears to be safe in the treatment of malignant biliary obstruction. Gastrointest Endosc 2011;73(1):149–53.
34. Zheng X, Bo ZY, Wan W, et al. Endoscopic radiofrequency ablation may be preferable in the management of malignant biliary obstruction: a systematic review and meta-analysis. J Dig Dis 2016;17(11):716–24.
35. Pozsár J, Tarpay Á, Burai J, et al. Intraductal radiofrequency ablation can restore patency of occluded biliary self-expanding metal stents. Z Gastroenterol 2011; 49(05):A70.
36. Kadayifci A, Atar M, Forcione DG, et al. Radiofrequency ablation for the management of occluded biliary metal stents. Endoscopy 2016;48(12):1096–101.
37. Rustagi T, Jamidar PA. Intraductal radiofrequency ablation for management of malignant biliary obstruction. Dig Dis Sci 2014;59(11):2635–41.
38. Sharaiha RZ, Natov N, Glockenberg KS, et al. Comparison of metal stenting with radiofrequency ablation versus stenting alone for treating malignant biliary strictures: is there an added benefit? Dig Dis Sci 2014;59(12):3099–102.
39. Yang J, Wang J, Zhou H, et al. Efficacy and safety of endoscopic radiofrequency ablation for unresectable extrahepatic cholangiocarcinoma: a randomized trial. Endoscopy 2018;50(8):751–60.
40. Sofi AA, Khan MA, Das A, et al. Radiofrequency ablation combined with biliary stent placement versus stent placement alone for malignant biliary strictures: a

systematic review and meta-analysis. Gastrointest Endosc 2018;87(4):944–51.e1.
41. Tal AO, Vermehren J, Friedrich-Rust M, et al. Intraductal endoscopic radiofrequency ablation for the treatment of hilar non-resectable malignant bile duct obstruction. World J Gastrointest Endosc 2014;6(1):13–9.
42. Wang LW, Li LB, Li ZS, et al. Self-expandable metal stents and trans-stent light delivery: are metal stents and photodynamic therapy compatible? Lasers Surg Med 2008;40(9):651–9.
43. Laquiere A, Boustiere C, Leblanc S, et al. Safety and feasibility of endoscopic biliary radiofrequency ablation treatment of extrahepatic cholangiocarcinoma. Surg Endosc 2016;30(3):1242–8.
44. Xu X, Li J, Wu J, et al. A systematic review and meta-analysis of intraluminal brachytherapy versus stent alone in the treatment of malignant obstructive jaundice. Cardiovasc Intervent Radiol 2018;41(2):206–17.
45. Skowronek J, Zwierzchowski G. Brachytherapy in the treatment of bile duct cancer - a tough challenge. J Contemp Brachytherapy 2017;9(2):187–95.
46. Benjamin IS, McPherson GA, Blumgart LH. Iridium-192 wire for hilar cholangiocarcinoma. Lancet 1981;2(8246):582–3.
47. Mattiucci GC, Autorino R, D'Agostino GR, et al. Chemoradiation and brachytherapy in extrahepatic bile duct carcinoma. Crit Rev Oncol Hematol 2014;90(1):58–67.
48. Mukewar S, Gupta A, Baron TH, et al. Endoscopically inserted nasobiliary catheters for high dose-rate brachytherapy as part of neoadjuvant therapy for perihilar cholangiocarcinoma. Endoscopy 2015;47(10):878–83.
49. Chen Y, Wang XL, Yan ZP, et al. HDR-192Ir intraluminal brachytherapy in treatment of malignant obstructive jaundice. World J Gastroenterol 2004;10(23):3506–10.
50. Zoepf T, Jakobs R, Arnold JC, et al. Palliation of nonresectable bile duct cancer: improved survival after photodynamic therapy. Am J Gastroenterol 2005;100(11):2426–30.
51. Ortner ME, Caca K, Berr F, et al. Successful photodynamic therapy for nonresectable cholangiocarcinoma: a randomized prospective study. Gastroenterology 2003;125(5):1355–63.
52. Dumoulin FL, Gerhardt T, Fuchs S, et al. Phase II study of photodynamic therapy and metal stent as palliative treatment for nonresectable hilar cholangiocarcinoma. Gastrointest Endosc 2003;57(7):860–7.
53. Witzigmann H, Berr F, Ringel U, et al. Surgical and palliative management and outcome in 184 patients with hilar cholangiocarcinoma: palliative photodynamic therapy plus stenting is comparable to r1/r2 resection. Ann Surg 2006;244(2):230–9.
54. Kahaleh M, Mishra R, Shami VM, et al. Unresectable cholangiocarcinoma: comparison of survival in biliary stenting alone versus stenting with photodynamic therapy. Clin Gastroenterol Hepatol 2008;6(3):290–7.
55. Quyn AJ, Ziyaie D, Polignano FM, et al. Photodynamic therapy is associated with an improvement in survival in patients with irresectable hilar cholangiocarcinoma. HPB (Oxford) 2009;11(7):570–7.
56. Cheon YK, Lee TY, Lee SM, et al. Longterm outcome of photodynamic therapy compared with biliary stenting alone in patients with advanced hilar cholangiocarcinoma. HPB (Oxford) 2012;14(3):185–93.
57. Wang F, Li Q, Zhang X, et al. Endoscopic radiofrequency ablation for malignant biliary strictures. Exp Ther Med 2016;11(6):2484–8.

58. Alis H, Sengoz C, Gonenc M, et al. Endobiliary radiofrequency ablation for malignant biliary obstruction. Hepatobiliary Pancreat Dis Int 2013;12(4): 423–7.
59. Figueroa-Barojas P, Bakhru MR, Habib NA, et al. Safety and efficacy of radiofrequency ablation in the management of unresectable bile duct and pancreatic cancer: a novel palliation technique. J Oncol 2013;2013:910897.

Endoscopic Ultrasound-Guided Ablation of Liver Tumors

Tiffany Chua, MD[1], Douglas O. Faigel, MD*

KEYWORDS

- EUS-guided ablation • Hepatocellular carcinoma • Hepatic metastases
- EUS-guided fine needle injection (EUS-FNI)
- EUS-guided portal injection chemotherapy (EPIC) • Radiofrequency ablation (RFA)
- High-intensity focused ultrasound (HIFU) • Irreversible electroporation (IRE)

KEY POINTS

- Endoscopic ultrasound (EUS)-guided tumor ablation is a new experimental application that shows promise in treatment of difficult to reach lesions, including those in the caudate and left lobe of the liver.
- EUS-guided tumor ablation offers a variety of additional treatment options for difficult or refractory cases.
- EUS-guided access to the hepatic vasculature may allow infusion of high concentrations of chemotherapy, such as by using drug-eluting beads into the portal vein (EUS-guided portal injection of chemotherapy), to increase efficacy and decrease systemic toxicity.

INTRODUCTION

Introduced in the last 1970s and 1980s, endoscopic ultrasound (EUS) was initially introduced to allow detailed imaging of the gastrointestinal tract wall, pancreas, and biliary tract. Improvements in the technology with the introduction of linear array instruments and needles led to EUS-guided fine-needle aspiration (FNA), a valued tool in obtaining tissue for histology in pancreaticobiliary, luminal gastrointestinal, and mediastinal malignancies.[1] The ability to accurately target lesions with a needle led to the development of EUS-guided therapeutic interventions. Current therapeutic interventions include celiac plexus block/neurolysis, pancreaticobiliary access, and EUS cystgastrostomy.[2] EUS-guided tumor ablation is a new experimental application that shows promise in treatment of difficult to reach lesions.[3] In this review, the authors discuss the current developments on EUS-guided ablation of liver tumors (**Table 1**).

Disclosure Statement: The authors have no financial relationships to disclose.
Division of Gastroenterology and Hepatology, Mayo Clinic Phoenix, Phoeniz, AZ, USA
[1] 13400 East Shea Boulevard, Scottsdale, AZ 85259.
* Corresponding author. 13400 East Shea Boulevard, Scottsdale, AZ 85259.
E-mail address: Faigel.Douglas@mayo.edu

Gastrointest Endoscopy Clin N Am 29 (2019) 369–379
https://doi.org/10.1016/j.giec.2018.11.007 giendo.theclinics.com
1052-5157/19/© 2018 Elsevier Inc. All rights reserved.

Table 1
A summary of currently available ablative modalities and their endoscopic applications to the liver

EUS-Guided Ablation of Liver Lesions: Current Therapies						
	Mechanism of Action	**Device/Medication Used**	**Method of Application**	**Target Evaluated**	**Advantages**	**Disadvantages**
Fine-needle injection (FNI)						
FNI ethanol	Cell dehydration + chemical vasculitis	FNA needle (18–25 gauge), 95% ethanol	Percutaneous, EUS	Hepatic cysts, HCC, liver metastases	Cost-effective, accessibility	Nonselective
EPIC	Chemotherapy via portal circulation	Paclitaxel-, irinotecan-, and doxorubicin-loaded microbeads, Abraxane	EUS	Porcine liver only	Minimize systemic exposure to chemo, increase hepatic concentrations	Not yet characterized
Thermal therapy						
RFA	Heat	Habib-HPB[a]	Surgical, percutaneous, ERCP	Cholangiocarcinoma	Specifically adapted for endoscope	Thermal injury to adjacent organs/vessels, "heat-sink" effect
Cryoablation	Rapid freezing and thawing	ERBE cryotherm-RFA probe (no endoscopic monotherapy)	Surgical, percutaneous, EUS	Porcine liver only (with combination probe)	Specifically adapted for EUS	Cryoshock
LITT	Heat	Nd:YAG	Percutaneous, EUS	HCC, liver metastases	Greater precision	Limited treatment area
HIFU	Heat + acoustic cavitation	SU121 transducer[b] (3.73 MHz)	Extracorporeal, EUS	Gel phantom, ex vivo bovine liver only	Specifically adapted for EUS	Bleeding, perforation
PDT	Selective photosensitization	Chlorin e6 (photosensitizer)	EUS	Locally advanced pancreaticobiliary disease	Selective modality	Prolonged skin photosensitivity

Other						
Brachytherapy	Radioactive seed implantation	Iodine-125, palladium-103	Percutaneous, EUS, ERCP	Non-liver lesions only	Selective modality, role for palliation	Radiation fibrosis
IRE	Pore formation in cell membrane	NanoKnife[c]	Surgical, percutaneous	No EUS data	Nonthermal	Need for anesthesia, cardiac synchronization

Abbreviations: ERCP, endoscopic retrograde cholangiopancreatography; IRE, Irreversible electroporation; RFA, radiofrequency ablation.

[a] EMcision, London, UK.

[b] Sonic Concepts, Bothell, WA.

[c] AngioDynamics, New York, USA

ENDOSCOPIC ULTRASOUND-GUIDED FINE-NEEDLE INJECTION THERAPY

Percutaneous injection of ablative agents is one of the most common ablative therapies worldwide. Thus far percutaneous ethanol injection has been the most widely used method, although injection of acetic acid has been described in the literature.[4] Percutaneous image-guided modalities include US and computed tomography, to treat hepatocellular carcinoma (HCC) and benign renal and hepatic cysts as the most common targets.[5] Injection of 95% ethanol is thought to cause local nonselective tissue necrosis through protein denaturation and cellular dehydration.[4,5] A secondary effect of destruction of nearby blood vessels via chemical vasculitis is thought to decrease rates of same-site recurrence.[4,5] The volume of ethanol required per lesion is often estimated with the following equation: $V = 4/3(r+0.5)^3$, where V is the volume of ethanol in milliliters and r is the radius of the lesion of interest.[6] In the literature, the sizes of the needles used for injection have ranged from 18 to 25 gauge per the discretion of the proceduralist.[5–7]

Because of its simplicity, cost-effectiveness, and availability, this technique has been readily adapted to endoscopy in the form of EUS-guided fine-needle injection (EUS-FNI) of ethanol into pancreatic lesions, especially mucinous cysts.[3,8] Several case reports have also described EUS-FNI of ethanol into hepatic lesions. Nakaji and colleagues[9] described a case in which a patient with a 1.8 cm HCC in segment VIII underwent elective EUS-guided injection therapy. Although this patient had lesions elsewhere in the liver treated with transarterial chemoembolization (TACE) and radiofrequency ablation (RFA) in the past, endoscopic treatment was selected due to the lesion's proximity to the inferior vena cava and hepatic veins. Follow-up imaging 2 weeks later showed complete necrosis of the tumor. The authors also describe a significant improvement in the quality of their visualization of the liver via EUS compared with prior transabdominal images of the patient.[9,10]

The same group from Kameda Medical Center in Chiba, Japan published their experience using EUS-guided ethanol injection as salvage therapy for a ruptured HCC and hemorrhagic ascites after unsuccessful TACE of the left hepatic artery.[10] Fifty milliliters total of ethanol were injected into a 4.5 cm lesion in segment III over 5 injections with necrosis of the HCC and resolution of the hemorrhagic ascites on 4-week follow-up imaging.[9–11]

EUS-FNI may also have utility in the treatment of metastatic lesions to the liver. Barclay and colleagues[6] followed a single patient who underwent multiple EUS-guided ethanol injections for recurrent metastases to the liver, likely a pancreatic or colorectal primary. Over a period of 5.5 years, the authors report 5 separate liver metastases with dimensions ranging from 1.6 to 6 cm in maximal dimension. Ultimately, only 2 lesions were treated endoscopically, the index liver metastases (1.6 cm) and a 4 cm lesion that progressed despite systemic chemotherapy.[6] The patient underwent serial injections of ethanol (median 6 mL per procedure) over a period of months with only minor adverse events such as abdominal pain and one subcapsular hematoma that resolved with conservative management.[6] There was complete response in the smaller lesion and partial response in the larger lesion, as defined by evidence of necrosis on imaging, the size of the lesion on follow-up imaging, and decrease in carcinoembryonic antigen level.[6] At the time of publication, the patient's disease was stable and did not require systemic chemotherapy.[6]

Although EUS-guided ethanol injection has been performed in malignant lesions of the liver, this technique has been described in benign neoplasms as well. Although symptomatic hepatic cysts are traditionally approached in a laparoscopic or percutaneous manner, there is evidence that supports EUS-assisted ethanol lavage as an efficacious and less invasive treatment. A 2014 study reported 5/8 cysts treated endoscopically versus 0/10 treated percutaneously were completely resolved on imaging at 1-year follow-up.[5] Median length of stay post-procedure was shorter in the EUS group (4.5 vs 6.5 days),[5] a difference attributed to lack of external drains. However, median cyst diameter and volume of the percutaneous group were higher, requiring larger volumes of ethanol.[5]

Other nonhepatic and nonpancreatic lesions have been treated with EUS-FNI using ethanol. A German study reported complete resolution of a 4 cm gastric gastrointestinal stromal tumor after a single endoscopic injection of 1.5 mL absolute ethanol. The patient was followed for 2 years without recurrence of the tumor. Nongastrointestinal target lesions have included recurrent pelvic lymph node metastases as well as a metastatic adrenal lesion secondary to rectal adenocarcinoma.[10–14]

In addition to direct injection of sclerosing agents into tumors, EUS-FNI is also being explored as a novel method of administering chemotherapeutic or other antitumor agents. For example, EUS-FNI has been used to directly treat pancreatic adenocarcinoma.[15] Injectants have included chemotherapeutic drugs such as gemcitabine, paclitaxel for cystic lesions, immune therapy, gene therapy, and viral therapy (ONYX-015).[15,16] Advantages of a localized approach are that it may avoid the systemic side effects of standard chemotherapeutic regimens. Although direct EUS-FNI of liver tumors using such agents has not been described, the potential of EUS delivery of chemotherapy to treat patients with liver metastases is under development. EUS-guided portal injection chemotherapy or EPIC uses drug-eluting microbeads injected under EUS guidance into the portal vein as a potential new treatment of multiple, bilateral hepatic metastases. Once injected into the portal vein, the beads travel to the liver where they become lodged in hepatic sinusoids, delivering the drug to the liver in order to increase hepatic levels while sparing systemic exposure and toxicity (**Fig. 1**).

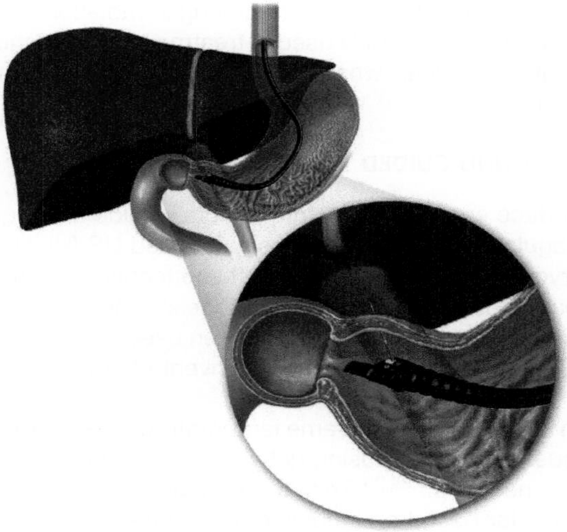

Fig. 1. EPIC involves identification of the portal vein under EUS and subsequent delivery of chemotherapeutic agents via FNI. (*From* Faigel DO, Lake DF, Landreth TL, et al. EUS-guided portal injection chemotherapy for treatment of hepatic metastases: feasibility in the acute porcine model. Gastrointest Endosc 2016;83(2):445; with permission.)

A 2016 study compared administration of irinotecan, doxorubicin, or albumin-bound paclitaxel nanoparticles (Abraxane, Celgene, Summit, NJ, USA) by EPIC versus systemic injection in porcine models.[17] For irinotecan and doxorubicin the drugs were loaded onto 75 to 150 μm LC Bead (Biocompatibles, London, UK) for EPIC versus unloaded drug of the same dose administered intravenously; Abraxane was administered unloaded onto beads in both groups. Results showed EPIC resulted in higher hepatic and lower plasma levels of each drug as compared with the control groups. A follow-up survival study in the porcine model demonstrated that EPIC with irinotecan- or doxorubicin-loaded microbeads was safe and well tolerated, with doxorubicin less myelosuppressive than systemic administration.[18] Cardiac levels were also obtained for doxorubicin in both studies and the concentration was significantly decreased compared with systemic administration, a potentially important result given the known cardiotoxicity of doxorubicin. A recent presentation at Digestive Diseases Week using a novel biodegradable microbead to deliver paclitaxel also achieved higher hepatic levels, lower blood levels, and less myelosuppression than systemically injected Abraxane.[19] Although human studies are not yet available, these results suggest that EPIC can decrease systemic exposure, potentially mitigating adverse effects associated with traditional administration of chemotherapy and possibly increase efficacy by delivering a higher concentration of drug to the liver.

ENDOSCOPIC ULTRASOUND-GUIDED BRACHYTHERAPY

Implantation of radioactive seeds to guide radiation therapy has been extensively studied in prostate cancer. EUS has been used as a delivery system to treat otherwise difficult to access lesions. Using the gastrointestinal lumen, EUS-guided radioactive seed placement with iodine-125 and palladium-103 have been performed in head and neck cancers, lung cancer, and recurrent esophageal cancer in several case reports.[20–22] More recently, 2 case series reported modest improvement in reduction of pain in advanced pancreatic adenocarcinoma with this modality.[20,22] Although this has not been described in the liver, EUS-guided brachytherapy may have theoretic utility in minimizing radiation fibrosis and structuring in radiation treatment of cholangiocarcinoma. Although Y-90 is widely used in treatment of HCC and occasionally hepatic metastases, it is unclear what additional benefit EUS may confer to its administration as yet.

ENDOSCOPIC ULTRASOUND-GUIDED THERMAL THERAPY

Therapies that introduce energy directly into tumors include techniques such as RFA, interstitial laser coagulation (ILC), high-intensity focused US (HIFU), irreversible electroporation, and cryoablation (CYA). Although these techniques have been evaluated for safety in the pancreas (primarily porcine models), only RFA and ILC have been applied to liver lesions. Although CYA has not been used in the liver as monotherapy, a combination RFA and CYA probe has been invented specifically for use with the echoendoscope.[3,23]

Similar to CYA in its utilization of extreme temperature, RFA delivers heat up to 50 to 100°C into the tissue of interest causing dehydration, protein denaturation, and subsequent coagulative necrosis.[3,24,25] This is a modality typically restricted to lesions less than 3.5 cm thus far based on studies of percutaneous applications of RFA.[3,26] The Habib EndoHPB (EMcision, London, UK) is an RFA catheter designed specifically for endoscopic use. Compatible with most RFA generators, the total catheter length is 1 Fr x 220 cm and probe lengths are available in 1 and 2 cm sizes. It has been used in the setting of pancreatic neoplasm as well as in the biliary tract via endoscopic retrograde cholangiopancreatography (ERCP) in the setting of malignant obstruction.[14] Although it has not yet been used in the liver, the recent success of EUS to access the biliary tree in malignancy inaccessible by ERCP provide interesting theoretic applications for bile duct tumors, or by direct placement within liver masses to affect RFA destruction.

CYA destroys tissue in situ via freezing and subsequent thawing. A probe is placed in the center of the lesion of interest and liquid nitrogen or argon circulated to an ideal temperature range of −20 to −60°C.[27] The sudden cycle of cellular ice formation and thawing causes osmotic dehydration and injury to the intracellular structures, resulting in cell death. Because of the larger size of the original probe, CYA has traditionally been used in open laparotomy although it has been adapted for laparoscopy and percutaneous approaches.[27] One major advantage is the ability to clearly assess the border between frozen and unfrozen tissue via ultrasound and use this modality in lesions near blood vessels with minimal risk of thrombosis.[27–29] However, CYA has been associated with a dramatic systemic inflammatory response and a "cryoshock" phenomenon, a rare but severe syndrome of multiorgan system failure and coagulopathy occurring in the first 48 hours post-procedure.[30] Chapman and colleagues[29] also documented a case complicated by acute respiratory distress syndrome.[31] EUS-guided CYA has not been described in humans but was performed successfully in a porcine model by Carrara and colleagues[23] using a combination cryotherm-RFA probe.

Laser interstitial thermal therapy (LITT) involves the placement of laser fibers into the center of a lesion whereupon local heat application destroys tumor cells in the target of interest. Nd:YAG is typically the type of laser used in LITT. In the past, treatment area size was limited to 15 mm based on fiber size although new developments could potentially allow treatment of larger areas.[32,33] The small caliber of Nd:YAG fibers lends itself readily to passage through an EUS scope and FNA needle.[7,34] Capitalizing on this advantage, more than one laser fiber can be passed through the FNA needle and customized to the size of the target lesion. Proponents of laser ablation also describe greater precision compared with other therapies, theoretically reducing risk for thermal injury to adjacent structures. A recent 2018 study showed that EUS-guided LITT successfully treated 4 men with 10 liver lesions secondary to HCC or metastatic colorectal cancer.[34] None of the patients experienced any complications at 2-month follow-up.

HIFU is a noninvasive technique that causes necrosis of the target tissue through heat generation as well as "acoustic cavitation," the formation and collapse of bubbles produced by intense ultrasound waves.[35] Primarily used in Asia, HIFU has been used externally in conjunction with TACE for treatment of HCC. A 2012 study comparing treatment of HCCs of TACE alone versus TACE + HIFU showed a significant increase in median survival time in the combination therapy group (57 months vs 36 months, $P = .048$).[35] Although no HIFU-related complications occurred in any of the 25 patients who underwent combination treatment, external administration of HIFU has been associated with skin burns, abdominal pain, bleeding, and perforation of nearby organs. To circumvent these potential adverse events, an EUS-guided HIFU transducer was designed to more closely target organs more commonly obscured by bowel.[35,36] This device successfully produced lesions in gel phantoms and ex vivo bovine livers in a feasibility study but has not yet been tested in humans.[35,36]

Photodynamic therapy (PDT) deserves a mention because of its ability to produce selective tissue necrosis through pretreatment with a photosensitizing agent. A laser catheter then delivers a controlled dose light at a specific wavelength that causes the photosensitizing agent to generate toxic singlet oxygen resulting in dose-dependent tissue necrosis in lesions anywhere from 6 to 40 mm in size.[5] In the past, utility of PDT was limited by the side effects of the photosynthesizing agents such as prolonged skin photosensitivity.[37] However, new photosynthesizing agents are more readily excreted and facilitate deeper tissue penetration of therapeutic wavelengths of light. EUS-guided PDT was shown to be technically feasible and safe in animal studies treating porcine pancreas.[5,37] More recently, Choi and colleagues[38] treated 4 patients with pancreaticobiliary malignancies using EUS-guided PDT; 2 of the 4 patients had lesions located at the caudate lobe of the liver. The median volume of necrosis was 4 cm^3, and patients had no disease progression at the time of follow-up (median: 5 months).

NONTHERMAL ABLATIVE TECHNIQUES

Irreversible electroporation (IRE), a novel nonthermal method of cancer treatment, has been trialed in liver lesions including HCC and liver metastases. Although it has not yet been adapted for endoscopic use, it provides an option that avoids many of pitfalls of thermal ablation. IRE uses high-frequency electric pulses to cause pore formation in the cell lipid bilayer, inducing apoptosis. Currently, NanoKnife (AngioDynamics, New York, USA) is the only commercially available device, and it allows up to 6 monopolar electrodes to be placed around the lesion of interest.[39] These electrodes are housed in a 19 gauge probe and can be used percutaneously or surgically. Placement of the individual electrodes is often confirmed by imaging and the amount of energy administered is determined by the Nanoknife device software.[39] Usage of IRE also must be accompanied by general anesthesia, paralysis, and cardiac synchronization to avoid muscle contractions and cardiac arrhythmias.[39–42]

Because of its nonthermal energy source, IRE is often considered an alternative for lesions not amenable to thermal ablation due to the risk of damage to adjacent organs and/or vasculature and masses that may be subject to the "heat sink effect", the inability of the target tissue to reach therapeutic temperature if large vessels are nearby. The rate of complications of IRE of malignant liver tumors has been described in the literature from 8% to 27.5%.[39] The most common complications included treatment-related abdominal pain, postablative abscess, hematomas, bleeding, and pneumothorax. A focused study evaluating the safety of surgical IRE in cirrhotic patients with HCC found that patients had a statistically significant shorter length of stay and 90-day readmission compared with similar patients who underwent microwave ablation.[40] Recurrence rates have been estimated as 29% at 6 months with worse outcomes for larger lesions.[41] IRE has also been used as a bridge to transplant in patients with HCC, with none of 6 patients treated with IRE showing viable tumor on explant.[42]

SUMMARY

EUS-guided ablative therapies have advanced significantly and have led to experimental applications in locations that have been difficult to image and/or reach with percutaneous approaches. EUS-guided treatments of the liver are under development. Regions of the left lobe of the liver and caudate are accessible to direct EUS-guided ablation. This could include injection of sclerosants or chemotherapeutic drugs or by the application of energy to destroy a lesion via RFA, cryotherapy, laser thermal ablation, etc. In patients with diffuse disease who are otherwise not candidates for liver-directed therapy, EUS-guided access to the hepatic vasculature may allow infusion of high concentrations of chemotherapy, such as by using drug-eluting beads into the portal vein (EPIC), to increase efficacy and decrease systemic toxicity.

The literature has shown that many percutaneous ablative techniques are readily adaptable for EUS. Although EUS-guided tumor ablation may not be first-line therapy, it does offer a variety of additional treatment options for difficult or refractory cases, because cancer has become a chronic illness to be managed. EUS provides access to lesions in the caudate and left lobe of the liver, which may be unreachable via percutaneous approaches. Combination percutaneous and EUS-guided approaches along with systemic and whole-liver chemotherapy may confer further survival benefit to patients with hepatic malignancies. Finally, as a minimally invasive approach, EUS treatment of liver lesions may improve quality of life as compared with other approaches by minimizing systemic side effects. The role of EUS-guided therapy for liver tumors has yet to be determined, preferably through well-designed prospective studies.

REFERENCES

1. Wiersema MJ, Vilmann P, Giovannini M, et al. Endosonography-guided fine-needle aspiration biopsy: diagnostic accuracy and complication assessment. Gastroenterology 1997;112(4):1087–95.
2. Siddiqui UD, Levy MJ. EUS-guided transluminal interventions. Gastroenterology 2018;154(7):1911–24.
3. Wallace MB, Sabbagh LC. EUS 2008 working group document: evaluation of EUS-guided tumor ablation. Gastrointest Endosc 2009;69(2):S59–63.
4. Schoppmeyer K, Weis S, Mossner J, et al. Percutaneous ethanol injection or percutaneous acetic acid injection for early hepatocellular carcinoma. Cochrane Database Syst Rev 2009;3:CD006745.
5. Chan HH, Nishioka NS, Mino M, et al. EUS-guided photodynamic therapy of the pancreas: a pilot study. Gastrointest Endosc 2004;59(1):95–9.
6. Barclay RL, Perez-Miranda M, Giovannini M. EUS-guided treatment of a solid hepatic metastasis. Gastrointest Endosc 2002;55(2):266–70.
7. Wacker FK, Reither K, Ritz JP, et al. MR-guided interstitial laser-induced thermotherapy of hepatic metastasis combined with arterial blood flow reduction: Technique and first clinical results in an open MR system. J Magn Reson Imaging 2001;13(1):31–6.
8. Yang D, DiMaio CJ. Endoscopic ultrasound-guided therapies in pancreatic neoplasms. Biomed Res Int 2015.
9. Nakaji S, Hirata N, Iwaki K, et al. Endoscopic ultrasound (EUS)-guided ethanol injection for hepatocellular carcinoma difficult to treat with percutaneous local treatment. Endoscopy 2012;44(S 02):E380.
10. Nakaji S, Hirata N, Kobayashi M, et al. Endoscopic ultrasonography-guided ethanol injection as a treatment for ruptured hepatocellular carcinoma in the left hepatic lobe. Endoscopy 2015;47(S 01):E558–60.
11. Livraghi T, Solbiati L, Meloni MF, et al. Treatment of focal liver tumors with percutaneous radio-frequency ablation: complications encountered in a multicenter study. Radiology 2003;226(2):441–51.
12. Artifon EL, Lucon AM, Sakai P, et al. EUS-guided alcohol ablation of left adrenal metastasis from non-small-cell lung carcinoma. Gastrointest Endosc 2007;66(6): 1201–5.
13. Masuda T, Beppu T, Mizumoto T, et al. Hybrid ablation using percutaneous and endoscopic approach for multi-nodular hepatocellular carcinomas. Hepatogastroenterology 2012;59:836–9.

14. Steel AW, Postgate AJ, Khorsandi S, et al. Endoscopically applied radiofrequency ablation appears to be safe in the treatment of malignant biliary obstruction. Gastrointest Endosc 2011;73(1):149–53.
15. Seo DW. EUS-guided antitumor therapy for pancreatic tumors. Gut Liver 2010; 4(Suppl 1):S76.
16. Levy MJ, Alberts SR, Chari ST, et al. 716 EUS guided intra-tumoral gemcitabine therapy for locally advanced and metastatic pancreatic cancer. Gastrointest Endosc 2011;73(4):AB144–5.
17. Faigel DO, Lake DF, Landreth TL, et al. EUS-guided portal injection chemotherapy for treatment of hepatic metastases: feasibility in the acute porcine model. Gastrointest Endosc 2016;83(2):444–6.
18. Faigel DO, Singh VP, Patel K, et al. Safety of endoscopic ultrasound-guided portal injection chemotherapy using drug-eluting microbeads in a porcine model. J Can Res Updates 2018;7(4):102–8.
19. Faigel DO, Fiala M, Pennington D, et al. Endoscopic-ultrasound-guided portal injection chemotherapy (EPIC) using a novel biodegradable microbead to deliver paclitaxel. Gastrointest Endosc 2018;87(6):AB84–5.
20. Lah JJ, Kuo JV, Chang KJ, et al. EUS-guided brachytherapy. Gastrointest Endosc 2005;62(5):805–8.
21. Martínez-Monge R, Subtil JC, López-Picazo JM. Transoesophageal endoscopic-ultrasonography-guided 125I permanent brachytherapy for unresectable mediastinal lymphadenopathy. Lancet Oncol 2006;7(9):781–3.
22. Sun S, Xu H, Xin J, et al. Endoscopic ultrasound-guided interstitial brachytherapy of unresectable pancreatic cancer: results of a pilot trial. Endoscopy 2006;38(04): 399–403.
23. Carrara S, Arcidiacono PG, Albarello L, et al. Endoscopic ultrasound-guided application of a new internally gas-cooled c ablation probe in the liver and spleen of an animal model: a preliminary study. Endoscopy 2008;40(09):759–63.
24. Curley SA, Izzo F, Delrio P, et al. Radiofrequency ablation of unresectable primary and metastatic hepatic malignancies: results in 123 patients. Ann Surg 1999; 230(1):1.
25. Dupuy DE, Goldberg SN. Image-guided radiofrequency tumor ablation: challenges and opportunities—part II. J Vasc Interv Radiol 2001;12(10):1135–48.
26. Pai M, Habib N, Senturk H, et al. Endoscopic ultrasound guided radiofrequency ablation, for pancreatic cystic neoplasms and neuroendocrine tumors. World J Gastrointest Surg 2015;7(4):52.
27. Jansen MC, Van Hillegersberg R, Chamuleau RAFM, et al. Outcome of regional and local ablative therapies for hepatocellular carcinoma: a collective review. Eur J Surg Oncol 2005;31(4):331–47.
28. Arcidiacono PG, Carrara S, Reni M, et al. Feasibility and safety of EUS-guided cryothermal ablation in patients with locally advanced pancreatic cancer. Gastrointest Endosc 2012;76(6):1142–51.
29. Chapman WC, Debelak JP, Pinson CW, et al. Hepatic cryoablation, but not radiofrequency ablation, results in lung inflammation. Ann Surg 2000;231(5):752.
30. Sadikot RT, Wudel LJ Jr, Jansen DE, et al. Hepatic cryoablation–induced multisystem injury: bioluminescent detection of NF-κB activation in a transgenic mouse model. J Gastrointest Surg 2002;6(2):264–70.
31. Washington K, Debelak JP, Gobbell C, et al. Hepatic cryoablation-induced acute lung injury: histopathologic findings. J Surg Res 2001;95(1):1–7.

32. Di Matteo F, Grasso R, Pacella CM, et al. EUS-guided Nd: YAG laser ablation of a hepatocellular carcinoma in the caudate lobe. Gastrointest Endosc 2011;73(3): 632–6.
33. Di Matteo F, Martino M, Rea R, et al. EUS-guided Nd: YAG laser ablation of normal pancreatic tissue: a pilot study in a pig model. Gastrointest Endosc 2010;72(2): 358–63.
34. Jiang TA, Tian G, Bao H, et al. EUS dating with laser ablation against the caudate lobe or left liver tumors: a win-win proposition? Cancer Biol Ther 2018;19(3): 145–52.
35. Kim J, Chung DJ, Jung SE, et al. Therapeutic effect of high-intensity focused ultrasound combined with transarterial chemoembolisation for hepatocellular carcinoma< 5 cm: comparison with transarterial chemoembolisation monotherapy—preliminary observations. Br J Radiol 2012;85(1018):e940–6.
36. Hwang JH, Farr N, Morrison K, et al. 876 development of an EUS-guided high-intensity focused ultrasound endoscope. Gastrointest Endosc 2011;73(4):AB155.
37. Yusuf TE, Matthes K, Brugge WR. EUS-guided photodynamic therapy with verteporfin for ablation of normal pancreatic tissue: a pilot study in a porcine model (with video). Gastrointest Endosc 2008;67(6):957–61.
38. Choi JH, Oh D, Lee JH, et al. Initial human experience of endoscopic ultrasound-guided photodynamic therapy with a novel photosensitizer and a flexible laser-light catheter. Endoscopy 2015;47(11):1035–8.
39. Zimmerman A, Grand D, Charpentier KP. Irreversible electroporation of hepatocellular carcinoma: patient selection and perspectives. J Hepatocell Carcinoma 2017;4:49.
40. Bhutiani N, Philips P, Scoggins CR, et al. Evaluation of tolerability and efficacy of irreversible electroporation (IRE) in treatment of Child-Pugh B (7/8) hepatocellular carcinoma (HCC). HPB (Oxford) 2016;18(7):593–9.
41. Niessen C, Igl J, Pregler B, et al. Factors associated with short-term local recurrence of liver cancer after percutaneous ablation using irreversible electroporation: a prospective single-center study. J Vasc Interv Radiol 2015;26(5):694–702.
42. Cheng RG, Bhattacharya R, Yeh MM, et al. Irreversible electroporation can effectively ablate hepatocellular carcinoma to complete pathologic necrosis. J Vasc Interv Radiol 2015;26(8):1184–8.

Moving?

Make sure your subscription moves with you!

To notify us of your new address, find your **Clinics Account Number** (located on your mailing label above your name), and contact customer service at:

Email: journalscustomerservice-usa@elsevier.com

800-654-2452 (subscribers in the U.S. & Canada)
314-447-8871 (subscribers outside of the U.S. & Canada)

Fax number: 314-447-8029

Elsevier Health Sciences Division
Subscription Customer Service
3251 Riverport Lane
Maryland Heights, MO 63043

*To ensure uninterrupted delivery of your subscription, please notify us at least 4 weeks in advance of move.

ELSEVIER

Printed and bound by CPI Group (UK) Ltd, Croydon, CR0 4YY
08/05/2025
01864745-0005